ANIMALIA

A Synthesis of Homeopathic Themes, Mappa Mundi, Provings & Clinical Cases

A practitioner's guide to the Homeopathic Themes
of 6 Animal families

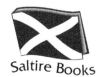

Saltire Books   *Saltire Books Limited, Glasgow, Scotland*

ANIMALIA

A Synthesis of Homeopathic Themes, Mappa Mundi,
Provings & Clinical Cases

A practitioner's guide to the Homeopathic Themes
of 6 Animal families

LUKE NORLAND

Saltire Books   *Saltire Books Limited, Glasgow, Scotland*

Published by Saltire Books Ltd

18–20 Main Street, Busby, Glasgow G76 8DU, Scotland
books@saltirebooks.com   www.saltirebooks.com

 is a registered trademark

First published in 2021

Typeset by Type Study, Scarborough, UK in 9/12pt Stone Serif
Printed and bound in the UK by TJ Books Ltd, Padstow

ISBN 978-1-908127-42-6

For Saltire Books
Project Development: Lee Kayne
Editorial: Steven Kayne
Design: Phil Barker

Original artwork for graphics on the title pages for Chapters 2 and 4 by Deborah McCarthy of Stroud.   debs.freefallco@gmail.com
Other images commercially sourced

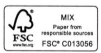

CONTENTS

Dedication

To my beloved wife; Alice,
Mother and father; Misha and Brigitte,
Brothers; Mani, Gabriel and Sam.
Your gifts of love and support are cherished . . .

FOREWORD

On a number of occasions that I have delivered lectures in the United Kingdom, I have met up with Luke Norland in the exhibition rooms adjoining various lecture halls. Here, he would be manning his RadarOpus table, promoting the company's superb homeopathic repertorising and materia medica software programmes. Often, he would be stationed next to the Saltire Books table. In gravitating to this 'home away from home', it was inevitable that Luke and I should meet. I was conscious of a warm, engaging, serious young man who evoked an empathetic sense of closeness in me although our lives had scarcely touched, since I live many miles away in Cape Town, South Africa. A mutual friend and colleague Geoff Johnson had always spoken highly to me of the Norland family and drew my attention to the excellent education and research programme being run through the School of Homeopathy in Stroud – an institute founded by Misha, Luke's father, and now lead by Mani, Luke's eldest brother. Luke was described to me as a gifted musician and avid student who in studying homeopathy steeped himself in every aspect of what Samuel Hahnemann termed 'this sublime science'.

In 2019, I received a kind invitation from Mani Norland to lecture on homeopathic archetypes to the School of Homeopathy in May 2020. I was delighted to accept the invitation but destiny in the form of the COVID-19 pandemic decreed otherwise. The possibility of me doing so in the future still regretfully hangs in the balance. However, release from the demands of lecturing in South Africa and abroad permitted me unlimited time to throw all my endeavour into completing my book *The Raven*. This unstinted largesse resulted in a book far longer and far weightier than either I or Saltire Books anticipated. Inevitably, I exceeded the deadline set for the submission of my manuscript and found *The Raven* having to cede precedence to another title that had arrived on Steven's desk – what can surely be regarded as the first work of a burgeoning, homeopathic literary talent – *Animalia* by Luke Norland.

Since my own title *The Raven*[i] had to be kept on pause by Saltire, whilst the complex typesetting exercise demanded by *Animalia's* format was completed, I was diligently kept appraised of its progress. Hence, long before I was asked whether I would be willing to write this foreword, I was well aware of the book's unique qualities, rich content and practical importance. I was sent the draft manuscript for my perusal and despite the current demands of my own writing and a welcome holiday that followed hot on the heels of *Animalia's* arrival, an initial cursory scanning of the text soon drew me back to partake of a little more – and then a little more – and eventually to become engrossed in reading about

---

[i] *The Raven* by David Lilley is due for publication by Saltire Books during 2021.

well-known friends of a homeopathic lifetime, and, in addition, animal archetypes that I have scant knowledge of or have never considered prescribing. All presented in a highly accessible and consistent format and enriched by essential insights into natural history, family relationships, archetypal symbolism and mythology. This is a book that serves many purposes – including homeopathic entertainment – the joy of reading about a beloved subject and savouring its wide-ranging connections to other fields of knowledge: scientific, philosophical, psychological and esoteric. It is a book for the bedside, for the study and for the desk – for the student, the young practitioner and the seasoned physician. It is a credit to Luke and to the School that nurtured him and a handsome feather in the Saltire publishing cap.

David Lilley
Cape Town
May 2021

ACKNOWLEDGEMENTS

I would like to take this opportunity to thank the countless provers who volunteered themselves to take part in the proving process, which is often arduous and shows a commitment to the art and science of homeopathy. I also wish to humbly thank the following teachers and homeopaths, to which this work is indebted:

Misha Norland, Rajan Sankaran, Jeremy Sherr, Massimo Mangialavori, Peter Fraser, Nancy Herrick, Janet Snowdon, Geoff Johnson, David Mundy, Jonathan Hardy, Louis Klein, Todd Rowe, Alastair Gray, Melanie Grimes, Anne Schadde, Farokh Master, Sachindra and Bhawisha Joshi, Mahesh Gandhi, Anne Vervarcke, Jonathan Shore, Elizabeth Schulz, Frederik Schroyens, Roger Van Zandvoort, Frans Vermeulen, David Lilley, Jo Evans.

I would also like to extend my warmest thanks to Steven and Lee Kayne and the entire editorial team at Saltire for giving the green light to this project, and for putting your faith in me as a first-time author. It has been a pleasure to work alongside you throughout the process.

Finally, I thank my good friend and colleague, Jo Magowan, for coming to my rescue with the final proof read.

ABOUT THE AUTHOR

Luke grew up sharing his family home with the School of Homeopathy and has been immersed in the homeopathic way of life since he was born into the world. Having first studied classical music in London, his career path eventually brought him back to his roots in the healing arts. Luke has a homeopathy practice in Frome, Somerset, combining this with his role as the UK coordinator for RadarOpus and teaching at the School of Homeopathy.

Luke's first training was as a classical musician; playing the French Horn since the age of 10. He is still a dedicated horn player as well as student of astrology, lover of nature and soon to be father. He enjoys playing in orchestras and spent much of his twenties composing experimental electronic music. He has also created a *Thematic Repertory* including new remedies and remedy families. Luke's approach to homeopathy is to blend together the different disciplines of repertory, materia medica, provings and systems so that each case can be explored from an appropriate anchor point to suit the individual.

Luke has gained valuable experience working with the school's provings, editing and assisting in the recent provings of Two-toed sloth, Spectrolite and Red campion. He also compiled the rubrics for Carbo fullerenum, Passer domesticus, Fulgurite, Galium aparine, Clupea harengus and Meles meles. This grounding in the repertory and provings has become an essential facet in Luke's process of finding a similimum for a diverse range of patients.

PREFACE

In the last 30 years, there has been a great proliferation of new remedies, especially from animal sources, that have entered the materia medica. I learned a great deal of this new material from my teachers at The School of Homeopathy and there are already a good number of high-quality books elucidating the themes of the main animal subkingdoms. So, in order to present something unique and hopefully of genuine use to the profession, I have compiled concise thematic information in a format which allows the busy practitioner (and inquisitive student) to quickly familiarise oneself with each animal subkingdom as required – all within the same volume. As a recent graduate, this is a book that I felt I needed for myself – one that I could quickly turn to when considering the prescription of an animal remedy. I was also quickly learning from my own practice that many patients appear to present qualities that belong to the animal kingdom.

The aim of the book is to simplify the process of researching animal remedies, both through the prism of kingdom analysis and when looking up lesser known remedies based on repertorisation. I have presented the information in a way that suits my approach to homeopathic practice; blending mythology, mappa mundi, provings, cases, repertory and materia medica.

The themes and polarities of each animal family are presented followed by quotations from provings and cases comprising of varied sources and remedies in that group. In this way, one gets a glimpse into the pure language of the prover and/or patient's raw experience – allowing them to speak for themselves. I want to thank both Jeremy Sherr and Peter Fraser for inspiring me to dig deep in the provings in order to present the material in this way.

When I first began the project, it was not my intention to provide a complete materia medica section of each remedy in every family, as there are already authors who have done sterling work in this area, particularly Frans Vermeulen. As I progressed, I gradually stumbled upon a way of gathering and synthesising remedy information that I felt would be a valuable contribution to the homeopathic community. Each remedy picture contains a distillation of characteristic rubrics (usually the smaller ones that are easy to miss when scouring the repertory) and an edited section of provers' statements speaking as one (thanks again to Jeremy Sherr for pioneering this invention). The format is adapted to suit the type of information that is available for what are often lesser-known remedies. My overall approach is to let the symptoms and provers speak for themselves and to add nuance by highlighting what I feel captures the essential qualities of each remedy. In this manner I hope to have avoided anything speculative.

My hope is that this work will find service in the hands of students, graduates and seasoned professionals alike, whilst shining a light on the amazing amount of material to come from the community, especially provings.

Tips on using this book

The use of Subscript refers variously to the proving / case of the particular remedy from which the section of text belongs. In certain sections of the book, quotation blocks are built from a composite of different remedy sources from within each family – helping to illustrate that the theme runs through several remedies. Here I put the remedy in subscript and the full reference in superscript in a nod to the reportorial formatting in Synthesis Repertory. Although this may be a somewhat unorthodox method, it means that one doesn't get distracted when reading the text – as it should be read as if it were from one person / or from one remedy. Where the quotation comes from a particular Homeopath rather than referring to a remedy case / proving, the author's name is in subscript (as in Synthesis repertory), with the numerical reference to the exact source in superscript.

The abbreviations used throughout this book are the same as in Synthesis repertory and RadarOpus.

Agg. = Aggravation
Amel. = Amelioration

A list of remedy abbreviations is available online at:
https://tinyurl.com/y4w366ot

Luke Norland
Frome, England
September 2020

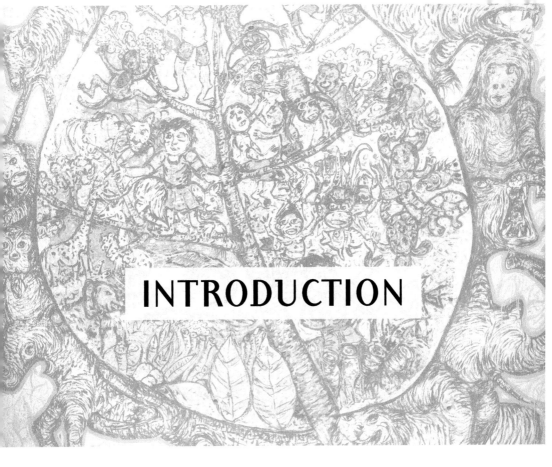

INTRODUCTION

HUMANS THAT RESONATE WITH ANIMAL REMEDIES

These people will seek out environments where they are able to go 'toe-to-toe' – with others, pitting their strength against the competition to prove they can come out on top. In minerals, there is also a need to prove their own strength to themselves, and failure means that they are lacking – the focus is turned inward. In Animal consciousness, the focus is on me versus a competitor, or me versus me. One will win and the other will fail. I believe that plants share this characteristic of competition for resources, but it is less explicit in terms of one versus another. Nux vomica is considered one of the most competitive 'types', so how to make sense of this? In evolutionary terms, plants were the first to colonise the land – they were pioneers. Animals such as insects had to evolve according to the marker set down by the first plant species, and so it is evident that there is a mutually dependent relationship between these two kingdoms. In fact, all animals (humans included) are totally dependent on the vegetable kingdom. Even the most ardent carnivore must feed on animals that themselves rely on plants to survive. So, although a lot of us will say that plants are at the bottom of the food chain, one can also see it the other way around; that plants have made themselves indispensable to animals to ensure their own survival.

One of the best examples of this is Wheat, as outlined by Yuval Noah Harari[1]. He describes how our quality of life has deteriorated since the days of hunting and gathering to becoming enslaved by the crops we farm. Essentially, wheat has made itself so central to human life, that our ancestors spent all their time performing back breaking labour to ensure its survival, so entwined was our own fate with that of this crop. Our diet, which used to be varied and healthy, became centred around monoculture, and we lived in fear of drought or pestilence damaging it which would mean starvation. We became the protectors of this otherwise unremarkable crop. Development of the now predominant cancer miasm has gradually and inexorably ensued; the cells which replicate themselves within malignant tumours bear a striking resemblance to our monocultural fields of crops.

Perhaps one could say that Plants are playing 'the long game' and Animals are playing 'the short game'. For example, many plants are perennials – meaning that they come back to life the next year. Many trees live for centuries and are incredibly durable, resisting death by recycling their own tissues to form new roots and growths. The accent is on collaboration between members of the species, whose roots share information and nutrients through the symbiotic relationship with Fungal networks. The violence in the Vegetable kingdom is characterised in the way that a plant's aggressive behaviour can be seen only when the film is sped up to reveal the gesture of the plant's growth. For example, Blackberry (*Rubus fructicosus*) that colonises space aggressively, using its backward pointing thorns to grip and climb over other species to quickly dominate territory.

Another key difference is in the simplicity of the plant's expression as compared to the complexity of an animal. Animals must adapt to a niche in order to survive so they become specialists at this mode of survival. Plants create their own food so are in a more stable position. They still need to compete for root and light space; the way in which they do so gives a characteristic that one can use to find resonance with human patterns of behaviour.

OVERVIEW OF ANIMALS IN NATURE

Animals exhibit a wide variety of behaviour revolving around the issue of survival of the fittest, especially when competition for resources are scarce. The right to reproduce is chiefly determined by strength in combat, ensuring the best chances of survival – i.e. the strongest genes are chosen.

Animals can live in *sociable groups* – usually prey – or are primarily *solitary* – often predators.

The animal patient's perception of their chief complaint is likely to be multi-faceted and stems from their perceived competitors; the problem is 'who rather than what' as Anne Vervarcke[2] succinctly puts it. Unlike plants, they cannot make their own food, so they must develop specialist hunting skills, or become adapted to a particular food source that is in abundance. For example, pandas

2   **Introduction**

and bamboo. Or, like badgers and pigs, become omnivorous. In other words, for animals it is very important to find a niche within which to survive and compete.

There is much more *action* and *reaction* than a plant rooted in soil can manifest. Animals are conscious beings, moving about freely within their territory – readily revealing their nature through their habits and appearance. Schumacher explains it very well:

> It is easy to recognise consciousness in a dog, a cat or a horse, if only because they can be knocked unconscious, a condition similar to that of a plant: the processes of life are continuing although the animal has lost its peculiar powers.[3]

The problem for animals may be that there is a bigger, more successful species taking over, or that there is someone higher up the food chain, to which there must be either submission or a fight to assert the dominant position. The options are to try to escape, or compete and fight. The loser must back down and go hungry, won't be able to mate and will must accept a weakened position as their lot.

Animals can make changes to their environment (whereas plants must adapt to it) in order to construct their own home and keep the family safe. Animals can also make many adaptations to behaviour and diet over time in order to evolve according to their habitat. Beavers are a very good example of a mammal who make extensive changes to their environment to create a safe and secure home. Their industry has a knock-on effect to the biodiversity of the whole area which they inhabit.

Animals rely on plants or prey animals for food, so problems arise when there is competition for scarce resources.

In the Avian realm, a partner is usually chosen based on creative abilities such as song or a colourful plumage. This animal theme is also like the Plant kingdom where attractiveness is important in ensuring survival through pollination.

COMMON ANIMAL THEMES

Plant cases tend to revolve around the way things feel for the patient; they will narrate the effect of the symptoms in detail, describing the sensation and finding it relatively easy to give modalities and concomitants. The mineral patient tends to focus on how their complaints impose limitations on them in each area of performance. In animal cases, there can be a mixture of both these types of presentation, with an accent on *describing their survival pattern*. They may spontaneously narrate their life-story (which could give hints to the entire lifecycle of the particular animal).

The patient perceives a conflict / split / duality within themselves

This may be expressed as the higher (human) self and the lower (animal) self.

Competitiveness can be felt as a "me against the world" attitude or may be internalised into "me against myself".

Self-esteem

In animal cases, the patient's sense of self-esteem is often lowered; they may feel injured, wounded or attacked by someone in a superior position. Conversely, they want to be well-liked, attractive and respected.

Competition for scarce resources

The experience of animal patients is a fight for survival; one must compete with others to stake their claim or find their niche, becoming a specialist in a certain environment. There is an increased risk of resources running out (compared to plants who make their own food), *so a greater competitive edge is required.* A competitive spirit does not necessarily point to animal remedies but needs to be taken as part of the whole pattern in the case.

Polarity – Victim / aggressor | Predator / prey

Within the Animal kingdom, the dipoles of victim and aggressor, prey and predator are played out in the most dramatic fashion. A patient may identify at different times with one or both roles. Animal cases can focus much more on being the victim than the aggressor so one might mistakenly rule out animal remedies where there is a victim mentality. The more overtly animal character-istic can be very subtle (or projected), particularly in birds, milks and sea animals. There can also be marked aggression and malicious behaviour. This is more likely to come through in children who are often less compensated, but it may be expressed through the subconscious of adult patients in the form of dreams, fears or projection onto others.

Sexual displays – there is a need to be attractive to ensure survival

In the animal kingdom, violence erupts most strongly at times when the females of the species become fertile. Males must compete to prove they have what it takes to pass on the strongest genes.

Need to be different, talented and special *vs.* feeling ugly, abused and worthless

To be successful, animals must find their niche in the environment. All species have a particular talent which they use to survive in even the most extreme circumstances. Human patients requiring animal remedies want recognition for their talents and to be noticed for their uniqueness. When decompensated, or moving into a 'failed state', animal remedies can express an inferior feeling of subjugation, submission, feeling ugly, unattractive, used, abused and worthless. This is contrasted with the polarity of feeling confident, that they are a great person and should be accorded respect by others. Like the metals, there is an accent on performance, a desire to be the best and prove oneself. Alongside this there is a strong desire to avoid humiliation and shame.

Fear of being attacked and outbreaks of violence
This is met with aggression or submission. If the vital force is imprinted with an animal pattern, then the interior world of the patient is attuned to threat and violence. It will be assumed that the world out there is also a violent, threatening one.

Whole life cycle / life story
The themes in animal cases tend to be too broad and complex to fit into a plant or mineral case. This may be because they are telling us about a whole unique lifecycle. The patient spontaneously talks about life situations, giving (often colourful) anecdotes of when the 'other' has wronged them, abused them, belittled them etc. The problem is perceived as coming from the outside rather than from a lack within (as with minerals). Plant patients are also greatly affected by external factors, but with animals there is a focus on 'who' is doing this to them, as opposed to their feeling about it and subsequent response (plants). In terms of presentation, animal patients can express themselves vividly, maintaining eye contact and engaging readily with the Homeopath.

Transformation
The life cycle of each animal goes through different stages of transformation which are characteristic to each sub-kingdom. For example, birds are born in an egg and must break their way out of this shell in order to hatch. The polarity of feeling trapped versus free is therefore evident from the very beginning of the life cycle. Insects metamorphose from a lengthy stay as earth-bound grubs through the pupal stage to become winged adults who have a very short window in which to reproduce. There is a sudden revolutionary change in their life which leads to an intense period of busy restlessness and increased sexuality. In mammals, the feeling of being suspended or floating comes from the embryonic stage which could easily be confused with the experience of a sea animal. In the oceanic realm, eggs are often abandoned so that the young must fend for themselves from an early age. Each sea animal devises a unique approach to survival; the hard protection of a shell, the ability to camouflage themselves, the safety and anonymity of a shoal etc. Many snakes are born equipped with venom and ready to meet the world without any parental supervision – they already know exactly what they need to do without any learning. Spiders are also born possessing a hardwired knowledge of how to construct their web – this puts them at the centre and in control of their surroundings through their great sensitivity to any vibrational change on the web. Each animal patient tells the story of their life cycle through the events that have had the most impact upon them, shaping their unique pattern of *dis-ease*.

Hierarchy; who is top in the pecking order?
Dominance versus submission. Knowing one's place in the structure; being accepted for one's gifts or being cast aside, unwanted and unloved.

Projection

Because the focus of the interview is often on how the patient perceives others to have injured them, it is natural that a lot of projection may be involved. The less-desirable animal qualities are projected onto the partner, co-worker, sibling, parent etc.

Animal patients may talk about 'humans' as if they themselves are not human

Examples of expressions are:

"They persecute me, oppose me, think they are better . . ."

"They're not fit to be humans . . ."

"I am not good enough; she is better than me . . ."

"I'll bring them down . . ."

"I feel split, divided, they hit me I hit him back . . ."

Evolutionary development

This is a very interesting area of Homeopathy and one in which I hope to see further development. For instance, it is my hope that we will eventually be seeing links between different animals and plants that evolved through the same periods. For example, the Devonian period saw the development of corals and echinoderms in the sea, whilst on land the ferns, seed plants and trees began to evolve. More research through the medium of provings is needed to establish meaningful connections for homeopathic practitioners.

Coming back to the animal kingdom specifically, one can make a broad distinction between the invertebrates (no backbone) and the vertebrates (Chordata). The mammals sit at the top of the evolutionary tree in terms of their capacity for adaptation and differentiation; each species adopting unique and divergent behaviours with diverse survival strategies. Whereas many arthropods, molluscs and other invertebrates are more undifferentiated from one another; following similar habits forged over the millennia, imparting an ancient or primeval quality. However, within this rather broad classification, there are most certainly exceptions and it is rather simplistic to say that the invertebrates are underdeveloped in comparison to vertebrates. Cephalopods – such as Sepia and Octopus – show an incredibly diverse range of behaviours and high intelligence in surviving and thriving in the dangerous and unforgiving oceanic realm. They could be said to represent the pinnacle of underwater invertebrate design and possess the most advanced nervous system in this grouping. However, the common pattern in invertebrates is to have a simple nervous system – equating to an over – reactivity to stimuli and to feel easily overwhelmed by too much input from the environment.

The earliest Chordata to develop were the fish, whose basic design and habit patterns are very similar between different species – so, although they made an evolutionary leap to provide a blueprint for backboned lifeforms, they are actually quite basic compared to the highly sophisticated cephalopods. For another exception, one can look to the highly complex behaviours of parasitic wasps, who possess an impressive array of genetic engineering skills, enabling them to transform the larvae of another species into one of their own. The process of moulting the exoskeleton or metamorphosizing from the larvae through a pupal stage to the imago also shows a highly evolved system of growth and change. Thus, whilst a division between invertebrate and vertebrate animals may be helpful in some cases, I would suggest its more fruitful to look at the elemental realm which each animal family inhabits – Sky, Water, Earth, Under-world – combined with an appraisal of their life-cycle, survival strategy and unique behaviours. Of course, provings remain the fundamental backbone of Homeopathy and the best way to uncover the subjective human experience of any remedy.

COMPARATIVE STUDY WITH MINERALS AND PLANTS

Minerals

As the building blocks of larger organic and artificial structures, the mineral remedies represent archetypal and mythological forms, constitutional 'types' and are well-suited to addressing deep-seated physical and psychological suffering.

Themes

Fundamental to existence, building blocks, focus on one's sense of purpose or lack of it
When unwell; question whether they are still able to perform their task / their role well enough?

Alchemy / Archetypal / Fundamental / Mythological / Logical / Precise / Order / Structure.

Cation and Anion
A need to bond for stability, otherwise a lack of bond creates instability and volatile reactivity.

Left side periodic table;
Dependence / Weakness / Needs support / Fragile ego / Hopeful beginnings / Impulsive / Reactive / Adaptable / Trampled / Cardinal.

Right side periodic table;
Independence / Trapped / Escape / Betrayed / Left to do it themselves / Accepting that things come to an end / Selflessness / Dissolving / Decaying / Transmuting / Neglected / Mutable / Changeable.

Metals (middle);
Shining / Performance / Attack and defence / Durability / Resistance to corrosion / Unreactive / Unchanged / Reliability / Stability / Fixed.

Introduction   7

Gemstones;
Precious beauty and spiritual power that is trapped underground (in the sub-conscious); transformed under extreme forces; going from darkness into light.

Plants

Plants can survive off very little, photosynthesizing sunlight directly into energy. In turn, they provide a platform for the entire food-chain, for even the most ardent carnivores predate upon plant-eating animals. Plants can also be very toxic; being both deadly killers and intoxicating drugs, used to expand consciousness, numb pains or act medicinally in myriad ways within the human body.

Themes

Polarities are in the foreground of the case
Fundamental polarity: Nurturing, nourishing and healing *vs.* Poisonous, intoxi-cating and threatening. Each plant family has different themes and polarities and the case revolves around these.

Attractiveness, sexuality and beauty; making oneself desirable
Flowers are the plant's reproductive organs, providing vivid displays to attract pollinating insects. Plants adopt a multitude of survival strategies ranging from attractiveness, through to outright aggression, deceit, parasitism, overgrowth, climbing, rambling, colonising inhospitable environments . . . the list could go on. Keynotes for the kingdom are ***adaptability*** and ***diversity***.

Threatened *vs.* threatening
Plants can respond effectively to threats and challenges by making sudden changes in their physiology; For example, making their leaves more toxic, exuding a foul smell etc. These ***reactions to stimuli*** allow them to defend themselves despite being rooted to the spot and therefore unable to escape or engage in outright combat. They can however adopt aggressive growth habits; sprouting thorns, prickles and poisonous barbs. Thus, plant remedies are often indicated in transient 'states' that we move through more quickly than the constitutional pictures of mineral remedies. However, 'plant-like' states can, and do, also become fixed chronic patterns.

Underground intelligence (*ruled by subconscious reactivity*)
The whole plant incorporates the roots, bulb or rhizome as well as the stem, leaves and flowers that we see above ground. Perennials come back to life each year by investing energy in their underground storage centre; the bulb. This is a control hub containing the information for the complete life cycle of the plant and collaborating with mycelium in the soil. Minerals tend to be more rational / objective and focused on their lack of capacity as a result of the dis-ease. Whereas Plant patients focus on the subjective / subconscious (underground)

experience of the way something feels, spontaneously describing the way they are affected by the problem.

The patient describes how it feels and their reaction to it
They are often attuned to sensations, modalities, concomitants, and aetiological factors.

In addition to the sensation and it is opposite, Sankaran points out that there is both an active and passive response to the varied stimuli that touch upon the patient's sensitivity / susceptibility. This is very much in-line with the principles of primary and secondary action, whereby the active reaction may be a state of euphoria followed by a passive reaction of sedation, stupor and torpor.

Specific states and organ affinities
From the Materia Medica, it is clear that many plant remedies are well-suited to specific states that affect a particular target organ(s) or body system. The form of the plant above ground represents the specific state of dis-ease that arises as a response to the information in the bulb (constitution), the type of soil in which it grows (miasm) and the environmental changes it faces (situations / challenges / stress factors).

Collaboration and communication; give and take
Collaboration between Minerals (structure, shape, solidity), Fungi (sugars), Earth (soil), Water and Fire (sunlight – photosynthesis).

MAPPA MUNDI

The Mappa Mundi provides a map with which to navigate, understand and make use of polarity – acknowledging the essence of dualism in nature, epitomised by the concept of primary and secondary action. It organises the 4 elements and temperaments onto a circle, plotting pertinent Homeopathic information along-side each aspect so that we can perceive where our patient's disturbance and its opposite compensation are chiefly manifested. It can be of practical use in case analysis, allowing you to see which polarity is highlighted by the patient's food cravings, modalities, organ affinities and psychological characteristics. It can also help to differentiate remedies that all seem to cover the case symptomatically, thus tying in with a 'Genius' approach; matching the affinities and sphere of action of a remedy with the patient's disease state. For example, If the seat of the pathology is in the Bladder and Digestive system, then you would expect to see remedies with an 'Earth – Water' polarity coming through in the Case Analysis.

Also known as the Circle of Elements, the Mappa Mundi is designed to bring a focus to the archetypal / inherent forces in nature and how they are expressed through humans. This is especially useful in states of sickness – when **homeo-static balance** is often replaced by a **tension of opposites** in which the patient expresses symptoms that see-saw from one pole to another, For example, from chill to fever. It can be used as a guide to the salient Homeopathic information as presented by the patient, highlighting the **dynamic and characteristic symptoms** that might otherwise get lost in the sea of data of the case.

It also lends itself to being used alongside traditional medicinal practices – For example, Chinese medicine, Greek Unani Medicine, Ayurveda and Medical Astrology as there is considerable crossover among the various approaches informed by Elemental forces. The simplicity of seeing ourselves as a part of nature, and therefore subject to its forces, is a real positive for practitioners employing an Elemental Map such as this.

Observing nature and the way it behaves

- Man is a part of nature and cannot behave in ways that contravene natural laws; according to Newton's Third Law of Thermodynamics, every action has an equal and opposite reaction. In homeopathy, Hahnemann calls this the principle of primary and secondary action.
- Every 'state' a human embodies, perceived through the characteristic signs and symptoms of his dis-ease and expressed through the universal language of the vital force, will have a correspondence within the macrocosm of nature. Therefore, every human pattern of behaviour is mirrored in form by something else in the natural world, sharing that type of behaviour through the law of similars.

Polarity – within every action exists the equal and opposite action

The Vital Force (VF) acts by dynamically and appropriately responding to fluctuations in the external and internal environment. As Hahnemann writes in aphorism 64 of the *Organon*:[4]

> *The life force brings forth the exact opposite condition-state (counter-action, after-action) to the impinging action (initial action) that has been absorbed into itself. The counter-action is produced in as great a degree as was the impinging action (initial action) of the artificial morbific or medicinal potence on it, proportionate to the life force's own energy.*

A homeopathic remedy (or any medicinal agent / stimulus, for example, cold wind) acts upon the Vital Force and causes a primary action in which the Vital Force remains passive and receptive. It then rouses itself to produce the exact opposite / secondary action in the same proportion to the degree of the primary action.

> *A hand bathed in hot water is at first much warmer than the other unbathed hand (initial action), but once it is removed and thoroughly dried, it becomes cold after some time, and then much colder than the other hand (after-action).*
>
> Organon (aphorism 65).[4]

More examples from *Organon* (aphorism 65):[4]

- A person heated by vigorous exercise (initial action) is afterwards assailed with chilliness and shivering (after-action).

- To someone who yesterday was heated by drinking a lot of wine (initial action), today every light breeze is too cold (counteraction of the organism, after-action).
- An arm immersed in the coldest water for a long time is at first far paler and colder than the other one (initial action), but once it is removed from the cold water and dried off it becomes not only warmer than the other but hot, red and inflamed (after-action of the life force).
- Excessive liveliness results from drinking strong coffee (initial action) but sluggishness and sleepiness remain for a long time (counteraction, after-action) unless this is taken away repeatedly by drinking more coffee (palliative for a short time).

Symptoms try to restore balance

Being stuck in a state of dis-ease means that your body is unable to effectively meet the demands of the internal imbalance. The Vital Force, or *symptom-maker*, instinctively tries to rebalance itself by producing the opposite set of symptoms that would nullify the dis-ease. But, when the Vital Force is weakened, the ability to respond effectively is dampened – leading to stasis, immovability, rigidity and sickness, often expressed clinically in a tension of opposites. For example, *Posture: a stance that is too rigid topples easily.*

Too many conditions must be met in order to keep that person in their exact position of comfort. For example, a chronic migraine sufferer may must avoid lots of foods that trigger the condition, taking medication to ward off attacks, and retreating to a dark room to lie completely still during an attack. A stance that is dynamic and ready for action responds to stress through constant adaptation to different circumstances. The healthy Vital Force or immune system keeps the body in perfect harmony without us even being aware of it!

The tension of opposites

This is an important aspect in case taking and analysis. Homeopaths are always looking for the most dynamic aspects of the case, where symptoms are highly polarised or even contradictory. When a person is sensitive to a certain situation or feeling, they can often express one pole or the other, or fluctuate between the two. For example, Molluscs – the animal has a shell in which they can feel both safe, cosy and protected or at other times trapped, suffocated and closed-off from the world – isolated and forsaken.

Health means that you are not bound by your complexes. Your whole self is in a state of harmony rather than dissonance, so you can be free to explore your creativity and to fulfil the higher purposes of existence. An over-identification with one aspect of ourselves, and denial of others leads to a polarised state of susceptibility. For example, over-identification with the ego, which is an illusion created on the mental level of consciousness, seems to be key to the roots of becoming stuck in disease. The world of duality springs from the separation of ego and soul, solar and lunar, male and female archetypes. There is an illusion that these two parts are distinct and separate from one another, leading to a tendency to identify predominantly with only one aspect of ourselves and consign unwanted characteristics to our 'shadow' self. It is the Solar principle (ego) that drives us to individuate, seeking identification as a separate being through the way others perceive us; our possessions, career, values, creative exploits. The Soul or Lunar principle is often neglected – our subconscious is that which binds us together as humans and brings us back to our animal nature.

Perhaps this fundamental split plays an important role in maintaining ill health through chronic disease? Does not homeopathic prescribing work in such a way as to uncover the uncompensated / subconscious aspects of the being, allowing for better integration and wholeness of self? Dreams, delusions and sensations are ways in which we seek to find the aspects of ourselves that remain in the shadow. Perhaps that is the true meaning of a medical practice that is termed holistic – to unite the disparate parts that are vulnerable until unification occurs? This is what Jung termed individuation – the process of unifying the disparate elements of the psyche into the wholeness of the personality.

Polarity and Dualism – Yin and Yang

In Chinese Medicine, treatment plans are made based on deficiency, stagnation or over-abundance of one or other of these ancient archetypal energies – assertiveness (Yang) / receptiveness (Yin). The well-known glyph depicts a circle within which are two identical interlocking forms, like two whales – one is white, Yang, while the other is black, Yin. In the dark of Yin, there is a little spot of light, much as in the darkest night there are still stars to be seen. In the light of Yang exists a spot of darkness, like a solar spot on the surface of the sun or a black hole at the centre of a galaxy. Each state contains within it the seed potential for the development of the opposite state. Yin and Yang are in constant flux. Change is inevitable.

Organs and their meridians are classified according to whether they are Yin (consolidating energy) / Yang (expending energy). They represent fundamental polarities, although each contains the seed of the other. The Mappa Mundi conforms to this same principle – within each Element / Temperament, the seed of the opposite is present. For example, Fire is expressed in terms of the heavenly, spiritual fire, the spark of existence associated with the Sky realm. The purity of Fire descends from the Heavens to the Underworld, represented by the hellish realm of Hades. This form of fire is destructive and damaging, wreaking havoc. Hence the vertical axis in Mappa Mundi goes from light to dark, hot to cold, and from connection to disconnection.

In Astrology, there are polarities between:

Sun (Identity / rational / father) and **Moon** (Subconscious / reflective / mother)

Mars (Dominant / active / male) and **Venus** (Receptive / passive / female)

Jupiter (Faith / optimism / growth) and **Saturn** (Restraint / criticism / limitation)

Some examples of psychological polarities in the Mappa Mundi

Mirth, liveliness, hilarity, desires company *vs.* Solitary, absorbed in thought, misanthropic (*Sanguine – Melancholic*)
Dominated, victimised, abused *vs.* Dictatorial, aggressive (*Phlegmatic – Choleric*)
Leadership, duty, responsibility *vs.* Seeking approval (*Choleric – Phlegmatic*)
Euphoric, elated, joyful *vs.* Depressed, melancholic (*Sanguine – Melancholic*)
Confident, bragging *vs.* Yielding, mild, timid (*Choleric – Phlegmatic*)
Active and assertive *vs.* Restful and receptive (*Choleric – Phlegmatic*)
Connected, sociable *vs.* Shut-off, closed (*Sanguine – Melancholic*)
Pride, egotism, *vs.* Humble, loyal (*Choleric – Phlegmatic*)
Jealousy, envy *vs.* Acceptance (*Melancholic – Sanguine*)

The following figures (1.1–1.5) demonstrate how versatile the Mappa Mundi can be in synthesizing a variety of information and serve to illustrate in graphical form what has already been discussed. This leads into the next section which outlines each element and temperament in greater detail.

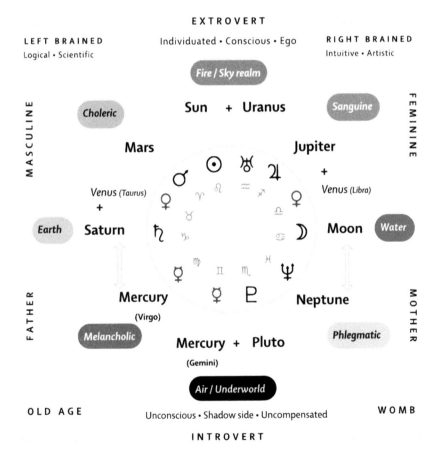

Figure 1.1 Astrological Planetary connections to the Mappa Mundi

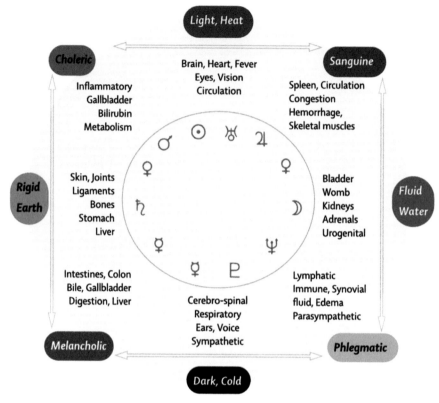

Figure 1.2 *Physical affinities mapped onto the circle of elements*

Incorporating the Realms into Mappa Mundi

Peter Fraser introduced a useful concept of the *Realms in Homeopathy*[5]. This was explored in a very interesting way in his books on the animal families – Spiders, Snakes, Insects and Birds. He also introduced the concept of each group needing to transform from one realm to another. For example, birds seek the freedom of the sky, and are most vulnerable when coming to the Earth realm – the feeling expressed by patients is often of being weighed down, trapped or tethered. Insects are rooted in the Earthly realm with a desire to transcend this to the Sky. Snakes draw their insight and power from underworld energy. Spiders are suspended in disorientation between the Earth and Sky on their web.

I have endeavoured to synthesise the Realms and the Mappa Mundi with Astrological themes to unify these models into one that I can use in my practice. I have found that it is useful to adopt a schema whereby Fire and the Sky realm are combined. The uppermost position of Fire in the Mappa Mundi brings to mind the heavenly connection – we turn our gaze upwards when contemplating Spirit, or the life-giving radiant energy of the Sun. By plotting the Sun and Uranus in this position, one combines Astrological Fire and Air and a pair of opposing signs – Leo and Aquarius. Uranus, often thought of as electrical fire,

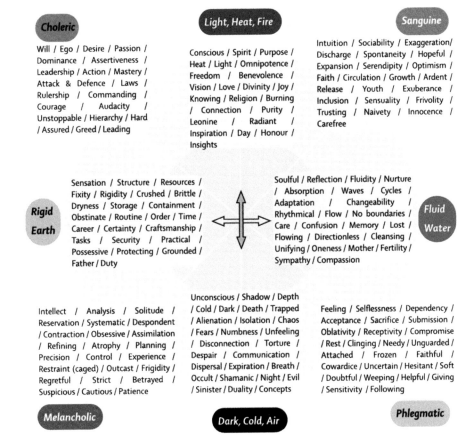

Choleric

Will / Ego / Desire / Passion / Dominance / Assertiveness / Leadership / Action / Mastery / Attack & Defence / Laws / Rulership / Commanding / Courage / Audacity / Unstoppable / Hierarchy / Hard / Assured / Greed / Leading

Light, Heat, Fire

Conscious / Spirit / Purpose / Heat / Light / Omnipotence / Freedom / Benevolence / Vision / Love / Divinity / Joy / Knowing / Religion / Burning / Connection / Purity / Leonine / Radiant / Inspiration / Day / Honour / Insights

Sanguine

Intuition / Sociability / Exaggeration/ Discharge / Spontaneity / Hopeful / Expansion / Serendipity / Optimism / Faith / Circulation / Growth / Ardent / Release / Youth / Exuberance / Inclusion / Sensuality / Frivolity / Trusting / Naivety / Innocence / Carefree

Rigid Earth

Sensation / Structure / Resources / Fixity / Rigidity / Crushed / Brittle / Dryness / Storage / Containment / Obstinate / Routine / Order / Time / Career / Certainty / Craftsmanship / Tasks / Security / Practical / Possessive / Protecting / Grounded / Father / Duty

Soulful / Reflection / Fluidity / Nurture / Absorption / Waves / Cycles / Adaptation / Changeability / Rhythmical / Flow / No boundaries / Care / Confusion / Memory / Lost / Flowing / Directionless / Cleansing / Unifying / Oneness / Mother / Fertility / Sympathy / Compassion

Fluid Water

Melancholic

Intellect / Analysis / Solitude / Reservation / Systematic / Despondent / Contraction / Obsessive / Assimilation / Refining / Atrophy / Planning / Precision / Control / Experience / Restraint (caged) / Outcast / Frigidity / Regretful / Strict / Betrayed / Suspicious / Cautious / Patience

Dark, Cold, Air

Unconscious / Shadow / Depth / Cold / Dark / Death / Trapped / Alienation / Isolation / Chaos / Fears / Numbness / Unfeeling / Disconnection / Torture / Despair / Communication / Dispersal / Expiration / Breath / Occult / Shamanic / Night / Evil / Sinister / Duality / Concepts

Phlegmatic

Feeling / Selflessness / Dependency / Acceptance / Sacrifice / Submission / Oblativity / Receptivity / Compromise / Rest / Clinging / Needy / Unguarded / Attached / Frozen / Faithful / Cowardice / Uncertain / Hesitant / Soft / Doubtful / Weeping / Helpful / Giving / Sensitivity / Following

Figure 1.3 *Keywords, themes and character traits*

rules convulsive, spasmodic movements which correspond to the physiological action of Fire in the Mappa Mundi, and the affinity to the central nervous system. Breaking free from constraints is also an important theme of Uranus, which fits with the well-known sensation in Bird remedies.

Jupiter is also an important Sky god. However, the faith, optimism, openness and adventurousness of Jupiter aligns it more closely with the Sanguine pole of the Mappa Mundi. Physiologically, Jupiter rules over arterial circulation, whilst Venus (Libra) is placed alongside Jupiter, bringing qualities of fairness, sexuality, pleasure-seeking and venous circulation.

The other significant adaptation that I have made to the Mappa Mundi is to combine elemental Air and the Underworld realm. There is a subtle difference to be made between the Sky and Air in this schema. The Sky realm refers to freedom, seeing the big picture and gravitating towards spiritual enlightenment. Elemental Air refers to the dark, cold of night, when the light of the Sun has disappeared. Sleep brings us into the domain of the subconscious, where nightmares and fears can be more prominent. The oxidising, tarnishing effect of

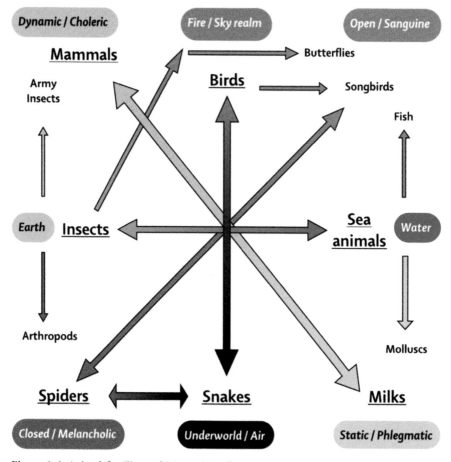

Figure 1.4 *Animal families and Mappa Mundi*

oxygen also refers to the corruption of the Underworld realm ruled by Pluto (Hades). Astrological Pluto rules the subterranean impulses, the urge to go deeper into one's inner experience through exploring subconscious motives. The Snakes are one of the most archetypal inhabitants of this realm, along with the syphilitic remedies.

Western Astrology

Western Astrology incorporates Greek Mythology (and the corresponding planetary associations); the 4 Elements; Jungian Psychology; the 4 Seasons and more. It offers an elegant and comprehensive system by which to study Psychological, Physiological and Pathological traits.

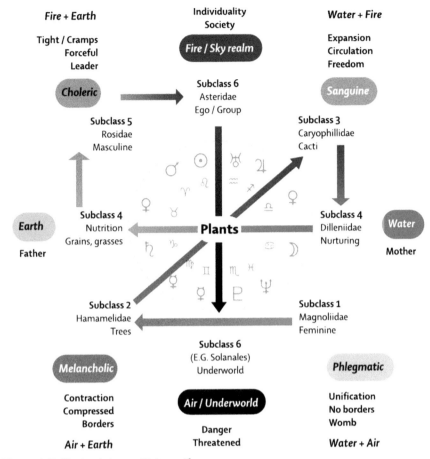

Figure 1.5 *Plant subclasses (Columns)*[6]

The Four Elements in Astrology

Pairs of opposites are formed between harmonising elements, such as Fire and Air / Earth and Water. Squares are formed between incompatible elements, such as Fire-Earth, Fire-Water, Air-Water, Air-Earth. In the Mappa Mundi, there are **oppositions** between:

- Fire – Air
- Earth – Water
- Sanguine – Melancholic
- Choleric – Phlegmatic

There are also **squares** (or right angles) between the following temperaments:

- Melancholic – Choleric
- Choleric – Sanguine
- Sanguine – Phlegmatic
- Phlegmatic – Melancholic

Some remedies and patients tend to express symptomatology through a tension of **opposites**, displaying obvious polarities evidenced in the subjective experience of their illness. Whereas others tend to express their suffering through a **square** (or right angle), with themes from two adjacent temperaments emerging. Both Choleric and Melancholic themes may be expressed through the characteristic signs and symptoms. For example, the affinities in the case may correspond to the Melancholic pole, manifesting in the Intestines, but the physiological action is Choleric (heat / inflammation / cramping / burning pains). Another example could be a person who is naturally optimistic and expansive (Sanguine), but when they are at work, the pressures force them into a more choleric mode of forceful industriousness, shouting at and criticising their colleagues who can't keep up with the pace. It is the Homeopath's job to be alive to these possibilities, diligently noting which dynamics hold the most intensity for the patient. It may be easy to discern a Phlegmatic temperament and therefore expect to see Choleric aspects too, but it is important as always, not to be biased and to be open to what arises spontaneously in the consultation.

VERTICAL AXIS: FIRE – AIR

Fire / Light and Heat / Spirit / Sky Realm

Creativity / Images of God / Brilliance / Luminosity
Spiritual impulse / Imagination / Inspiration
Sex and libido, love
Time: Midday
Flavour: Sweet
Season: Summer

Affinities: Brain, heart and arterial circulation, nervous system, eyes and vision.

Qualities: Conscious / Spirit / Purpose / Heat / Light / Omnipotence / Freedom / Benevolence / Vision / Love / Divinity / Joy / Knowing / Religion / Burning / Connection / Purity / Leonine / Radiant / Inspiration / Day / Honour / Insights

Astrological Fire
Universal radiant energy – excitable, enthusiastic, dynamic, spontaneous.
Wild, turbulent, uncontrolled, passionate, reckless, extravagant.
Conscious, wilful, overpowering, causing destruction.
Self-centredness, pride, self-esteem, directness.
Need to use energy – leading to burn-out.
Over-enthusiastic, vigorous.
Impulsive, unrestrained.
Over-confident.

Sun / Uranus (Leo / Aquarius) – The Circulatory system

Leo – Heart disease, Angina pectoris, Locomotor ataxia, Hyperaemia, Spinal disease, Spinal meningitis, Fevers.

Sun; *Affinities* – Vital fluid, Spleen, Distribution of heat, Pons varolii, Oxygen, Heart.

Uranus; *Sensations* – Spasmodic, Electric, Explosive, Convulsive, Disorganizing.

Aries (Fire and Head); *Affinities* – Brain, Cerebral hemispheres, Cranium, Eyes, Internal carotids, Neuralgia, Insomnia, Cerebral congestion, Brain fever.

Astrological Planetary Influence

Sun
Extrovert, Yang.
Sense of purpose, Conscious.
Role in society, Outward disposition.
Rational, Father, Integration, Core.

Uranus
Need for excitement.
Originality, Inventiveness.
Need for freedom, Purposeless rebellion.
Trapped, Independence from tradition.

Mind

- Ailments from
  - Egotism
  - Responsibility
- Ambition – increased
- Antics; playing
- Ardent
- Clairvoyance
- Confusion of mind
  - Dream; as if in a
  - Intoxicated – as if
- Confident
- Coquettish – too much
- Courageous
- Dancing
- Delirium – fever – during
- DELUSIONS
  - Body – out of the body
  - Christ; himself to be
  - Divine; being
  - Great person; is a
  - Humility and lowness of others; while he is great
  - Music – hearing music
  - Superiority; of
  - Tall – he or she is tall
- Despair – religious despair of salvation (Air pole)
- Dictatorial – power; love of
- Duty – too much sense of duty
- Eccentricity
- Ecstasy

- Egotism
- Energised feeling
- Excitement – religious
- Exhilaration
- Extravagance
- Freedom
- Haughty
- Honest
- Impulsive
- Insanity – religious
- Joy
- Lascivious
- Laughing
- Light – desire for
- Love – exalted love
- Music – amel.
- Music – desire for
- Nymphomania
- Pompous, important
- Praying
- Prophesying
- Religious affections – too occupied with religion
- Responsibility – taking responsibility too seriously
- Satyriasis
- Singing
- Temerity
- Wildness
- Will – strong will power
- DREAMS

- Clairvoyant
- Dancing
- Joyous

- Lascivious
- Music
- Sexual

Physicals

- **HEAD**
  - <u>Brain</u>; complaints of
  - Inflammation – Meninges
- **EYE** – Complaints of eyes
- **VISION** – Complaints of vision
- **CHEST**
  - Angina pectoris
  - <u>Heart; complaints of the</u>
- **MALE** – sexual desire – increased
- **FEMALE** – sexual desire – Increased
- **BACK** – Inflammation – Spinal cord
- **FEVER**
  - <u>Fever – Burning heat</u>
  - Fever – heat
  - Fever – intense heat
- **PERSPIRATION** – Odour – sweetish

- **GENERALS**
  - Noon
  - Congestion – blood; of
  - Circulation
  - Complaints of the blood
  - Convulsions
  - Energy – excess of energy
  - Food and drinks
    - § Alcoholic drinks – desire
    - § Sweets – desire
  - Heat
    - § Flushes of
    - § Sensation of
  - Heated; becoming
  - Locomotor ataxia
  - Moon – new moon – agg.

Related remedies and families

Primary

androc. arg-n. aur. bell. fire-el* helium hydrog. ignis-alc. lach. lampro-sp. sulph. tarent.

Bold

acon. adam. agar. aloe. ang. ant-c. apis. arg-met. ars-i. aur-m. aur-s. aves* cact. cann-i. cann-s. canth. carb-ac. carb-an. carbn-s. carbo-f. caust. cham. chel. cimic. cina. cinnb. coff. con. crat. croc. crot-h. cupr. cycl. dig. dulc. elaps. euph. falco-pe. gels. glon. grin. haliae-lc. hep. hyos. iod. kali-s. kalm. lac-c. lac-leo. lil-t. lycps-v. lyss. mag-s. merc-c. milks* naja. nat-s. olib-sac. ox-ac. ozone. par. petr. phos. phys. plat. podo. positr. sec. sol. spig. stage-11*$_{minerals}$ stage-9*$_{minerals}$ stram. sul-ac. syph. valer. verat. zinc.

Italic

Adon. Ail. Aml-ns. Anac. Argon. Ars. Arum-t. Aur-ar. Aur-m-n. Bar-s. Bism. Calc. Calc-ar. Calc-s. Caps. Carb-v. Caryophyllales* Cench. Chin. Cob. Colch. Coll. Column-6$_{Plants}$* Conv. Crot-c. Crot-t. Digin. Drugs* Elec. Eup-per. Ferr-i. Ferr-p. Gamb. Gink-b. Hydr-ac. Iber. Ign. Imponderables* Insecta* Irid-met. Jade. Kali-c. Lanthanides* Liliales* Lux-f-n. Lyc. Merc. Merc-i-f. Merc-i-r. Nat-m. Neon. Nit-ac. Nux-v. Phase. Prun. Psil. Pyrog. Ran-s. Raph. Rosales* Row-7$_{Plants}$* Saroth. Sars. Sep. Series-6$_{Minerals}$* Spong. Staph. Stront-c. Stroph-h. Stry. Sul-i. Tab. Vip. Visc. Zirc-met.

Air / Cold and Dark / Underworld

Dark, destruction and images of death
Indifference, alienation, suicidal despair
Seeking meaning – the formation within – thoughts and thinking – information
Fears – suffocation, falling, night, the dark, death, damnation, evil, the devil,
ghosts.
Oxidation and acidity
Cold reason and logic
Time: Midnight
Flavour: Sour

Affinities: Lungs/ Respiratory System, Cough, Ears, Hearing.

Qualities: Unconscious / Shadow / Depth / Cold / Dark / Death / Trapped /
Alienation / Isolation / Chaos / Fears / Numbness / Unfeeling / Disconnection /
Torture / Despair / Communication / Dispersal / Expiration / Breath / Occult /
Shamanic / Night / Evil / Sinister / Duality / Concepts

Astrological Air
Realm of abstract ideas, rational thinking, theorising and logical reasoning.
Want to rise above mundane routines, emotional needs and responsibilities.
Analytical, intellectual, detached, objective, wide perspective.
Eccentricity, fanaticism, unbalanced, lacking deep emotion.
Lacking stability, head in the clouds.

Mercury (Gemini) – The Respiratory and Nervous System

Gemini – Bronchitis, Asthma, Pneumonia, Consumption, Pleurisy, Corrupted
blood.

Mercury – Nerves, Bronchial Tubes, Pulmonary circulation, Thyroid gland, Right
cerebral hemisphere, Cerebro-spinal system, Sensory nerves, Vital fluid in nerves,
Vocal cords, Ears, Sight, Tongue, Sense perception, Breath.

Astrological Planetary Influence

Pluto – Underworld
Tyranny, Destructiveness, Chaos.
Underworld, Death, Annihilation.
Transformation, Rebirth, Taboo,
    Occult.
Obsessive-compulsive,
Perversion, Depth.
Suicidal, Psychosis, Criminal,
    Genius.

Mercury – Air
Networks, Ideas, Making connections.
Communication, Expression and
    Dispersal.
Cleverness, Duplicity.
Shape shifting, Shadow side.
Borders, Trade, Merchants.
Commerce, Short journeys.

Mind

- Night
- Ailments from
  - Fright
  - Reproaches
- Anguish
  - Night
  - Restlessness; with
- Antagonism with herself
- Anxiety
  - Night – midnight – before
  - Night – midnight – after
- Aversion
  - Everything; to
  - Family; to members of
  - Persons – all, to
- Company – aversion to – sight of people; avoids the
- Confusion of mind – identity; as to his – duality, sense of
- Death – desires / thoughts of
- Deceitful
- Delirium
  - Dark; in
  - Death; talks about
  - Devils; sees
  - Frightful
- Delusions
  - Alone; being – world; alone in the
  - Confidence in him; his friends have lost all
  - Criminal; he is a
  - Dead
    - § everything is
    - § he himself was
    - § persons, sees
  - Devil
  - Die
    - § about to die; one was
    - § time has come to
  - Division between himself and others
  - Dogs – black
  - Doomed; being
  - Friend – affection of; has lost the
  - Friendless; he is

- Horrible – everything seems
- Identity – errors of personal identity
- Mutilated bodies; sees
- Outcast; she were an
- People – behind him; someone is
- Possessed; being – *evil* forces; by
- Pursued; he was
  - § Devil; by
  - § Enemies; by
  - § Ghosts; by
- Repudiated; he is – relatives; by his
- Separated
  - § Body – mind are separated; body and
  - § Body – soul; body is separated from
  - § Himself; he were separated from world; from the – he is separated
  - § Specters, ghosts, spirits
  - § Talking – dead people; with
- Desires – nothing; desires
- Despair
  - Religious despair of salvation
- Detached
- Disconnected feeling
- Disgust
  - Everything; with
- Eccentricity
- Estranged
- Fanaticism
- Fear
  - Night
  - Dark; of
  - Death; of
    - § impending death; of
  - Devil; of being taken by the
  - Devils; of
  - Dogs; of
  - Evil; fear of
  - Falling; of
  - Ghosts; of
  - Imaginary – things; of imaginary

- ○ Narrow place; in
- ○ Sudden
- ○ Suffocation; of
- ○ Wind; of
- Forsaken feeling – isolation; sensation
- Frightened easily
- Inconstancy
- Indifference
- Intellectual
- Laughing – aversion to
- Liar
- Mania
  - ○ Demonic
- Moral feeling; want of
- Music – aversion to
- Remorse
- Scratching with hands
- Starting

- Striking
- Suicidal disposition
- Theorizing
- Thinking – logical thinking
- Thoughts
  - ○ Persistent
  - ○ Persistent – evil; of
  - ○ Two trains of thought
- Unfeeling
- Wicked disposition
- Will
  - ○ Contradiction of
  - ○ Two wills; sensation as if he had
- DREAMS
  - ○ Funerals
  - ○ Graves
  - ○ Intellectual
  - ○ Outsider – being an outsider

Physicals

- **EAR**
  - ○ Complaints of ears
- **HEARING**
  - ○ Acute
  - ○ Impaired
- **RESPIRATION**
  - ○ Asphyxia
  - ○ Asthmatic
  - ○ Complaints of respiration
- **COUGH**
  - ○ Cough In general
- **CHEST**
  - ○ Inflammation – Bronchial tubes
  - ○ Inflammation – Pleura
  - ○ Lungs; complaints of the
- Perspiration – odour – sour
- **GENERALS**

- ○ Night – midnight – after
- ○ Apoplexy
- ○ Cold – air – agg.
- ○ FOOD AND DRINKS
  - § Fruit – desire – *sour*
  - § Sour drinks – desire
  - § Sour food, acids – desire
- ○ Heat – lack of vital heat
- ○ Moon – full moon – agg.
- ○ Numbness
- ○ Pain – neuralgic
- ○ Painlessness of complaints usually painful
- ○ Pulse – slow
- ○ Shock
- ○ Warm – amel.

Related remedies and families

Primary

acon. *agar. air-el* am-m. anac. arg-n. ars. bell. cact. camph. cann-i. carb-an. carb-v. carbo-f. crot-h. dendr-pol. drugs* falco-pe. haliae-lc. hyos. merc. ophidia* ph-ac. plb. plut-n. positr. solanales* stram. syph. syphilitic-miasm* valer. zinc.*

Bold

adam. am-c. androc. ant-c. ant-t. apiales* argon ars-i. ars-met. ars-s-f. asaf. asar. aur. birds-prey* borx. bov. bry. calad. calc-p. carbons* carb-ac. chinin-ar. coc-c. coff. con. conifers* crot-c. cupr. dros. euphr. ferr-p. fungi* graph. hep. heroin. hippo-k. hydrog. ignis-alc. imponderables* ip. kali-ar. kali-n. kali-p. lac-c. lac-e. lach. lampro-sp. laur. lob. lsd. lux-f-n. lyc. mang. merc-c. mosch. nat-ar. nat-m. nat-p. nat-sil. nicc. nit-ac. nux-m. ozone. phos. plat. reptiles* row-9*plants rumx. sabad. sal-fr. seneg. sep. series-7*minerals spong. squil. stage-12*minerals stage-15*minerals stann. tab. tarent. tax-br. ther. tubercular-miasm* zinc-p. zirc-met.

Italic

Acer-sc. Agath-a. Aloe. Alum-p. Anacardiaceae* Animals* Arachnida* Asc-t. Aspidin. Asterales* Aur-ar. Aves* Bism. Brom. Cadm-s. Calc. Calc-ar. Capparales* Caps. Card-m. Caust. Chin. Chlor. Choc. Cimic. Cinnb. Clup-hr. Coca. Cocc. Column-6*Plants Cur. Dilleniidae* Dulc. Dys. Fagales* Ferr-ar. Gal-met. Germ-met. Granit-m. Hafn-met. Ham. Hamamelididae* Hura Hydr. Hydr-ac. Iod. Kali-c. Kali-i. Lac-h. Lanthanides* Lat-h. Latex-v. Leguminosae* Lil-t. Mag-c. Mag-p. Malvales* Matridonals* Meph. Merc-i-f. Merc-i-r. Milks* Naja Nat-s. Noble-gases* Nux-v. Olib-sac. Oncor-t. Op. Oryc-cn-s. Papaverales* Pass-d. Plan. Psor. Ran-b. Row-8*Plants Salicales* Samb. Sang. Scrophulariales* Scut. Sea-an* Sec. Series-1*Minerals Sil. Spect. Spig. Sulph. Sumb. Tell. Vacuum. Verat. Verat-v.

HORIZONTAL AXIS: EARTH – WATER

Water / Fluidity / Adaptability

**Seeking unity, blending, dissolving time and structure in feelings
Change, Adaptation, Flexibility, Fear of drowning
Weeping and Unsure, Fluid and mobile**
Flavour: Salty
Time: 6am

Affinities: Kidneys, Bladder, Speech, Mouth and Lower Lip

Qualities: Soulful / Reflection / Fluidity / Nurture / Absorption / Waves / Cycles / Adaptation / Changeability / Rhythmical / Flow / No boundaries / Care / Confusion / Memory / Lost / Flowing / Directionless / Cleansing / Unifying / Oneness / Mother / Fertility / Sympathy / Compassion

Astrological Water
The realm of feelings, intuition, deep emotion, overwhelming fears, passions.
Compulsive, irrational, lacking solidity and structure. Desires protection.
Secretive, hidden undercurrents, turmoil beneath a calm exterior.
Needs to be channelled / contained / held otherwise it is formless.
Sensitivity, fluidity, empathy, responsiveness.
Connection, oneness, acceptance, love.

Venus / Pluto (Libra / Scorpio) – The Generative Organs and fluid systems

Scorpio: Bladder, Urethra, Genitals, Descending colon, Prostate gland, Sigmoid flexure, Nasal bone, Pubic bone, Womb and Uterus, Prostate, Nasal catarrh, Mucous membranes, Nasal cartilage.

Libra: Kidneys, Adrenals, Lumbar region, Skin, Ureters, Vasomotor system. Bright's disease (Inflammation of kidneys), Lumbago, Suppression of urine, Nephritis, Diabetes, Renal calculi, Uraemia.

Astrological Moon
Uterus, Ovaries, Mammae.
Cyclical, Reflective, Soulful, Fertile.
Caring, Sensitive, Moody, Waxing and Waning.
Uncompensated, Feelings, Responsive, Receptive, Reactive.
Yin, Emotional, Sense of self, Home. Inward, Mother, Union, Subconscious.
Creature comforts, Habitual, Instinctive. Flowing, Oversensitivity, Family,
Nurture.

Mind

- Affectionate
- Ailments from – grief
- Bathing – desire to bathe
- Buoyancy
- Cares, full of – others; about
- Caring
- Confusion of mind – Identity; as to his – boundaries; and personal
- Content
- DELUSIONS
  - Dissolving; she is
  - Floating
  - Protection, defense; has no
  - Water
  - Weight – no weight; has
- Dependent of others
- Dream; as if in a
- Emotions – strong; too
- Fear – drowned; of being
- Grounded – not grounded
- Helplessness; feeling of
- Hiding – himself
- Home – desires to go
- Homesickness
- Impressionable
- Independent – lack of independence
- Insecurity; mental
- Intuitive
- LOVE
  - Exalted love – humanity; for
  - Family; for
  - Love-sick
  - Openness; and
- Maternal instinct; exaggerated
- MENSES
  - Before
  - During
- Merging of self with one's environment
- Mood – changeable
- Mother complex
- Nurturing theme
- Oneness – sensation of
- Reflecting
- Sadness – alone – when
- Sadness – weeping – with
- Secretive
- Selflessness
- SENSITIVE
  - Emotions; to
  - Everything; to
  - External impressions; to all
- Sensual
- Sentimental

- Spirituality
- Stability – desire for stability
- Suggestible
- Sympathetic
- Thinking – aversion to
- Thinking – logical thinking – inability for
- Tranquillity
- Unification – sensation of unification
- Water – loves
- WEEPING

  - Involuntary
  - Sad – thoughts; at
  - Sobbing; weeping; with
- Withdrawal from reality
- DREAMS
  - Drowned; being
  - Drowning
  - Ocean
  - Rain
  - River
  - Sea
  - Water

Physicals
- **EYE**
  - Lachrymation
- **NOSE**
  - Catarrh
  - Discharge – watery
- **FACE** – Complaints of face – Lips – Lower
- **MOUTH** – Complaints of mouth
- **STOMACH** – Thirst
- **BLADDER**
  - Complaints of bladder
  - Retention of urine
  - Urinary complaints
  - Urination – dysuria
- **KIDNEYS**
  - Complaints of kidneys
  - Inflammation
  - Suppression of urine
- **URETHRA** – Complaints of urethra
- **URINE**
  - Copious
  - Watery, Clear as water
- **FEMALE** – Uterus; complaints of
- **GENERALS**

  - Morning – 6 h
  - Bathing – sea; bathing in the agg. / amel.
  - Catarrh
  - Constitution – hydrogenoid
  - Diabetes mellitus
  - Food and drinks
    § salt – agg.
    § salt – desire
  - Moon – waning moon – agg.
  - Mucous membranes; complaints of
  - Mucous secretions – watery
  - SEASIDE; AT THE
    § agg.
    § amel.
  - SWELLING
    § General; in
    § Puffy, edematous
  - Wavelike sensations
  - Weather – cold weather – wet – agg.
  - Wet – applications – amel.

Related remedies and families

Primary
alum. aqua-nv. canth. carc. ign. lys. lyss. nat-m. neon oncor-t. spong. stram. thuj. water-el*

Bold

agn. alum-sil. alumn. am-c. am-m. ambr. amer-n. ant-c. ant-t. aq-mar. aq-pur. arg-n. argon aur-m. bar-c. berb. borx. bov. bufo. calad. calc. calc-p. calc-sil. calop-sp. cann-s. chin. cic. clem. coc-c. colch. cor-r. dig. dros. dulc. foll. gal-met. galeoc-c-h. gast. gav-im. grat. hell. insecta* irid-m. kali-n. kali-sil. kalm. kreos. lac-del. led. lux-f-n. magnesiums* mag-c. mag-m. mag-s. matridonals* med. melal-alt. meny. merc. merc-c. milks* mur-ac. murx. natrums* nat-c. nat-sil. nit-ac. ox-ac. pic-ac. puls. pycnop-sa. rhod. rhus-t. sabin. samb. sars. sea-an* sel. sep. sil. siliciums* squil. stage-13*$_{minerals}$ stage-2*$_{minerals}$ staph. stront-c. stych-gig. taosc. teucr. trach. urol-h.

Italic

Abrot. Acet-ac. Aids. All-c. Alum-p. Androc. Apis Apoc. Ars. Aster. Aur. Aurums Aur-m-n. Aves* Bar-i. Bar-m. Bar-s. Benz-ac. Bry. Cact. Calc-ar. Calc-f. Calc-i. Calc-s. Camph. Cann-i. Cann-xyz. Carb-ac. Caust. Chlor. Cimic. Cina Cist. Cocc. Column-4* Com. Cop. Crot-h. Crot-t. Cupr. Cypra-eg. Eup-per. Falco-pe. Ferr. Form. Graph. Halogens* Hep. Hyos. Ind. Kali-c. Kali-chl. Lach. Lil-t. Lyc. Mag-p. Manc. Olnd. Op. Oryc-cn-s. Pall. Ph-ac. Phel. Phos. Phosphoricums* Plan. Plat. Podo. Pyrog. Row-2*$_{Plants}$ Ruta Sabal Sanic. Syc. Tax. Ust. Verat. Vinc. Vip.*

Earth / Dryness / Form / Function

Sensation, Solidity, Stability and Limitation
Seeking Containment, Memory and Structure
Fixed and Rigid. Hard and assured
Fear of dirt and germs, being crushed / trapped
Flavour: Bitter/ Rancid

Affinities: Bones, Digestive Tract, Mouth, Liver, Anus, Stiff Upper Lip.

Qualities: Sensation / Structure / Resources / Fixity / Rigidity / Crushed / Brittle / Dryness / Storage / Containment / Obstinate / Routine / Order / Time / Career / Certainty / Craftsmanship / Tasks / Security / Practical / Possessive / Protecting / Grounded / Father / Duty

Astrological Earth
Physical realm of sensation, materials, resources and structure.
Practical, disciplined, patient, earning a living, basic needs.
Efficient, factual, conventional, dependable.
Secure, routined, reserved, cautious.
World of form and function.

Moon / Saturn (Cancer / Capricorn) – Nutrition, Digestion and Structure

Capricorn: Skin, Knees, Joints, Hair, Dislocation of Bones, Eczema.

Saturn – Gallbladder, Vagus Nerve, Teeth, Skin, Joints, Ligaments, Sigmoid Flexure.

Moon: Indigestion, Dipsomania, Gastric Catarrh, Hiccough, Flatulency.

Astrological Saturn

Suppressive.
Desires recognition.
Constriction / contraction.
Revolts then conservative.
Castrates father; Tyrannical.
Rigid ruler; Hard task-master.
Critical of oneself and others.
Demands structure and imposes limitations;
working very hard to perfect your routine.

Mind

- Activity – desires activity
- Ailments from – business failure
- Amusement – aversion to
- Answering – aversion to answer
- Anxiety – business; about
- Anxiety – money matters; about
- Avarice
- Business – desire for
- Cares; full of – business; about his
- Cautious
- Change – aversion to
- DELUSIONS
  - Fail; everything will
  - Home – away from home; he is
  - Past – living in the past
  - Past – long past events
  - Poor; he is
  - Ruined – is ruined; he
  - Starve – family will
  - Want – he will come to
  - Work
    - § accomplish her work; she cannot
    - § hard; is working
    - § hindered at work; is
    - § too much work; he has
- Dogmatic
- DWELLS
  - Disappointments; on
  - Grief from past offenses
  - Past disagreeable occurrences; on
  - Recalls – disagreeable memories
- Recalls – old grievances
- Efficient, organised

- FEAR
  - Business failure; of
  - Poverty; of
  - Undertaking anything; of
  - Work; of
- Grumbling
- Home – desires to go
- Irritability – questioned; when
- Materialistic
- Mistakes; making – work; in
- Monomania
- Obstinate
- Patience
- Perseverance
- Practical
- Prejudiced – traditional prejudices
- Prostration of mind – business; from
- Protected feeling
- Recognition; desire for
- Reserved
- Serious
- Slowness
- Stability – desire for stability
- Talking – business; of
- Taste agg.; bitter
- Time – slowly, appears longer; passes too
- Tough
- Trifles – important; seem
- Truth – telling the plain truth
- Weeping – cannot weep, though sad
- DREAMS
  - Work

Physicals
- **HEAD** – Hair
- **MOUTH**
  - Complaints of mouth
  - Dryness
  - Saliva – bitter
  - Speech – wanting
  - Taste – bitter
  - Dryness
    - Thirst – without
- **STOMACH**
  - Complaints of the stomach
  - Disordered
  - Indigestion
  - Vomiting; type of – bitter
- **ABDOMEN**
  - Complaints of abdomen – Intestines
  - Inflammation
    § Cecum
    § Colon
    § Gastroenteritis
    § Intestines
    § Small intestine
  - Liver and region of liver; complaints of
- **RECTUM** – Anus; complaints of
- **STOOL** – Hard
- **URINE** – Scanty
- **EXTREMITIES**
  - Contraction of muscles and tendons
  - Dislocation

- Knees; complaints [Extremities]
- Nails; complaints of – brittle nails
- **SKIN**
  - Complaints of skin
  - Dry
  - Eruptions – eczema
- **GENERALS**
  - Evening – 18 h
  - Bones; complaints of
  - Brittle bones
  - Discharges – scanty
  - Dryness of usually moist internal parts
  - Flexibility – want of – Joints
  - Food and drinks
    § bitter drinks – agg.
    § bitter food – desire
  - Injuries – Bones; fractures of
  - Joints; complaints of the
  - Moon – waxing moon – agg.
  - Motion – aversion to
  - Mucous membranes; complaints of – dryness
  - Muscles; complaints of
  - Pain – Ligaments
  - Shortened muscles and tendons
  - Softening bones
  - Stiffness
  - Weather
    § cloudy weather – amel.
    § dry – agg.

Related remedies and families

Primary
bamb-a. bry. calc-f. caust. con. earth-el* fl-ac. graph. insecta* kaliums* kali-c. marb-w. meli. nat-c. psor. ruta sapph. series-4*_{minerals} sil. stann. thuj. verat.

Bold
bapt. bar-c. borx. brom. calc. calcareas* calc-p. calc-s. carb-an. carbn-s. chin. chinin-ar. chinin-s. cucurbitales* cycl. eup-per. ferr. form. gels. graminales* / poales* guaj. ham. hecla. helx. hydr. hyper. ip. jade jup. kali-ar. kali-bi. kali-br. kali-i. kali-n. kali-s. kali-sil. lyc. mag-c. nat-ar. nat-m.

nit-ac. nux-m. nux-v. op. oxyg. phyt. plb. rhus-t. samb. siliciums* stage-4*_{minerals} stage-6*_{minerals} stram. stront-c. symph. techn. valer. zinc-p.

Italic

Bar-m. Bar-s. Bell-p. Bism. Bor-pur. Cadm-s. Calad. Calc-ar. Calc-i. Calen. Canth. Carbons Carb-ac. Carb-v. Carbo-f. Cedr. Cham. Cimic. Cina. Cladon-ra. Cocc. Column-4* Cortiso. Cupr. Cupr-f. Dulc. Dys. Fabales* Fel. Ferrums* Fl-pur. Fluoratums* Helon. Hep. Ign. Iris. Kali-chl. Kali-m. Kali-p. Lac-d. Lact. Leguminosae* Lith-c. Lith-f. Loganiaceae* Merc. Merc-i-r. Mill. Morph. Mur-ac. Nat-f. Petr. Ph-ac. Plat. Puls. Raph. Rheum. Rhod. Row-3*_{Plants} Sacch. Sanic. Sec. Sep. Series-6*Minerals_{Staph.} Stront-m. Stront-met. Sulphuricums* Syph. Tell. Til. Zinc. Zing.*

SANGUINE – MELANCHOLIC AXIS
(DILATION – CONTRACTION)

Sanguine

**Open, Innocent, Childlike, Hopeful and Singing, Adolescent
Optimistic and Ardent, Sociable and Open characters
Open, Dilated, Growth, Expanding**
Fear of loneliness
amel. discharges > company
Tropical rain forest
Congestion / Haemorrhage
HOT and WET
Time: 9am
Season: Spring

Affinities: Blood, Heart and Arteries, Skeletal muscles, Spleen.

Qualities: Intuition / Sociability / Exaggeration/ Discharge / Spontaneity / Hopeful / Expansion / Serendipity / Optimism / Faith / Circulation / Growth / Ardent / Release / Youth / Exuberance / Inclusion / Sensuality / Frivolity / Trusting / Naivety / Innocence / Carefree

Venus / Jupiter: The Sanguine temperament

Jupiter – Liver, Glycogen, Suprarenals, Arterial circulation, Fibrin of blood, Fats.

Sagittarius – Hips, Femur, Ilium, Thighs, Sciatic nerve.

Venus – Throat, Kidneys, Thymus gland, Venous circulation, Homeostasis, Warm, Lymphatic, Relaxing, Sedentary.

Astrological Planetary Influence

Jupiter

Urge to connect with the spiritual
  realm through openness to the 'big
  picture'.
Spirit, Faith, Optimism, Freedom.
Joy, Vision, Expanding awareness.
Belief, Imagination, Exploration.
Adventurous, Scattered energy, Long
  journeys.
Seeing the big picture, view from the
  sky, over-extending oneself.

Venus

Co-operation, Giving, Compromise.
Beauty, Love, Comparison, Taste,
  Exchange.
How we make ourselves and others
  happy.
Pleasure, Sharing, Values, Socialising.
Expressing affection for others.
Seduction, Attraction.
Balance, Harmony, Sexual Lust,
  Flirtatious.
Conciliation, Friendship, Beauty,
  Desire.
Reaction, Sensation, Relationship,
  Partner.

Mind

- Adventurous
- Affectionate
- Amativeness
- Amorous
- Amusement – desire for
- Benevolence
- Brotherhood; sensation of
- Capriciousness
- Carefree
- Change – desire for
- Cheerful
  - Foolish; and
  - Lightness; with sensation of
- Childish behaviour
- Communicative
- Company – desire for
- Contact; desire for
- Curious
- Dancing
- Delirium – gay, cheerful
- Delusions
  - Beautiful
  - Friend – surrounded by friends;
    being
  - Visions; has – beautiful
- Desires – full of desires
- Elated

- Ennui
- Euphoria
- Exaggerating
- Expansive
- Extravagance
- Fancies – exaltation of
- Fear – alone; of being
- Foolish behaviour
- Frivolous
- Freedom
- Gossiping
- Grounded – not grounded
- High-spirited
- Home – leave home – desire to
- Hopeful
- Idealistic
- Ideas – unconnected
- Impulsive
- Inconstancy
- Innocent
- Injustice; cannot support
- Jesting
- Joy
- Kissing – everyone
- Laughing
- Laughing – immoderately
- Libertinism

- Loquacity
- Mirth
- Mood – changeable
- Naive
- Naked; wants to be
- Open
- Optimistic
- Perfume – loves to use perfume
- Persisting in nothing
- Pleasure
- Playful

- Restlessness – excitable
- Shameless
- Sociability
- Thoughts – wandering
- Time – fritters away his time
- Travelling – desire for
- Undertaking – many things, persevering in nothing
- Vivacious
- DREAMS
  - Adventurous / Parties

Physicals
- **CHEST** – Enlarged sensation – Heart
- **ABDOMEN** – Spleen; complaints of
- **GENERALS**
  - Apoplexy
    - § Haemorrhagic, sanguine
  - Forenoon – 9 h
  - Circulation; complaints of the blood
  - Congestion – blood; of

- Discharges – amel.
- Energy – excess of energy
- Expansion; sensation of
- Haemorrhage
  - § Arterial
- Muscles; complaints of
- Orgasm of blood
- Seasons – spring – agg.
- Tension – Arteries; of

Related remedies and families

Primary
cact. cactacae* cean. chin. glon. hyos. lach. phos. sanguine*

Bold

acon. apis aran. arn. cann-i. caryophyllidae* cench. cic. coff. ferr. fungi* hydr-ac. labiatae* lepidoptera* mang. naja nitricums* nitro. op. ophidia* phosphoricums* pisces* pyrog. rubiales* sacch-a. stage-5*_{minerals} stage-7*_{minerals}

Italic

Agar. Agath-a. Aloe Alumin. Amer-n. Aml-ns. Ant-c. Ant-t. Arg-n. Argon Aur. Aves* Bapt. Bar-m. Bell. Bov. Bufo Camph. Cedr. Cent. Cham. Chlor. Choc. Clup-hr. Cocc. Column-3*_{Plants} Con. Croc. Crot-h. Dulc. Eup-per. Ferr-p. Fulg. Gels. Gink-b. Glyc. Ham. Hamamelididae* Hydrog. Ictod. Ign. Ip. Kali-i. Kali-p. Kola Kreos. Lac-c. Lampro-sp. Med. Meli. Mill. Myric. Myrt-c. Nat-c. Nat-m. Nat-s. Neon Nux-m. Nux-v. Ol-an. Olib-sac. Olnd. Oryc-cn-s. Piperaceae* Plat. Psor. Ran-b. Ranunculaceae* Row-4*_{Plants} Row-6*_{Plants} Rub-t. Sabad. Samb. Sea-animals* Sec. Seneg. Sep. Spig. Stram. Stroph-h. Stroph-s. Sul-ac. Sulph. Talp-eu. Tarax. Ther. Usn. Verat. Verat-v. Verb. Zinc. Zinc-n.

Melancholic / Nervous

Moaning, Complaining, Holding on, Consolidating
Philosophical, Introspective, Detached, Wise
Heavy, Resentful, Jealous, Brooding
Restrained, Shuns company, Melancholic, Closed, Repressed
Contracted, Atrophy
Fear of loss, > solitude
Withdrawn and Closed/ Pessimistic Types
COLD and DRY
Flavour: PUTRID
Season: Autumn
Time: 9pm

Affinities: Black Bile, Liver, Colon, Constipation, Marasmus, Atrophy.

Qualities: Intellect / Analysis / Solitude / Reservation / Systematic / Despondent / Contraction / Obsessive / Assimilation / Refining / Atrophy / Planning / Precision / Control / Experience / Restraint (caged) / Outcast / Frigidity / Regretful / Strict / Betrayed / Suspicious / Cautious / Patience

Mercury / Saturn: The Melancholic temperament

Virgo / Mercury – Peritonitis, Malnutrition, Dysentery, Colic, Constipation, Diarrhoea, Cholera, Typhoid, Appendicitis, Tapeworm, Abdominal, Large and Small Intestine, Liver, *Spleen (opposite pole – sanguine)*, Duodenum, Chymification, Peristalsis of bowels.

Capricorn / Saturn – Erysipelas, Leprosy.

Aquarius / Saturn – Gloom, Endurance, Nervousness, Sensitivity.

Astrological Planetary Influence

Mercury (Virgo)
Digestion, absorption and elimination.
Obsessive over details.
Discerning, fussy about nutrition.
Analytical, sorting, refining.
Purity, perfectionism; has to be just right. Harvesting (Autumn).
Health-conscious (anxiety about disease).
Practical selfless service to others.
Organised *vs.* Chaotic (Pisces opposition).

Saturn
Constriction / contraction.
Rigid ruler; Hard task-master.
Critical of oneself and others.
Desires recognition.
Castrates father; Tyrannical.
Revolts then conservative.
Suppressive – eats his children.
Demands structure and imposes limitations; working very hard to perfect your routine.

Mind

- Ailments from – friendship; deceived
- Anxiety – health; about
- Aversion
  - Everything, to
  - Family; to members of
  - Persons – all; to
  - Persons – certain; to
- Brooding
- Censorious
- Closed character
- Company – aversion to
  - Desire for solitude
  - Sight of people; avoids the
- Complaining
- Confidence – want of self-confidence
  - Failure; feels himself a
  - Self-depreciation
- Conscientious about trifles
- Deceitful
- Deception
- Delusions
  - Betrayed; that she is
  - Cheated; being
  - Conspiracies – against him; there are conspiracies
  - Despised; is
  - Division between himself and others
  - Forsaken; is
  - Lost; she is – salvation; for
  - Oppressed; he were
  - Outcast; she were an
  - Outsider; being an
  - Poisoned – he – about to be poisoned; he is
  - Poisoned – he – has been
  - Trapped; he is
  - Unfortunate; he is
  - Worthless; he is
- Wrong – suffered wrong; he has
- Desires – suppressing his desires
- Despair
- Despair – recovery; of
- Discontented
- Discontented – himself; with
- Disgust
- Excitement – nervous
- Fastidious
- Fear
  - Betrayed; of being
  - Disease; of impending
  - Loss; of suffering a
  - Poisoned – being poisoned; fear of
- Hiding – himself
- Introspection
- Jealousy
- Jesting – aversion to
- Loathing
  - General loathing
  - Life
- Looked at; to be – cannot bear to be looked at
- Meditating
- Melancholy
- Misanthropy
- Mocking – sarcasm
- Mood – repulsive
- Muttering
- Perfectionist
- Pessimist
- Philosophy – ability for
- Plans – making many plans – revengeful plans
- Suspicious
- Suspicious – solitude; desire for
- Taciturn
- Thoughts – compelling
- Unfortunate; feels
- Unfriendly humour
- Weary of life

Physicals
- **STOMACH** – Digestion – impeded
- **ABDOMEN**
  - Complaints of abdomen – Intestines
  - Duodenum; complaints of
  - Inflammation
    - § Appendix
    - § Colon
    - § Duodenum
    - § Peritoneum
  - Pain – cramping
  - Peristalsis – reversed
- **RECTUM**
  - Cholera
  - Constipation
  - Diarrhea
  - Dysentery
- Worms – complaints of worms – tapeworm
- **FEMALE** genitalia/sex – menses – suppressed menses
- **PERSPIRATION** – suppression of discharges – agg.
- **SKIN**
  - Eruptions – leprosy
  - Erysipelas
- **GENERALS**
  - Evening – 21h00
  - Atrophy
  - Contractions
  - Discharges – suppressed
  - Emaciation
  - Hardness, induration
  - Mucous secretions – suppressed
  - Old age – premature
  - Perspiration – suppression of perspiration; complaints from
  - Seasons – autumn – agg.

Related remedies and families

Primary

alum. araneae* ars. ars-s-f. aur-ar. aur-s. carc. chin. germ-met. graph. guaj. melanch* myric. nat-c. nit-ac. ozone. sapph. thuj. verat.

Bold

alum-sil. am-c. anac. ant-c. arg-n. arsenicums* aur. aurums* aur-m-n. bar-c. bar-s. borx. brom. cact. calc-ar. calc-p. calc-sil. carb-an. carb-v. carbn-s. chinin-ar. chinin-s. con. crot-t. dulc. ferr-p. gink-b. heroin. hyos. ip. kaliums* kali-ar. kali-bi. kali-i. kali-n. kali-s. kali-sil. lach. lyc. m-arct. mag-s. merc-c. nat-m. nat-p. nat-s. nat-sil. nicc. par. phos. plut-n. pseuts-m. sel. sep. stage-14*_{minerals} stage-16*_{minerals} stann. stront-c. sul-ac. tax. tub. vanil. zinc-p.

Italic

Abrot. Acids* Acet-ac. Adam. Agn. Alum-p. Ambr. Bism. Bov. Bry. Bufo Cadm-s. Calc. Carbo-f. Chloram. Cinnb. Coca Cocc. Column-2*_{Plants} Cupr. Earth-el* Ferr-ar. Ferr-i. Fl-ac. Gamb. Gels. Grat. Halogens* Hamamelididae* Hell. Hydr. Hydr-ac. Ign. Iod. Kali-chl. Kali-p. Lac-c. Lanthanides* Lith-c. Mag-c. Mag-p. Med. Merc. Mur-* Naja Op. Ph-ac. Plb. Plb-act. Plb-m. Puls. Rhus-g. Row-8*_{Plants} Sabal Samb. Sanic. Sars. Sil. Staph. Streptoc. Sul-i. Sulph. Sulphuricums* Syc. Syph. Tell. Vip. Zinc.

CHOLERIC – PHLEGMATIC AXIS (ASSERTIVE – RECEPTIVE)

Choleric / Forceful / Dominant

**Dynamic, Dictatorial, Tight, Forceful and shouting, Action with bravery
Courageous, Decisive, Formal Rulers, Law Enforcement**
Intolerant of contradiction, Irritable, Aggressive
Focused, Passionate, Intelligent, All or nothing
Hungry, Critical, Hot tempered
Explosive, Fear of failure
> activity (occupation amel.)
HOT and DRY
Season: Summer
Time: 3pm
Flavour: SPICY

Affinities: Gall, Ducts in liver, Bilirubin in blood, Stomach, Inflammatory process, Fast metabolism.

Qualities: Will / Ego / Desire / Passion / Dominance / Assertiveness / Leadership / Action / Mastery / Attack and Defence / Laws / Rulership / Commanding / Courage / Audacity / Unstoppable / Hierarchy / Hard / Assured / Greed / Leading

Sun / Mars: The Choleric temperament

Mars – Iron in blood, Genitals, Motor nerves, Left hemisphere, Muscular movements, Desire body.

Scorpio – Rupture, Scurvy, Fistula, Piles, Red pigmentation in blood.

Astrological Planetary Influence

Mars
Energetically setting targets.
Making maximum effort to reach the goal.
Going on the attack or being attacked.
Brave, Conquest, Battles, Heroic, Blood lust.
Attack, Warrior, Anger, Inflammation.
Action, Audacity, Boldness, Courage.
Masculine strength and bravado.
Conflict with others, asserting oneself.
Impulsive, Rash, Impatient.

Sun
Extrovert, Yang.
Radiating the self.
Sense of purpose, Conscious.
Rational, Father, Integration, Core.
Role in society, Outward disposition.

Mind

- Abrupt
- Abusive
- Ailments from
  - Ambition – deceived
  - Ambition – excessive
- Ambition – increased – competitive
- Anger
  - Contradiction; from
  - Violent
- Answering – dictatorial
- Ardent
- Attack others; desire to
- Audacity
- Busy
- Contradiction
  - Disposition to contradict
  - Intolerant of contradiction
- Courageous
- Cursing
- Defiant
- Delusions
  - General; he is a
  - Officer; he is an
- Strong; he is Determination
- Dictatorial
- Fastidious – prove himself; he has to
- Fear – failure; of
- Fearless
- Fight, wants to
- Firmness
- Heedless
- Hurry
- Impatience
- Impetuous
- Industrious
- Insolence
- Irritability
- Obstinate
- Occupation – amel.
- Passionate = choleric
- Pertinacity
- Quarrelsome
- Quick to act
- Rage
  - Contradiction; from
- Rash
- Violent
- Will – strong will power

Physicals

- **STOMACH**
  - Appetite – increased
  - Pain – violent
- **ABDOMEN**
  - Complaints of abdomen – Gallbladder and ducts
  - Gallstones
- **MALE** genitalia/sex –
  - Complaints of male genitalia
- **FEVER** – Dry heat
- **SKIN** – Inflammation
- **GENERALS**
  - Afternoon – 15h00
  - Circulation; complaints of the blood
  - Cold – applications – amel.
  - Food and drinks
    § coffee – desire
    § spices – desire
    § stimulants – amel.
    § stimulants – desire
  - Heated, becoming
  - Inflammation
  - Pain – Muscles – cramping
  - Stiffness – Muscles
  - Tension – Muscles; of

Related remedies and families

Primary

androc. apis apisin. arg-met. aur. bry. canth. castor-eq. caust. cham. chel. choleric* coca cocain. coff. cupr. dama-da. falco-pe. ferr. ferrums* fl-ac. form.

hep. ign. iod. kola lac-e. lach. lil-t. lyc. nux-v. plat. polys. rhus-t. stage-10*_{minerals} stage-8*_{minerals} sul-ac. tarent. verat.

Bold

adam. agar. aloe apis-rg. aur-m-n. aur-s. bell. calop-sp. carc. column-5*_{plants} cur. dendr-pol. dulc. ferr-p. gels. ham. insecta* kali-br. lac-leo. lac-lup. lac-o. m-ambo. m-arct. mammalia* med. merc. nat-ar. nat-s. nicc. op. pip-m. plut-n. predators* sapph. schist-am. sep. staph. tung-met. uran-met. valer.

Italic

Acon. Anac. Ang. Animals* Araneae* Arn. Ars. Berb. Bism. Bov. Calad. Calc-met. Camph. Cancer-miasm* Caps. Carbo-f. Card-m. Chinin-s. Chion. Coloc. Crot-c. Cupr-ar. Dios. Droseraceae* Dyspr-met. Ferr-ar. Ferr-i. Fulg. Fungi* Geraniales* Hed. Hydr. Hyos. Iris Kali-c. Lac-c. Lac-d. Lept. Lyss. Mag-lac. Mag-met. Mag-n. Mag-s. Mag-sil. Merc-d. Mez. Nat-p. Oryc-cn-s. Pall. Pass-d. Plb. Podo. Puls. Rheum Rhus-g. Rosales* Row-5*_{Plants} Sea-an* Series-6*_{Minerals} Solanaceae* Stage-11*_{Minerals} Stage-12*_{Minerals} Sulph. Sulphuricums* Test. Thuj. Tub. Typhoid-miasm* Verat-v.

Phlegmatic / Yielding / Mild

Static, submissive, loose. Patience and depth, Soft and slow
Faithful, indecisive, craving security and order, shape and structure
Qualities: Soft, Compassionate, Overweight, Forgiving, Loyal, Memory of the past,
Fear of domination, being engulfed, loss of identity
Pleading and entreating
Yielding types > rest
Mist, Fog, Drizzle,
FRESH/ FROSTY
COLD and WET
Season: Winter
Time: 3am

Affinities: Lymphatic System, Synovial Membranes, Capsules, Cartilage, Conjunctivae, Tears, Edema / Dropsy, Waterlogged, Rheumatism, Phlegm.

Qualities: Feeling / Selflessness / Dependency / Acceptance / Sacrifice / Submission / Receptivity / Compromise / Rest / Clinging / Needy / Unguarded / Attached / Frozen / Faithful / Cowardice / Uncertain / Hesitant / Soft / Doubtful / Weeping / Helpful / Giving / Sensitivity / Following

Constitution: Hydrogenoid

Moon / Neptune: The Phlegmatic temperament

Cancer – Oesophagus, Uterus, Ovaries, Lymphatics, Sympathetic nervous system, Synovial fluid, Alimentary canal, Lymph, Chyle, Nerve sheaths, Dropsy.

Pisces – Bunions, Gout, Deformed feet, Tumours, Dropsy, Toes, Fibrin of blood.

Neptune – The Pineal gland, Dreaming, Sleep / Wake cycles. Immune vulnerabilities, Lymphatic toxicity. Psychic sensitivity, Vulnerability. Poor boundaries. Victim / Rescuer relationships.

Astrological Planetary Influence

Neptune
Escapism, Idealism, Sacrifice, Oblivion.
Selflessness, Devotion, Martyrdom.
Oceanic Feeling, Fantasy, Illusion.
Rescuing / needing to be rescued.
Dissolving of form, Addiction.
Evasion of responsibilities.
Collective unconscious.
Dreams, Turbulence.
Victim or victimised.

Moon
Caring, Sensitive.
Receptive, Reactive.
Moody, Waxing and Waning.
Cyclical, Reflective, Soulful, Fertile.
Yin, Emotional, Sense of self, Home.
Inward, Mother, Union, Subconscious.
Uncompensated, Feelings, Responsive.
Creature comforts, Habitual,
    Instinctive.
Flowing, Oversensitivity, Family,
    Nurture.

Mind

- Ailments from
  - Abused; after being
  - Discords – friends; between one's
  - Domination
  - Embarrassment
  - Reprimands
  - Reproaches
  - Rudeness of others
- Bed – remain in bed; desire to
- Caressed; being – desire to be caressed
- Clinging – children; in
- Comply to the wishes of others; feeling obliged
- Confidence – want of self-confidence – support; desires
- Consolation – amel.
- Cowardice
- Delusions
  - appreciated; she is not
  - neglected – he or she is neglected
- Discouraged Harmony – desire for
- Held – amel. / desire being held

- Helplessness; feeling of
- Lamenting
- Laziness – morning
- Longing – repose and tranquillity; for
- Mildness
- Pities herself
- Quiet disposition
- Quiet; wants to be
- Rest – desire for
- Selflessness
- Sensitive
  - opinion of others; to the
- Servile
- Sympathy from others – desire for
- Timidity
  - Bashful
- Unfortunate; feels
- Weeping
- Will – weakness of
- Yielding disposition
- DREAMS
  - Embarrassment

Physicals

- **FEMALE** genitalia / sex – <u>ovaries</u>; complaints of
- **EXTREMITIES**
  - Inflammation – Joints – <u>synovitis</u>
  - Pain – rheumatic
- **SLEEP** – Sleepiness – lying – inclination to lying down
- **PERSPIRATION** – <u>Clammy</u>
- **GENERALS**
  - Night – midnight – after – 3 h
  - Children; complaints in
  - Constitution – <u>hydrogenoid</u>
  - <u>Dropsy</u>
  - Exertion; physical – agg.
- <u>Flabby</u> feeling
- Inflammation – <u>Lymphatic</u> vessels
- Joints; complaints of the – <u>Synovial</u> membranes
- <u>Lie down – desire to</u>
- Lying – amel.
- Motion – amel. – slow motion
- Seasons – winter – agg.
- <u>Sluggishness</u> of the body
- Touch – amel.
- Weakness – exertion – agg. – slight exertion
- Weather – cold weather – wet – agg.

Related remedies and families

Primary

aids. ambr. anac. bamb-a. bar-c. brom. calc. calc-p. calc-s. carc. choc. cocc. dulc. lac-c. lac-d. lac-o. lyc. lys. lyss. mag-c. milks* molluscs* muriaticums* ol-eur. phlegmatic* podo. puls. sanic. sep. sil. staph. thuj.

Bold

acet-ac. am-m. ars-i. aur-m. barytas* bism. bufo calcareas* camph. caps. carbons* carb-v. chlor. cycl. euphr. ferrums* fl-ac. foll. hell. hura hyper. ign. kali-c. kali-i. kali-m. kreos. mag-m. mang. matridonals* moni. mur-ac. musca-d. nat-c. nat-m. nat-s. niob-met. olnd. petr. ph-ac. phyt. plac. plb. prey* rhus-t. row-1*_{plants} ruta sapph. stage-17*_{minerals} stage-3*_{minerals} telop-sp. zinc-p.

Italic

Acon. Adon. All-c. Am-c. Ant-c. Anthraci. Aur-m-n. Bar-i. Bar-m. Bell. Blatta-a. Bry. Buth-a. Cain. Calc-f. Calc-i. Carneg-g. Caust. Cedr. Cench. Cere-b. Chinin-ar. Colch. Column-1*_{Plants Com.} Con. Conv. Crat. Croc. Crot-c. Cupr. Dama-da. Dendr-pol. Dig. Echi. Falco-pe. Ferr-i. Germ-met. Graph. Gunp. Halogens* Heroin. Hydrog. Hyos. Iod. Kali-br. Kali-chl. Kali-met. Kali-n. Kali-s. Lac-d-i. Lac-del. Lac-e. Lac-eleph-m. Lac-f. Lac-h. Lac-h-m. Lac-lam. Lac-loxod-a. Lac-lup. Lac-mat. Lac-sui. Limen-b-c. M-arct. Magnoliidae* Merc. Merc-c. Merc-i-f. Merc-i-r. Myris. Nit-ac. Op. Oxyd. Phase. Plat. Plut-n. Pop-canes. Psor. Pyrog. Ranunculales* Sabin. Samb-c. Sarcodes* Sea-animals* Sel. Squil. Stroph-h. Sul-i. Tarent. Tarent-c. Ter. Ver-ca. Verat.

ASTROLOGICAL MYTHOLOGY IN THE ANIMAL KINGDOM

Mars and Venus relate to the Male and Female archetypes respectively. When there are stressful aspects to Mars in an Astrological birth chart, it could indicate

'Animal' tendencies to go into conflict with others, problems with asserting oneself, going on the attack or being attacked. Mars aspects may denote a predatory animal whereas stressful aspects to Venus might suggest a herd / prey animal. The themes of Venus relate to the attractiveness of the animal kingdom – the desire to be alluring, and to attract a mate. There is also a desire to maintain balance and harmony within the group which relates to gregarious animals – such as herd mammals, flocking birds and hive insects.

MARS / Ares

Attack, Warrior, Anger, Inflammation
Brave, Conquest, Battles
Enemies, Heroic, Blood lust
Action, Audacity, Bold, Impulsive

VENUS / Aphrodite

Seduction, Attraction, Balance,
 Harmony
Sexual lust, Flirtatious, Conciliation
Friendship, Beauty, Desire, Reaction
 Sensation, Relationship, Partner

The chart of a patient needing an Animal remedy is likely to contain difficult aspects *from* –

Mars = Predator (also warm blooded, burning pains).
Or
Venus = Prey (cold, lack of vital heat).
To
one of the following planets:

- **Mercury – Aves, Flying insects.** *Networks / Communication / Flight*
- **Moon – Milks, Molluscs.** *Nurture / Nourishment / Support / Sensitivity / Family*
- **Jupiter – Aves.** *Optimism / Growth / Expansion / Sky view / Philosophical*
- **Saturn – Araneae.** *Restriction / Recognition / Cannibalism / Doubtful / Structured*
- **Uranus – Insecta.** *Collective / Metamorphosis / Electrical fire / Dissatisfaction / Revolution*
- **Neptune – Sea Animals.** *Escapism / Sacrifice / Illusion / Victimised / Oneness*
- **Pluto – Ophidia.** *Depth / Intensity / Transformation / Death / Conspiracies*

More detailed explanation on these correspondences is provided in each chapter.

References

1 Harari YN. *Sapiens – A Brief History of Humankind*. London: Harvill Secker; 2014.
2 Vervarcke A. *Family Finder Module*. Ghent, 2018. (Accessed in RadarOpus.)
3 Schumacher EF. *A Guide for the Perplexed*. New York NY: Vintage; 1995.
4 Hahnemann S. *Organon of the Medical Art Practitioner* (trans. O'Reilly WB). Palo Alto CA: Birdcage Press LLC; 2001. (Originally published in 1810.)
5 Fraser P. *Using Realms in Homeopathy*. Bristol: The Winter Press; 2006.
6 Yakir M. *Wondrous Order – Systematic Table of Homeopathic Plant Remedies*. Kandern: Narayana Verlag; 2017.

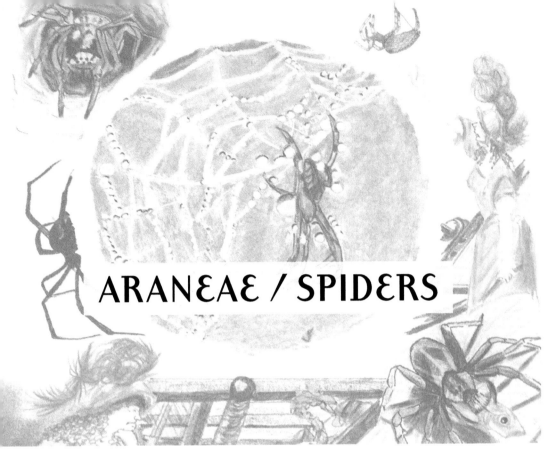

ARANEAE / SPIDERS

MYTHOLOGY

Kronos / Saturn

Arachnids (like Kronos) are known to indulge in cannibalism – mothers can eat their young, or their offspring might indeed eat the mother just as Kronos castrated his father and then ate his own progeny to ensure the same would not happen to him. He ruled the Titans and is the god of time (which is a feature of disorientation in spider remedies). Saturn demands recognition for one's hard work (which is also a key aspect of Spider remedies and one of the ways to differentiate them from insects who will often work more collectively). The element of deception and duplicity is also part of the myth; Kronos plotted with Gaia to overthrow his father. When caught in the web, one becomes tight and constricted; bound up. The psychological and physiological effects of Saturn are to constrain and constrict like the rings encircling the planet itself. Catching prey requires structure and a disciplined approach; spinning the web and maintaining this perfect order each and every day. It also requires great patience in waiting for the trap to be sprung. These are all Saturnian qualities.

Constriction / Contraction / Rigid ruler / Hard taskmaster
Critical of oneself and others / Desires recognition
Castrates father / Tyrannical / Revolts then conservative
Suppressive – eats his children as does the female spider or scorpion
Demands discipline, structure and imposes limitations / working very hard to
perfect your routine
Classical Music (particularly string instruments) and Ballet

Mars – Saturn

Fighting authority. Fighting for recognition. Fear of competition.
Testing your strength. Courage, hard work and control.
Ailments from domination.

Qualities

Cold, dry, chronic, contracting, binding, restricting, centripetal, obstructive.

Affinities of Saturn

Gallbladder, vagus nerve, teeth, skin, joints, ligaments, sigmoid flexure, eczema, erysipelas, leprosy, dislocation of bones, weak knees.

Arachne

Arachne in Greek mythology was a weaver who challenged Athena and was consequently transformed into a spider. There are three versions of the myth. One version has it that she was a shepherd's daughter that was particularly skilled at weaving. Boasting about her skill, she infuriated Athena, who appeared and contested her. Athena weaved four scenes in which the gods punished those humans that considered themselves equal to gods and committed hubris; Arachne, on the other hand, weaved scenes in which gods abused humans. Arachne's work was clearly better than Athena's; the goddess even more enraged due to what the weaving depicted, threw Hecate's potion onto Arachne, transforming her into a spider and condemning her to weave for eternity.[35]

SPIDERS IN HOMEOPATHY

One of the chief characteristics of Spiders as a group is their use of silk to survive. Although not all Spiders use silk, it is a strong part of the archetype that we as humans associate with them. The silk is used to trap their prey or to provide shelter (or both). Some spiders produce a very intricate and beautifully artistic design whilst others line their underground homes with silk and sit in their lair until an unsuspecting prey walks past their trap-door and they leap out to make the kill.

Silk can be adapted in so many different ways; making webs, nets and glue, wrapping up their prey, or making a cocoon for their young. The web is their means of communication and interaction with the external world. The strongest sensory field for the spider is the sense of touch; they are hyper-aware of the slightest movement – the web transmits vibrations of the caught insect to the waiting spider. If the vibrations are too strong it may hold back, suspicious that there may be something there which it can't tackle. Spiders are involved and in-tune with what is going on out there through their web.

Spider silk has greater tensile strength than steel and is so precious that the spider always eats it back up again. They never let their silk go to waste. Certain spiders can project silk out of their spinneretts into the wind, achieving lift off into gusts that allow them to travel thousands of miles.

Human patients who respond to Spider remedies have been reported by varied sources, such as Ververcke and Hardy to have a love of knitting, weaving and / or string instruments.

By contrast, most Insects only use silk when in the larval / chrysalis form.

MAPPA MUNDI

Melancholic

Secretive, cunning and solitary
Trapped / Constricted / Bound-up
Enclosed in a silk cage
Dominated, suffering

Choleric

Defiant, rebellious, destructive
Fearless / Fighting / Rage / Industrious / Dictatorial

Air

Manipulative, deceitful and cruel
Sensitive to vibration / Hearing acute
Nervous system affinity / Necrosis / Venomous / Toxic

Fire

Sexuality, dancing, playing antics, lascivious and wild
Angina pectoris and heart affinity / Locomotor ataxia / Jerking / Convulsive

Choleric

ACTIVITY - desires activity
AILMENTS FROM - position; loss of
AMBITION - increased - competitive
CONTRADICTION
disposition to contradict
intolerant of contradiction
DEFIANT
DICTATORIAL - power, love of
FEARLESS
FIGHT, WANTS TO
HURRY
IMPATIENCE
INDUSTRIOUS
OBSTINATE
POWER - sensation of
QUARRELSOME
QUICK TO ACT
RAGE
VIOLENT
WILL - strong will power
EXERTION; PHYSICAL – amel.

Fire / Sky Realm

ACTIVITY - desires activity - creative
AILMENTS FROM - love; disappointed
AMBITION - increased
AWARENESS HEIGHTENED
DANCING
LASCIVIOUS
NYMPHOMANIA
SATYRIASIS
WILDNESS

WILL - strong will power
MALE - SEXUAL DESIRE - increased
FEMALE - SEXUAL DESIRE - increased
CHEST - ANGINA PECTORIS
HEART; COMPLAINTS OF THE
DREAMS - FLYING
ENERGY - excess of energy
LOCOMOTOR ATAXIA

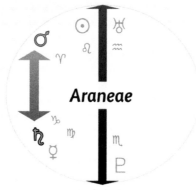

Araneae

Melancholic

ANOREXIA NERVOSA
COMPANY - aversion to - desire for solitude
COMPLAINING
DECEITFUL
DECEPTION
DELUSIONS
betrayed; that she is / cheated; being
trapped; he is / wrong - suffered wrong; he has
EXCITEMENT - nervous
HATRED
HIDING - himself
MANIPULATIVE
PLANS - making many plans - revengeful plans
SUSPICIOUS
TOUCHED - aversion to be
DREAMS - SPIDERS
EMACIATION
PARALYSIS

Air / Underworld

COMPANY - aversion to
CONFUSION OF identity, as to his
CRUELTY
DEATH - thoughts of
DECEITFUL
DELUSIONS - persecuted - he is
DESTRUCTIVENESS
FEAR
death, of / evil; fear of / insanity
FORSAKEN FEELING
isolation; sensation of
HATRED
LIAR

MALICIOUS
MANIA
MANIPULATIVE
SENSITIVE - noise, to
STARTING
STRIKING
SUICIDAL DISPOSITION
WICKED DISPOSITION
HEARING - ACUTE
DREAMS - FRIGHTFUL
HEAT - lack of vital heat
PULSE - slow

Figure 2.1 *Mappa Mundi dynamics for the Spiders*

THEMES

Silk Spinners

Spiders use their spinnerets to weave a web; a strategy which is essential to survival at all times of their lives. In the company of spider energy, you can feel wrapped-up and trapped by their intrigues; caught or stuck in the web that they weave. A spider patient's anamnesis could be an amazing narrative, capturing and fixating your attention on them.

Human Spider patients are quick to react and will note and magnify slight emotional changes in the environment (as if picking up on the vibrational change of the web). It is often to their advantage to wrap up others in their web of intrigue, so the Homeopath may note attention-seeking antics, deceitfulness and trickery, especially in children. They easily feel threatened and have got to be on the lookout. Think of the spider at the centre of his web, feeling for the slightest change.

cf. Snakes – sensitive to vibrations, underworld, venomous, toxic.

Spiders use silk to wrap up their prey – keeping it alive but in a shallow state of animation, returning to eat it later. The experience is nightmarish; binding you up tightly, disarming you so you can't attack or run away. Enclosing and engulfing you in a semi-conscious state.

Rubrics

Attention-seeking behaviour | Cruelty | Deceitful | Deception | Intriguer | Quick to act / react | Sly | Tricky | Threatened / Threatening | Delusions – trapped; he is | Suspicious | Senses – acute | Sensitive – emotions; to / touch; to / noise; to | Hearing – acute

Recognition

Patients needing spider remedies feel special, creative, and desire recognition for their talents. They often feel that the recognition they deserve is not forthcoming and this can be an aetiological factor for mental and physical complaints. The resulting sensation may be one of resentment, powerlessness, feeling small, inferior and abused by others who treat them unfairly (*cf. insects*). The desire to be seen and noticed, although a common feature in animal remedies, is particularly important in Spiders.

> *Needs attention, feels as if he is being ignored.* lampo-cy.[13] *I am not recognised for my strengths – Feel I am dying inside because of it. Makes me feel hollow, sad and empty. . . . They don't recognise my strengths, they don't recognise my gifts; I am very dynamic and then I am shat on* tarent.

Rubrics

Activity – desires activity – creative activity | Ailments from – abused; after being | Attention-seeking behaviour | Competitive | Delusions – abused / insulted, he is | Delusions – appreciated, she is not | Delusions – misunderstood; she is | Delusions – small – he is | Delusions – wrong – suffered wrong; he has | Demanding | Powerless | **Recognition; desire for** | Resentment |

Forsaken and neglected

Strong attachment to the partner (especially in Theridion) whilst easily feeling **neglected and misunderstood**. However, dependency on loved ones creates a great deal of ambivalence for Spider patients who are very sensitive to feeling dominated; they hate the feeling of being too tightly bound up in the relationship. The spider traps its prey by wrapping it tightly in a silk cage; they are themselves most sensitive to this feeling of being bound-up, tight and restricted.

Felt resentful and abused. Had no control over her temper. Bellowed and lashed out at everyone androc.[8] *Depression . . . alone and forsaken . . . like in a dark cavern . . . as if tightened up . . . like buried in a dome of glass, without feelings, I do not hear anything anymore, I do not participate in life anymore* tegen-at.[34] *A feeling of being completely forsaken, alone completely, and I will not be able to survive without that person. . . . I am a person who knows what she wants, I know exactly what I want to do, do things alone. I am strong enough. But in this relationship, I was completely crazy; I felt forsaken.*ther.[4]

Rubrics
Dependent of others | Forsaken feeling – isolation; sensation of | Delusions – neglected; he or she is neglected | Delusions – trapped; he is | Delusions – understand – being understood; she was not | Pities herself | Possessiveness

Complaining, attention-seeking, cunning, deceit and manipulation

There can be hypochondriacal tendencies, as has often been observed in Tarentula and Aranea children. Health problems may be blown completely out of proportion, with much complaining, attention-seeking antics, feigning illness or using deceit and trickery to get their way.

Tarentula has *attention-seeking behaviour resulting from feeling **forsaken** or **neglected**, where the parents are too busy in their profession or in conflict between themselves.* Master[12] *Mischievousness, desire for attention, manipulativeness, activity, love / hate relationship with bugs and spiders, a tendency to hide, to make up stories to cover his transgressions, and a history of cutting things.* aran-ix.[20] *She is better behaved with adults, then becomes suddenly manic. If she is pulled up for lying, she will go mental about it.* tarent.

Rubrics
Complaining | Cunning | Feigning – sick; to be | Hiding – himself | Hypochondriasis | Liar | Intriguer | Manipulative | Mischievous | Sly | Tricky

Highly strung, hurried, busy, hyperactive, manic, wild dancing

Hurried, busy and industrious; having a sense of *not enough time.* Arrive late for appointments. This tendency to operate on hyperdrive can also have its positives, as this prover of Lampona cylindrata describes *"More awake, more active, cleaning, organizing, vacuuming, very efficient, very elated, I feel amazing."* lampo-cy.[13]

Manic behaviour / ADHD
She gets a manic look and can't stop it. Over-excited. Rough and tumble play fighting, manic look and manic laugh. Energy is impossible to handle. . . . Feels really shocking, like your space is invaded tarent.

Wild rhythmical dancing releases pent up energy.

Danced all night in a frenzy, could not keep still, and was frustrated when the music finished. androc.[8] *Tarantism, which was impossible to control could be suppressed and cured by music with a fast and strong rhythmic beat. The victims on hearing the music became excited and danced faster and faster till they fell down tired and sweating and got rid of the poison.* Master[11]

Highly strung nervous energy – noise / vibration reverberates in their whole body.

They have a great deal of energy held ready to keep them in balance and to spring into action whenever their trap is sprung and their prey is caught. Fraser[2]

Rubrics
Concentration – difficult – attention; cannot fix | Dancing – wild | Excitement – nervous | Industrious | Frantic, frenzy | Hurry | Hysteria | Mania | Generals – energy – excess of energy – children; in |

Persecution complex; unfairly treated, taken advantage of, wronged by others

Feel different, misunderstood and mistreated.

> *Popular conception classes the spider purely as a **lurking** menace that deals horrible death to the unwary. The other half shows a wee, timorous, cowering beastie, a creature so **perse-cuted** and **preyed** on that it is a wonder it survives* Shore[19] *They resent those who want to put them into a **cage** like their family did. . . . Avoidance of close contact and terri-torial feeling leads to isolation.* Mangialavori[1] *I kind of feel **cheated**, or taken advantage of – really? This is what I am? People's perception is that you're a **nothing** . . . is that my own **inferiority** complex – I am kind of like nothing, I have no earning potential. I don't exist, am considered **obsolete**.* tarent. *Arsenicum and Bromium share suspiciousness with spiders. Bromium has the guilt of having done something wrong whereas spiders often **feel that something wrong has been done to them**, or that they want to do something tremendously **destructive** or **malicious**.* Joshis[16]

This can of course be expressed another way, where there is guilt for having mistreated others oneself, expressed here by a prover of Loxosceles reclusa; *"Sadness but can't cry. Want to provoke someone to get me crying. Sentimental. Guilty for things done in childhood to take attention away from siblings."* loxo-recl.[10]

Rubrics
Delusions – cheated; being | Delusions – looked down upon; she is | Delusions – misunderstood; she is | Delusions – persecuted; he is persecuted | Delusions – wrong – suffered wrong; he has

Defiant and rebellious, intolerant of contradiction or authority

There is a strong aversion to domination or authority, leading to rebellious acts and *indifference to all reprimands.* lat-h[32] Spider patients hate being dependent so they tend to manipulate situations to assert themselves; they are most comfortable lying at the centre of their own web of intrigue!

If you push my buttons, I am not going to take it. . . . She is used to bossing people around – but can't do that at school – she has to be polite. She is mean to people she adores, she wasn't talking to me and said she didn't care. When someone is mean she wants to do the same back to them tarent. *Have been feeling hostile towards people lately. . . . Anger that was boiling inside of me. . . . A deep irritability in the gut, a violent form which could lead to aggression. . . . I felt that my irritability was violent and had to exercise restraint to keep myself 'nice'* lat-h.[32]

Rubrics
Anarchist | Anger – authority; against | Ailments from – domination | Contradiction – intolerant of contradiction | Defiant | Dictatorial – power; love of | Domineering | Rebellious | Violent

Extreme sensitivity

Spiders have an extremely delicate sense of touch which enables them to detect their prey by vibrations of the threads of their silk webs. The least disturbance to any sense, especially sounds, are noted and magnified. This extreme sensitivity is also expressed on the psychological plane and may lead to cutting oneself off from the emotional world altogether.

The remedy made me more sensitive and since then I have been able to counteract this by becoming harder and by being able to detach from emotion. . . . I felt no emotional involvement with my actions. lat-h.[32] *I feel a sense of waiting and am hyper-vigilant. I am constantly scanning my world for an awareness of what might happen.* loxo-recl.[10] *Spiders are emotionally and mentally very sensitive . . . pick[ing] up on the mood and the sensitivities of others but they have no real understanding of what this means or how to react to it appropriately.* Fraser[2] *She is sensitive to everyone's moods. She will pick up on a tiny grouch or tone of voice. Being talked about, laughed at or told off will really upset her. If pulled up for lying, she will go mental about it.* tarent.

Rubrics
Awareness heightened | Senses – acute | Sensitive – emotions; to / touch; to / noise; to | Hearing – acute | Starting

Secretive, hiding, solitary, wary

They are passive hunters, they wait by the web – waiting in the cold is like having a nameless fear, inspiring an ever-watchful attitude. lampo-cy.[13] *They are also secretive, having to hide any emotions or feelings lest these become a weapon that can be used against them. This is often in contradiction to their urges to seek attention and be noticed.* Fraser[2] *Don't want to interact with anyone. Feel isolated like I have a secret.* loxo-recl.[10] *I retreat, I want to be alone, to run away. Friends say 'tell me what's going on'. And I just want to hibernate and disappear . . . my feelings are very true and very real. Consolation does not help – this is how I feel. It is embarrassing to show what your true emotions are because you always need to keep the exterior that everything is fine. To express the true being is embarrassing, because people judge you – they look at you differently.* tarent.

Rubrics
Company – aversion to – desire for solitude | Consolation – agg. | Emotions – strong; too | Hiding – himself | Secretive

Suspiciousness, fear or contemplation of death, fear of evil

The mind symptoms of Latrodectus mactans correspond to the feelings of a person facing death; an extreme state of nervous irritation accompanied by fear of going mad, losing breath and dying.

Another hit of depression. Suicidal thoughts. Felt, what's the use . . . a desire to escape my life here as it is. . . . Thoughts of how easy it would be for me to die. . . . Didn't seem like a big deal to have such morbid thoughts (this is a very strange thought for me to have – hope it is the remedy). **"It is easy to die. You could just die today."** loxo-recl.[10] *I had a loose, putrid, black bowel movement, which smelt of decay and death. As if the devil, evil came out. I have never before experienced anything like this. It was most ugly. It was as if all the bad feelings about myself and all the bad things that I have done over my life passed.* lat-h.[32]

Rubrics
Death – thoughts; of | Suicidal disposition | Fear – death / evil / insanity

Destructiveness, violence, fighting, conflict

There may be violence, biting and striking which often happen in paroxysms. Tendency to tear things up, break household objects and generally *create crises, conflict and chaos*!

Strikes her body, continues threatening; deep anguish, her clothes annoy her; continual restlessness, **threatening words of destruction and death***; she believes she is insulted; a mocking laughter, and joy expressed in her countenance.* tarent.[9] **Assertive, impatient, aggressive.** *Desire to break things. Became excited to anger and confrontation.* **Could not appreciate anyone else's feeling.** *Later she reflected on her actions and felt ashamed. Argumentative.* **Pursued conflict almost with relish.** *. . . Increased irritability, a "how dare you!" feeling. Felt like tearing offenders to pieces with his bare hands. He felt an* **enormous surge of violent emotions** *at trifles and had to exercise great control to stop outbursts of violence and impulses to hurt someone. . . . In the evening,* **furious for no apparent reason.** *Wanted to kill her husband and children, banged doors and threw things. By bedtime, she felt fine but the intensity of her evil thoughts was very frightening.* androc.[8] *His lifelong love of being of service to people was entirely annihilated, he felt agitation and hatred, before he felt god will reward me. "I want the reward now, give me the reward".* lampocy.[13]

Rubrics

Biting | Brutality | Destructiveness | Fearless | Fight; wants to | Hatred – revengeful; and hatred | Malicious | Plans – making many plans – revengeful plans | Threatening | Violent |

Intensity; magnetic state

A feeling of great energy and confidence, a magnetic state. His emotions were more intense than ever before. In his love affair, he surrendered to his feelings for the first time, and his girlfriend commented that this was the most intense relationship she had ever had. . . . Very changeable moods. One moment extremely friendly, nice and amiable, then irritable. Incredible upsurge of energy, laughing, felt very high, then low, then high again. . . .Very strong liking and disliking to people. Very intense, ranging from immense sexual attraction to extreme hatred. Spoke with hatred and maliciousness about colleagues. androc.[8]

Rubrics

Emotions – strong, too | Hatred | Magnetic state | Malicious | Mood – changeable | Power – sensation of

Heart affinity, unrequited love

Ailments from unrequited / disappointed love. Compensating with attractive / attention-seeking behaviour.

The situation of Tarentula is that of a person who wants to be noticed but is not, such as could happen when a person tries unsuccessfully to attract the attention of another especially from the opposite sex. This is not a situation of disappointed love, but one of unrequited love. Sankaran[5] Dream: *My partner was sitting on a bench when an ex-girlfriend walked past very seductively. She went down and sat on another bench with two men. I was seeing all of this through a hessian or a gauze partition. I was very jealous, sad and angry.* lat-h.[32]

The proving of the remedy derived from *Latrodectus haselti* has the title '*Deadly Romance*' alluding to the importance of the heart and love relationships in the remedy, whilst hinting that this may be an important feature for the group given the heart affinity and 'unrequited love' theme.

Discussion with friend over relationship ending makes me sad. I have an emptiness in the stomach. . . . I feel I am not attractive enough. . . . We started kissing but I was overcome with tiredness, my lips wouldn't work. . . . Dream: Fighting with ex-wife and her partner, running away from them. I was hit on the forehead and an old wound opened up. (This injury was inflicted 20 years ago during a fight at the end of our relationship.) I was bleeding profusely from the wound. . . . I felt lonely and realised that my partner was away, I couldn't contact her. I tried to phone her. lat-h.[32]

Heart affinity:

*A few hours after the bite the patients have great **anguish of the heart**, **great dejection**, but greater **difficulty in breathing**; they complain in a mournful voice, roll their eyes,* *and when asked by bystanders where they suffer, they either do not reply or point out the affected region by placing the hand upon the chest, as if the heart were affected more than all else.* tarent.[9]

Strong chest pains on left side with shortness of breath. Compressions under the clavicle – I must compress my left breast for it to release and let go. . . . My breath just feels short – can't have full respiration. It feels compromised, not what it would normally be. Like I can't breathe . . . the shortness of breath, the anger and despair come together and are unleashed. tarent.

Rubrics

Ailments from – love; disappointed | Attracting others | Angina pectoris | Anxiety in – Heart; region of | Chest – Constriction | Heart; complaints of the | Chest – Oppression | Chest – Pain – Heart – extending to – Arm – left | Chest – Palpitation of heart

Strong sexuality but love can kill

High interest and desire in sex (without love or communication). Emotions are dangerous and need to be kept under control, hence there may be a strong sexual drive but with a lack of feeling. Arachnid mating rituals often involve a display of dancing to try to impress the female, and convince her to mate. Mating is a dangerous activity for the male who may be killed and / or cannibalised after performing the act.

Sexuality is important as a means of display and attention. . . . However, it also involves touch and should include some sort of emotional dimension; all of which tend to be anathema to the Spider. Fraser[2] *To arouse the senses by having physical contact becomes dangerous, caus(ing) a violent reaction.* Mangialavori[1] *This evening for the first time in many months I felt strong sexual feelings . . . a sense of personal ownership and power in my ability to be sexual. . . . I was imagining a virgin planning a big night out to lose her virginity – does not go right. Catches a taxi cab in a huff and does it with the cabbie. Puts engaged sign on taxi cab.* lat-h.[32] *Dream; It was like sex in slow motion. He said, "be careful, I don't want to have another stroke." We were wearing silky black clothes.* loxo-recl.[10] *Strong sexuality. 'I was feeling impotent, but on the remedy now have increased desire'.* lampo-cy.[13]

Rubrics

Lascivious | Nymphomania | Satyriasis | Touched – aversion to be | Male / Female Genitalia / Sex – Sexual desire – increased

The feminine dominates; the matriarch *vs.* the spinster

Female spiders are dominant. As mothers they may be very dominating over their children. They don't give their children much freedom. Mothers who try to control their children too much may end up pushing them away, leading to a feeling of isolation in their elder years (*spinster*).

The classic image of the aged matriarch controlling her children and grandchildren with any means necessary . . . one bitten by the vampire becomes in turn a vampire" Shore[19]

My daughter – she's so lovely and wants to give me a hug but I push her away. Why don't I engage in that sort of comfort, why do I push it away? Even my own daughter who is the most intuitive, amazing human being on this planet? tarent.

Some spiders carry their offspring on their back even if there are 400 of them! Baby scorpions have great trouble leaving their mother, because once they leave her back, she thinks they do not belong to her and could kill them.

Ungrounded; Suspended and disorientated in the web

For a being that spends its time in a state of balance on a finely constructed web, it is perhaps understandable that a feeling of disorientation should be prominent in Spider cases. When this balance is disturbed, there can be problems with Vertigo and feeling very unsteady or out of balance. Theridion is known for its curative effects in Meniere's Disease, Labyrinthitis and Vestibular problems.

*The web hangs suspended in the Sky but in order to function it must be anchored to the Earth. . . . At the centre of the web sits the spider motionless but **in a state of tension and awareness, sensitive to the tiniest movement** anywhere on the web. . . . The confusion and disorientation of being neither in one place nor the other is widespread. . . . A **disconnection from time, disorientation and clumsiness**, making mistakes . . . and even confusion of identity* Fraser[2]. *Wonder what my family would think if they came home to find me hanging from a rope (strange thought will try to keep my mind away from that). This morning when boys going off I thought "You boys can come home and find me hanging by the rafters".*

That is not me. "That is crazy". loxo-recl.[10]

Rubrics
Mistakes; making – time; in | Orientation; sense of – decreased | Vertigo – Fall; tendency to

Eating Disorders, liquid food

Spiders eat only what is necessary to stay alive – they can go for long periods without food. They are known to reduce their metabolic rate in response to starvation and can distend their abdomens to store large amounts of food. In human patients this may be expressed as anorexia or evolve into other eating disorders. Eating disorders can be used as a weapon against suffocating parents.
Desire to take food in liquid form. *Feeds by sucking juices from its victim.* (Lat-m., Lat-h.)
Desires: fruit, milk and liquid.
Desire for, and amelioration from: smoking tobacco.

The mygale, like most spiders, has a very small oesophagus, so it is not capable of real eating. It kills its prey quickly with its enormous jaws, bites the prey in pieces, then makes a web around it like a cocoon and pours out its stomach juices over the prey. Then after a while it sucks the resulting liquid food. woutman[25]

Rubrics
Anorexia nervosa | Bulimia | Indifference – eating – to eating | Food and drinks – liquid food – desire / solid food – aversion

Energy vampires

Feeling as if I am being sucked out of the present. I need to get out of the room. lampo-cy.[13] *Dream about vampires and humans. We are trying to kill the vampires first (before they get us) with a stake. A van picked us up: four vampires and four people acting like vampires. A vampire inquired about how we are so lightweight and asked us how we are able to walk on small branches. I kept silent, fear I would be discovered and harmed.* tela.[24] *The spasms and rigor mortis seem to visit you like Dracula at night.* mygal.

Altered sense of rhythm; tics, Tourette's and paroxysms

In nature, spiders go from being completely still to springing into action at the slightest change in vibration on the web. Thus their movements tend to be exaggerated or extreme. Or they may be aggravated by sudden / extreme movements and noises (vibrations). *"Lots of sudden things, sudden elation, sudden desire for sleep."* lampo-cy.[13] Impulsive pattern of movement. Parkinsonism, Dyspraxia, Chorea, Locomotor ataxia, jerks, tics, convulsions, paralysis. *"I scream and cry. I have tourette's! Say the fuck word all the time."* tarent.

Rubrics
Tourette's syndrome | *Extremities* – incoordination / Jerking / Tottering gait | *Generals* – chorea / Convulsions – tetanic rigidity / Jerking / Locomotor ataxia / Paralysis agitans / Restlessness / Sudden manifestation

Distortions in time – moving too quickly

Theridion has this symptom in a marked way, and could hint at a tubercular miasm for the spider group. Tarentula (the Homeopathic archetype for the family) is a wolf spider and does not construct a web. Its bite is known to produce tarentism; a form of wild dancing to release pent-up energy. But many spiders spend most of their time lying completely still in wait of their prey so this miasmatic classification may be rather basic. *"My mind escalates and goes on the treadmill; it can't keep up. I just go into overdrive and it takes me a while to calm down"* tarent.

Rubrics
Time – quickly, appears shorter; passes too | Dancing – wild

Toxicology

E. A Farrington's Clinical Materia Medica makes the following statement on Arachnida spider poisons. There is one two-fold action, they all **poison the blood**, all act prominently on the nervous system producing **spasms; chorea, hysteria.** Among other symptoms are trembling, great **restlessness**, oversensitiveness and nervous prostration. There is also **periodicity.** Tics, prominent dancing, assuming the attitude of prayer with fervent expression and clasped hands, sexual violence, spasmodic unavoidable erections, nausea, dizziness, variable pulse. There may be rapid changes, self-exaltation, diarrhoea, fevers, mental confusion, hilarity, loquacity and lasciviousness. Gray[13]

Differential diagnosis – Snakes

*There are many similarities in the expressions of patients who need a snake or a spider remedy. Both can feel small and **vulnerable** and **hide in ambush, waiting for a victim to pass. Then they suddenly attack and kill.** Both can be **poisonous,** and both can **scheme, plot and mislead**. But snakes tend to be talkative, attractive, inciting, and kill when provoked. Spiders have insect qualities like restlessness, dirty dancing, and either the **web** with its stickiness, the **hunt** or the **trap** (trapdoor spiders). It is not too surprising to have **ropes or strings in a spider case** as well (often they play string instruments, while birds prefer wind instruments).* Vervarcke[7]

Common Spider qualities

- Deceit
- Cunning
- Suddenness
- Rhythmic music amel. Love of dancing
- **Tobacco** amel.
- Restlessness. Need to keep the hands busy. For example, knitting.
- Dyskinesia, lack of coordination (tarentism).
- Periodicity.
- Stinging pains.
- *cf.* Insects, the sensation language of spiders may be expressed as caught and trapped.
- Vampire association.
- Spiders are generally very chilly and better for warmth.

Keywords

Caught, trapped in the web. Web of lies / deceit. Trap-door.
Entangled. Intricacy. Maintaining structure.
Glue, wrapping up / binding their prey.
Lying in wait. Sudden activity. Highly strung, tensioned, taught, vibration.
Poisonous, hairy. Cocoon.

Differential Diagnosis

- Cancer – Tubercular Miasm
- Stage 5 and 6 (proving yourself)
- Fungi (invaded)
- Anacardiaceae (caught)
- Cactaceae (Bound, trapped)

- Rosaceae (impulsive, sudden)
- Rubiaceae (senses acute)
- Ranunculaceae (nerves)
- Insecta

REMEDIES

Araneae (Spiders) aran. aran-cv. **aran-ix**. aran-sc. **atra-r**. avic. brachy-st. hadrn-for. hadrn-mod. **lampo-cy**. **lat-h**. lat-hp. lat-k. **lat-m**. lat-td. loxo-ga. loxo-lae. loxo-parr. **loxo-recl**. loxo-refr. **mygal**. phol-pl. portia-fi. sicar-a. sicar-h-k. sicar-t. *TARENT*. tarent-c. tegen-ag. tegen-at. tegen-do. tegen-gi. tegen-pa. **tela. ther**. ther-na.

Aranea diadema (Papal Cross Spider)

Phylum: Arthropoda.
Class: Arachnida.
Order: Araneae.
Suborder: Araneomorphae.

The legs of orb-weaver spiders are specialised for spinning orb webs; the well-known circular, flat, wheel-like webs. They are cannibalistic; preying upon each other before, during or after sexual activity. They attack based on their size, sexual experience and hunger levels. They are naturally reclusive, only biting humans if cornered or provoked. They can respond to disturbances by vibrating rapidly on their web until becoming a blur, a reaction that is assumed to confuse potential predators. Spiders of this genus clearly present the sexual dimorphism inherent in the orb-weaver family, with males being normally a quarter to a third the size of females.

Proving by: **Central Council for Research in Homeopathy, India (1987).**
Earlier provings were performed using tincture or low potencies.

Keywords
Swollen / Rhythmical / Dramatic / Fiery / Intense / Formication / Darting / Griping / Icy / Shocks / Spleen / Necrosis / Periodicity / Trigeminal nerve / Smoking / Knitting / Intricate / Precise

Strange, rare and peculiar

- **Delusions**
  - Falling – he is
  - Hearing – talk seems distant
  - Large – parts of body seem too large
  - *Swollen; is*
  - Unreal – everything seems unreal

- **Death – desires**
- **Fear**
  - Crowd; in a
  - Death; of
  - Narrow place; in
- Sensitive – **rhythmical music**

Mind

- Aversion – family; to members of
- Ardent
- Dramatic
- Fiery temperament
- Intense personality
- Loquacity – changing quickly from one subject to another – important matters about; on
- Passionate

Pathogenetic _{Ward}[26]

Asleep, fingers / Bowels, stone / Fingers, formication / Forearms, large / Head, darting / Jaws, darting / Swollen, hands / Temples, pressive

Clinical _{Ward}[26]

Ants, body / Arms, swollen / Asleep, extremities / Asleep, fingers / *Boring*, heel / Boring, tibia / Colic, daily / Confusion, head / Crawling, external / *Creeping*, skin / Dead, weakness / *Digging*, arm bones / Drop, weakness / Faintness, epigastrium / Faintness, stomach / *Formication*, body / Formication, diarrhoea / Fullness, bowels / Griping, abdomen / Hands, swollen / Heaviness, abdomen / Heaviness, bowels / Heaviness, thighs / Heavy, forearms / *Icy*, bones / Large, forearms / Lie dead / Lying necessary / Numbness, extremities / Pressive, temple / Recurring, colic / Stone, bowels / Strong, arms / *Swollen*, cheeks / *Swollen*, hands / *Swollen*, head / Thighs, heavy

Sensations, as if _{Roberts}[27]

- Eyes and vision – Mist – before eyes
- Mouth – **Shocks** – Electric; through tongue
- Abdomen – Fermenting; bowels were
- Upper extremities – **Ice** – bones were made of

Clinical _{Roberts}[27]

Nervous exhaustion. Neuralgic pains. Enlargement of spleen. Diarrhoea. Asthma. Quotidian fevers. Necrosis of bones, esp. of os calcis. One of the coldest remedies; coldness even of bones. Marked periodicity.

Materia medica Julian[22]
- Head numbed, head pains, improved by smoking.
- Daily headaches improved by fresh air.
- Vertigo, even when in bed.
- Feeling of ants on the nape of the neck.
- Pain in the *trigeminal nerve and occipital nerve.*
- Face pale, yellowish colour.

Themes
Less hysterical than Tarentula, but equally as passionate, intense and fiery. Paralytic symptoms – difficult to write.

> *The sensation of swelling is typical for this remedy, especially of the upper limbs. This can be a subjective ('sensation as if') or an objective. Writing is difficult. A forsaken feeling is symbolised by the delusion that the voice of the one they love sounds far away. Their own voice can seem unreal (hearing; illusion; talk seems distant).* Mangialavori[1]

Natural behaviour
This spider produces the most amazing intricate web designs. Their activity is less fruitless and they may produce wonderful works of art or be interested in handicrafts or knitting. They can be very precise.

Aranea ixobola (Wheel-web Spider)

Phylum: Arthropoda.
Order: Araneae.
Class: Arachnida.
Family: Araneidae [Orb weavers].

This spider is commonly found in Europe after being imported from America. It is an orb weaver spider spinning a classic wheel shaped web.

Proving by: **Julius Mezger, Germany (1958).**

Keywords
Teasing / Deceitful / Mischievous / Witty / Addictive / Sadomasochistic / Neurotropic / Vascular / Shaking / Contracture / Disquiet / **Smoking** / Charming / Cunning / Extremes; goes to / Malicious / Seduction / Impulsive / Violent, in secret / Hypertension / **Hyperactivity** / Parkinsonism

Themes
- Keynote: **Loves to tease**, pleasure in teasing others. Julian[22]
- Children can be deceitful, cunning, mischievous, witty and uncooperative.
- Frantic anxiety about loved ones.
- Compulsive, addictive especially sexually – extra marital affairs, pornography, sadomasochistic sex. *cf. Fl-ac.* Klein

- Night owl – up until 2 am. (*Medorrhinum*).
- Sleep – disturbed by frightful dreams.

Materia medica _{Julian}[22]

- *Neurotropic* and *vascular* action, both central and peripheral.
- Action directed to the digestive system, principally the liver and gall bladder.
- Extreme inner *disquiet*.
- *Shaking*, sensation of inner *trembling; need to move* about.
- Spasmodic **contracture** of the unstriped muscles (arterial congestion; spasms of the digestive passages), and of the striped muscles (cramps, tremors, clonic spasms).
- *Overwhelming need to smoke.*
- Euphoric state, as if he had drunk wine, *teasing disposition*, and need to speak, followed by melancholy, weariness of life; irritable.
- *Has to make a great effort not to be impolite or rude.*

Peter Fraser[2] writes that they are concerned with order of the interpersonal environment and need to have it under their control (within the intrigue of the web). He astutely observes that it is the only spider in the rubric Dictatorial (courtesy of a clinical addition from Farokh Master). These types may therefore be very controlling of others around them, coming across as abrupt, rude, snappish and even hardhearted. On the other hand, they can be charming, curious and witty. In children, they may have the whole family wrapped around their little finger through their difficult and oppositional behaviour – demanding that things go their way. The parents may be forced to acquiesce to their wishes to maintain any sense of familial harmony.

Mind

- Abrupt
- **Addicted**; tendency to become
- Animals – love for animals
- Answering – snappishly
- Cares, full of – relatives; about
- **Charming** others
- **Cunning**
- Deceitful
- Dictatorial
- Dreams – dead; of the / frightful
- Envy
- Euphoria
- *Extremes; goes to*
- Hardhearted
- Hurry
- Impolite
- **Impulsive**
- **Lascivious**
- Loquacity – changing quickly from one subject to another
- Love – **perversity**; sexual
- Push – desire to; others
- **Malicious**
- **Restlessness** – move; must, driving from place to place
- Secretive
- **Seduction** – desire for
- Snappish
- **Teasing**
- Thoughts – rapid
- Throws – things around
- Time – loss of conception of
- Tobacco – smoking – amel.
- **Violent, in secret**
- **Witty**

Clinical
Behavioural problems in children. Attention deficit and hyperactivity disorder. Hypertension / Hyperthyroidism / Lupus / Parkinsonism / Sclerosis; multiple / Tetanus

Atrax robustus (Sydney funnel-web spider)

Phylum: Arthropoda.
Class: Arachnida.
Order: Araneae. *Suborder:* Mygalomorphae.

Atrax robustus is a species of venomous mygalomorph spider native to eastern Australia. They build burrows, spending most of their time in these silk-lined tubular retreats. When potential prey (such as insects, lizards or frogs) venture across the traps they set, they suddenly rush out to subdue them with a venomous injection. They become more active at night, seeking cover in their cool, moist hideaways during the extreme daytime heat of the Australian sun.

Provings by: **Dr P. Sankaran, India (1968).**[6]
Jonathan Shore, Austalia (1999).[19]

Keywords
Suspicious / Underhand / Invading / Venomous / **Armour** / Cunning / Jumping – frantically / outcast / Verminous / Goitre / Tubercular / **Vampire**

Dream themes (from Shore's Proving)
Paranoia / Meanness / **Suspicious** / Hostile / Accused / **Underhand** / I had to put on armour / Preparing for a battle / Turmoil / Hatred / Death / Venomous / Destroy / Avarice / **Invading**
   "The classic image of the aged matriarch controlling her children and grand-children with any means necessary . . . *one bitten by the vampire becomes in turn a vampire.*" Shore[19]

Rubrics
- Cunning
- Dancing
- Delusions – *outcast; she were an*
- Jumping – frantically
- Tourette's Syndrome – face – twitching
- Vertigo – Periodical – short time; for
- Eye – Agglutinated / Discharges – white – milk-white /
- **Eye – Protrusion – exophthalmos**
- Eye – Pupils – contracted – pinpoint; to

- External throat – Goitre – exophthalmic
- Extremities – Motion – Involuntary / Tingling / Twitching / Weakness – sudden
- Sleep – Comatose
- Perspiration – Clammy
- Skin – Eruptions – erythema
- Generals – Analgesia / Collapse / Haemorrhage – blood – dark / Hypertension

Clinical indications [Julian][22]

- Tubercular conditions.
- Exophthalmic goitre.
- Glaucoma.
- Neuralgia of the face and under the orbits.
- Earache.
- Verminous conditions.

Proving

The remedy appears to have a strong affinity to the eye; the following symptoms were reported during a proving by P. Sankaran[6]:

- Pain above left eye, aggravation at bedtime, in bed before sleep.
- Discharge, white or little yellowish at night, copious, eyelids stuck in the morning.
- Redness of eyes esp. left, in evening.
- Pain in eyeball esp. left as if it is pushed forward, with copious yellowish white discharge.

Other important symptoms were brought out in the urinary tract:

- Urine feels a little hot and slightly excoriating.
- Frequent urination at night.
- Sensation as if something remained after passing urine.
- Last drop very hot and feels as if it is very concentrated, excoriating.

Lampona cylindrata (White tailed spider)

Phylum: Arthropoda.
Class: Arachnida.
Order: Araneae.
Suborder: Araneomorphae.

White-tailed spiders are vagrant hunters; seeking out and poisoning prey rather than spinning a web to capture it. Therefore, they do not make a permanent home. Their preferred prey are web-weaving spiders. They position themselves at the outer edges of a web, and by plucking and strumming the threads they imitate the struggling of an ensnared insect to deceptively lure out the unsuspecting host spider.

Proving by: **Alastair Gray, Australia (2000).**[13]

Keywords

Bitten / Squashed / Vulnerable / Neglected / **Bewitched** / Beautiful / Watchful / Isolated / Desolation / Suddenness / *Kleptomania* / Gambling / Attacked / Defiance / Courageous / Superstitious / Mutilation / Invasion / Frozen / Grasping / Tenacious

SRP delusions

- Bewitched; he is
- Neglected; he is
- Poisoned; about to be; that he is
- Superhuman; control, is under
- Squashed; is
- Body parts; black; are
- Body, body parts; smaller
- Bitten; will be
- Influence; is under a powerful
- Insane; become; that one will
- Someone; grasps his neck

Mind

- Abrupt / Rashness
- Colours; aversion to; red
- **Compulsive disorders**
- Confusion of mind; location, about; loses his way in well-known streets
- Courageous
- Dance, desires to; amel.
- Death; desires
- **Defiant**
- Despair; pain, with
- Despair; sexual desire, from
- Escape, desire to; run away, to
- Estranged; family, from her and friends
- Fastidious
- Fear; panic attacks, overpowering
- **Fear**
  - Poisoned; being
  - Poverty; of
  - Robbers; of
- Fight; wants to
- Giggling
- Industrious, mania for work
- **Kleptomania**
- Praying / Prophesying
- Rashness
- Rest; cannot, when things are not in proper place
- Sighing
- Superstitious
- Talk; finish what he has to say, cannot

Dreams

Animals, of; black / Clairvoyant / Dancing / Danger / Driving a; car / Invasion / Murder; murdered; of being / Mutilation / Poisoned; of being / Pursued; of being / Stealing, theft / Vertigo / Vulnerable; he is

Physicals
- **Head**
  - Pain
    - § Frozen; as if head and brain are – occiput
    - § Grasping, gripping – Forehead
    - § Lancinating – Temples – extending to; Occiput
- **Eyes**
  - Discharges – sticky
  - Discharges – white
  - Ecchymosis
  - Hemorrhage
  - Light – agg. – artificial
- **Vision**
  - Accommodation – defective
- **Neck**
  - Hardness – lymphatic tissue
- **Stomach**
  - Alive sensation
  - Stomach – Appetite – ravenous, canine, excessive – eating – increasing hunger
  - Abdomen – crying of an animal; like
- **Urine**
  - Greenish – dark
- **Male**
  - Pain – Testes – sitting; while
- **Female**
  - Fullness – vagina
  - Menses – milky / Ropy, tenacious, stringy
- **Sleep**
  - Disturbed – itching; from
- **Generals**
  - Discharges – metallic taste
  - Food and drinks – thinking of food agg.

Themes from the proving Gray[13]

They are passive hunters, they wait by the web, waiting in the cold is like having a **nameless fear**, inspiring an **ever-watchful attitude**, they do not sleep. In friendship they may often be shallow, biting deeply emotionally in marital arrangements and losing their head. Spiders become what they eat, they have no name, no identity or ego, causing great despondency.

- *His lifelong love of being of service to people was entirely annihilated, he felt agitation and hatred, before he felt god will reward me.*
- Visual disturbances, heightened senses.
- **Sensitive to water, noise**, the sound of water, music, smell acute.
- Hates water and hates colours.
- Sense of smell amel., sensitivity to smell >
- **Desolation, alone, home isolated from family.**
- Lots of **sudden** things, sudden elation, sudden desire for sleep.
- The desire to steal things. (Kleptomania).
- **Addiction; wants to take more, gambling.**
- *Feeling feminine, feeling beautiful.*
- **Feels attacked** by people, spiritually.
- Desire to kill.
- Confidence, attraction, telling people what she thinks.
- I can do things, **defiance**, taking things against instruction.
- More awake, more active, very active, cleaning, organizing, vacuuming, very efficient, very elated, I feel amazing.
- Generally alert and focused becoming tired and falling apart.

- Difficulty sleeping. Talking, walking, sex, amel. chocolate, sweets, ice cream.
- Ice cream, sweets ameliorates.
- Chocolate amel.
- "I want the reward now, give me the reward" before impotent – now strong desire for sex.
- Brief cases, bags, dogs.

Latrodectus hasselti (Redback spider)

Phylum: Arthropoda.
Class: Arachnida.
Order: Araneae.
Suborder: Araneomorphae.

Latrodectus hasselti (Australian black widow) is a species of highly venomous spider in the Theridiidae family. They prey on insects, spiders and small vertebrates that become ensnared in their web, killing by injection of a complex venom through their two fangs. In order to first render their prey immobile, they squirt their victims with 'superglue' from the spinnerets. The prey is bound in a silk cage before having their liquefied insides sucked out. Male spiders and spiderlings often live on the periphery of the female spiders' web, stealing leftovers. The redback usually displays sexual cannibalism while mating. Their poison is neurotoxic to vertebrates, giving rise to the syndrome of latrodectism in humans. The female spins her web during the night, remaining in the same location for most of her adult life. Redback spiderlings cohabit on the maternal web for several days to a week, during which time sibling cannibalism can be observed. They leave the web carried on gusts of wind before dropping a silk thread upon which they can abseil down to a new location where they build their own web.

Proving by: **Julia Twohig, Australia (1997).**[32]

Keywords
Poisoned / Evil / Hollow / Identity – lost / Honour – wounded / Shame / **Body – ugly** / **Mutilating** / Sentimental / Stabbed / Hysterical / **Betrayed** / **Bitten** / Wounded / Herpetic / Putrid / **Old wound** / Decay and death / Devil / Hostile / Hijacking / Paralysed / Terror / Jumping / Dancing / Violate / Estranged / Touched; being – aversion to / Tightly bound / Tough / Survive / Cannibalism / **Devour own offspring** / Protecting when threatened

Fundamental delusions
- Friend – affection of; has lost the (*Aurum, Hura, Hydrogen, Thuja*)
- Identity – someone else; she is (*Alumina, Cannabis indica and sativa, Lachesis, Valeriana*)
- Head – strange head; his head were another (*Theridion*)
- Whispering to him; someone is (*Anacardium, Chironex fleckeri, Medorrhinum, Rhodium*)

SRP delusions

- Experienced – before; thought everything had been (*cf. Anhalonium, Crotalus cascavella, Positronium*)
- Poisoned – about to be poisoned; he is (*cf. Hyoscyamus, Lachesis, Rhus-tox*)
- Evil – done some evil; had (*cf. Cyclamen, Zincum*)
- Hollow – body is hollow; whole
- Forsaken – friend; she has been forsaken by a near (*cf. Rhus-tox*)
- Superhuman – control; is under superhuman (*cf. Argon, Ophidia, Thuja*)

Single remedy delusions

- Brain – swashing
- Brain – intoxicated
- **Ailments from**
  - Excitement – emotional
  - Grief
  - Honour; wounded (*cf.* Aurum sulph, Staphisagria)
  - Shame

Mind

- Anger
  - **destroy** things; with tendency to
  - **stabbed** anyone; so angry that he could have
- Carefree
- Cautious
- Checking – twice or more; must check (**OCD**)
- Dancing – amel.
- Dancing – wild
- **Delusions**
  - Alone, being – world; alone in the
  - Body – ugly; body looks
  - Evil – done some evil; had
  - Head – strange head; his head were another
  - Large – he himself seems too
  - Succeed, he does everything wrong; he cannot
- **Detached**
- Estranged – society; from
- Fear – disease, of impending – *incurable*; of being
- Fear – health – ruined; that she has
- Fearless
- Frightened easily
- Impulse; morbid – violence, to do
- Indifference – reprimands; to all
- Irritability – touch; by
- Mutilating his body
- Philosophy – ability for
- Sensitive – colours; to
- Sensitive – noise; to – talking, of
- Sentimental – moonlight; in (Ant-c)
- Thoughts – sexual
- Thoughts – violent
- Throwing things around
- Touched – aversion to be
- Undertaking – many things, persevering in nothing
- Weeping – hysterical
- Wrong; everything seems

Dreams
Accusations – crime; wrongful of / **Amputation** – arm; of / **Betrayed**; having been / **Bitten**; being / Buildings – demolition of public building / Court; judicial / Forsaken; being / Friendly; being / Killing – brother is; her – sister; her / Knives / Lost; being / Mother / Murder / Nakedness / **Pursued**, being – dogs; by / Pursued, being – man; by a – violate her; to / Religious / **Scientific** / Sexual / Shooting; about / Shopping / Snakes / Spiders / Thunderstorm / Violence / **Wounded**; being

Physicals
- **Skin**
  - Cicatrices – break open / Cracks / Ecchymoses /
  - **Eruptions**
    - § Desquamating
    - § *Herpetic* – itching
    - § Rash
    - § Red – *insect stings*; like
    - § Urticaria
    - § Formication – lice; as if from
    - § Itching – crawling
  - Swelling – dropsical – wound; around

- **Stomach**
  - Appetite – diminished – eating; when time for
  - Appetite – increased – accompanied by – nausea
  - Emotions – are felt in
  - Eructations – desire to eructate
  - Fullness, sensation of – water; after
  - Nausea – sleep – after – agg.
  - Tension
  - Thirst – extreme
  - Trembling

Female Genitalia/Sex
- Congestion – Uterus – irritation of bladder; with
- Leukorrhea
  - Alternating with – bloody discharge
  - Bloody – menses – appear; with sensation as if menses would
  - Brown – menses – before – agg.
  - Masturbation; disposition to
  - Menses – dark – clots; with / Traces of menses between the periods
  - Pain – Ovaries – left – extending to – uterus / Supports abdomen with hands – bearing down

Aside from Tarentula, this is one of the fullest Spider provings with many symptoms in the repertories, providing another useful template for this group of remedies.

Extracts from the proving
One prover reported the sudden appearance of eight strong white hairs on the top of her head, near the hairline. We were quite prepared to dismiss this as fanciful or at the very least unrelated to the proving until a patient whom I treated with Latrodectus haselti 30C reported that her prematurely grey hair was becoming dramatically darker, especially at the front. . . .[32]

Provers speaking as one

"I had a *loose, putrid, black bowel movement*, which smelt of **decay and death**. As if the **devil, evil** came out. I have never before experienced anything like this. It was most **ugly**. It was as if all the *bad feelings about myself and all the bad things that I have done over my life passed*. Something shifted. . . . I had a violent dream that I **reopened an old wound** on my forehead. I had originally *received this wound during a jealous fist fight over a woman*. I woke from my dream holding my penis and sleepily walked towards the door . . . split(ting) my forehead open at the site of the original wound. *I reopened the old scar*. There was **blood** everywhere. . . . Today while travelling on a train I thought of **hijacking** the train. I have no idea why. I have been feeling **hostile** towards people lately. . . . Anger that was **boiling inside** of me. . . . A *deep irritability in the gut*, a violent form which could *lead to aggression*. . . . I felt that my irritability was violent and had to exercise restraint to keep myself 'nice'. . . . I thought I could *hear somebody whispering* in the lounge, I then heard noises, creaks, down the hallway. With every noise my **terror** increased. I was **paralysed** with fear. My heart was in my mouth. I was hot. . . . I turned the stereo up to full blast and I started **dancing** to it. It wasn't my usual style of dancing. I was **jumping around** and swinging my arms . . . the remedy made me more sensitive and since then I have been able to counteract this by **becoming harder** and by being able to **detach from emotion**. . . . I felt *no emotional involvement with my actions*"[32]

- One prover who had previously been bitten by Lampona cylindrata, and whose wound had never healed or responded to treatment, had a curative response during the proving of Lat-h. "Within an hour of taking the proving remedy, the bite began to itch and came up in a blister with a watery discharge. It went away after a few hours and since then has completely cleared for the first time. One year after the proving there is still no sign of the old bite."[32]

Natural behaviour

"The Redback has an incredible ability to *survive* a wide range of vastly different and often *harsh* habitats. . . . This group of primarily ground dwelling spiders have the habit of throwing out **sticky trap** lines that form an irregular, tangled web of **fine** but incredibly **strong** silk . . . Latrodectus haselti is a *prolific breeder*. . . . It is possible for a female to lay thousands of eggs in one hatching. The sacs are made of **tightly bound** silk and are very **tough**. . . . Male spiders conduct an elaborate pre copulation **ritual** . . . including leg *flicking, lunging, abseiling, somersaulting, running* away, *bouncing* and cutting of the web . . . (After coitus) the female begins to ingest her mate. This **sexual cannibalism** is seen in relatively few other species. . . . Young spiderlings are highly cannibalistic and the **mother** may also **devour** some of her **offspring**. Cannibalism seems to be a growth strategy for the female, from the neonatal stage to adulthood the cannibalistic female grows quickly and in this **competitive** environment they **prey** on smaller siblings. . . . The female L. hasselti is not aggressive unless she is **protecting** her young, or otherwise **threatened**."[32]

Araneae / Spiders

Latrodectus mactans (Black widow spider)

Class: Arachnida.
Order: Araneae.
Suborder: Araneomorphae.
Family: Theridiidae.

The females are well known for their distinctive black and red colouring and for their proclivities towards post-coital cannibalism. When they detect prey ensnared by the web, they quickly dart out of their retreat, wrap the victim tightly in silk, then bite and envenom their catch. Their web is strong enough to catch animals as large as mice. Within ten minutes, the venom starts to take effect whilst the prey is held captive by the spider. When their movements cease, digestive enzymes are released into the wound, before the spider carries its catch back to the retreat for feeding

Provings by: **The Hering Proving Committee, USA (1932).
Jonathan Shore, Finland and Germany (1999).**[19]

Keywords
Infarction; myocardial / Angina pectoris / Agonizing / Lancinating / Radiating / Waves; in / Apoplexy / Chorea / Anorexia / Agony / **Sudden death** / Malicious / **Anarchistic** / Underground / **Entangled** / Clinging / Waiting for prey / **Outcast** / Deceit / Power / Struggle / Rejection / Frenzied / Sucking juices / **Silk cage**

Mind
- Mind symptoms correspond to the feelings of a **person facing death**.
- Extreme state of nervous irritation.
- Fear of going mad, losing breath and dying.

Physicals
- Shivers, profuse cold sweat and pain which is very similar to **angina pectoris**.
- The venom causes interference to the passage of the nerve impulse at the neuromuscular junction.

Themes
Anarchistic / Underground / Illegal / Separated / Fight / Freedom / Floating / Struggle / Power / Surrounded / Life or death / Kill / I am outside / No longer a member of the group / Outcast / Suddenness / Rejection / Sensitiveness to danger / Psychic awareness / *Deceit* / Manipulation / **Clinging** to the web / Waiting for prey / **Entangled** / Quickly attacks / Biting / **Sucking** its juices out / **Encloses her in a silk cage**

Clinical
Examination showed an area of muscular constriction along the lower spine with some- what accentuated but normal reflexes and undisturbed skin sensorium. However, the

*patient was in a state of **frenzied restlessness**, screaming and crying with pain, unable to lie still, yet aggravated by any motion.* Whitmont[31]

Rubrics

- **Mind**
  - Anorexia nervosa
  - Death – agony before death
  - Death – sensation of
  - Fear – death; of – angina pectoris; during
  - Fear – death; of – sudden death; of
  - Fear – suffocation; of
  - Malicious – hurting other people's feelings
  - Rolling – floor; on the – pain; from
  - Shrieking – dying; thinks she will be
  - Staring, thoughtless
- **Chest**
  - Angina pectoris
  - Constriction – Heart – extending to – Back
  - Infarction; myocardial
  - Inflammation – Lungs / Pleura
  - Murmurs – cardiac murmurs
  - Pain – Heart – Region of – tearing pain
  - Shocks
  - Spasms of
- **Generals**
  - Apoplexy
  - Chorea
  - Convulsions – isolated groups of muscles
  - Doubling up of the body
  - Emaciation
  - Food poisoning
  - Haemorrhage – blood – non-coagulable
  - Hypertension – sudden
  - Inflammation – Nerves – Peripheral
  - **Laboratory findings**
    § Erythrocytes – increased
    § Leukocytes – increased
    § Platelets – decreased
    § Spinal fluid pressure – increased
  - **Pain**
    § Agonizing / Appear suddenly / Bursting / Cutting / Lancinating / Radiating / Stinging / Tingling / Waves; in
    § Paralyzed parts
    § Paralysis – painful
    § Periodicity – year – every
    § Pulse – thready
    § Sick feeling; vague
    § Swelling – Glands; of
    § Tetanus
    § Wounds – bites – poisonous animals; of
    § Wounds – bleeding freely

Dreams

Proving conducted by Jonathon Shore – *Investigations into the Psyche of the Spider.*[19]

"She is in a group of people separated from another group who they must join in order to plan a revolution. **Anarchistic fight for freedom. Underground, illegal.** She is with an old girlfriend of hers, who was in reality an anarchist in Berlin. . . . They are trying to reach the others from whom they are **separated** by a concrete wall. The wall can be scaled by using the branch of a tree hanging over the wall. She climbs down the branch, but her feet do not actually step on the wood. It is as if she is **floating** and softly landing on the ground. At last, finally, finally they are together. *Happiness and joy* about this. . . . Then there develops a tension and a **struggle for power** between her and her friend. Friend is angry and upset. It is as if she is surrounded by a circle, like a magic circle which cannot be *penetrated. I cannot communicate with her because of the anger.* I want the contact, I try and try but it does not work. *Cannot get through to her. . . .* Suddenly the whole mood of the group changes. There is anger in the air. They look at me in a strange way, **I am surrounded.** Like *I am in the middle of a pack of wolves.* They use no words. It is a mind connection. They use their thought power. They don't must speak out aloud. I can hear their thoughts in my head. I knew immediately it was **life or death.** The danger coming towards me was absolutely clear. . . . **They could kill me.** Like wolves, if one starts to attack the others will follow. I thought we were all part of one group now **I am outside, no longer a member.**"

"This dream touches on many of the central features of spiders; the feeling of **being an outcast, the suddenness** with which it takes place and the inexplicability of the **rejection** and the terrible feelings consequent upon this have been clearly verified in a cured case. . . . The **sensitiveness to danger, psychic awareness of its presence and psychic sensitivity in general** are also strong currents. The imagery associated with **anarchy**, with lawlessness, with what is *underground, below the surface, about to break loose in revolution* speaks to the power and nature of the psychic forces at work. The currents of **deceit** and **manipulation** in their deeper aspects. . . ."

Natural behaviour

"Found in warm, dry, dimly lit protected corners, secluded places where it builds a large, irregular, funnel-shaped web, close to the ground or under debris. This web consists of straggly, uneven, *coarse viscous* threads running in all directions, in all three dimensions, with none of the geometrical exactitude which gives the orbwebweavers or sheetwebweavers their aesthetic charm. *The female spends virtually her entire life* **clinging to the web** *upside down* **waiting** *for* **prey** *to become* **entangled** *in the web.* The strands of silk making up the web are very strong. . . . The spider *quickly attacks* whatever touches its web, indiscriminately **biting** it, then waits for the prey to become paralysed before **sucking its juices out.** Despite this, it is not considered to be an aggressive spider, biting only in self-defence when provoked. . . . In preparation for mating, the male spins a delicate web upon which he deposits the seminal fluid to be gathered by the palpi. He then spins a very thin web, *surrounding the female with threads that tie down all her legs* and **encloses her in a silk cage.**" Bonnet[17]

Loxosceles reclusa (Brown recluse / Fiddleback spider)

Phylum: Arthropoda.
Class: Arachnida.
Order: Araneae.
Suborder: Araneomorphae.

The Brown recluse spider has a necrotic venom. They have markings on the dorsal side of their cephalothorax, with a black line coming from it that looks like the neck of a violin pointing to the rear of the spider. They are resilient, capable of tolerating up to six months of extreme drought and scarcity of food. When threatened they usually avoid conflict, preferring to flee or 'play dead'. They build asymmetrical webs with a shelter consisting of disorderly threads. Their webs are to be found in woodpiles and sheds, closets, cellars, and other places that are dry and mostly undisturbed. Unlike most web weavers, they leave these lairs at night to hunt.

Proving by: **Louis Klein, Canada (1997–98).**[10]

Keywords
Bewitched / Ugly / Criticised / Invaded / Invincible / Invisible / Sarcasm / Joyless / Courageous / Mutilation / Destructiveness / Remorse / Robbers / Criminals / Death / Guns / **Contracture** / Suicidal / Fleeing / Brushed off / **Old and unattractive** / Exposed / Cocoon / Hunting / Hibernation / Innocence / Fraud / Revenge / Malicious / Molested / Retreat / Grief – silent / Strange – crank

SRP delusions
- *Bewitched*; he is
- Body – *ugly*; body looks
- Criticised; she is
- Insects; sees
- *Invaded*; one's space is being
- Invincible; he is
- Invisible; she is
- *Old* – feels old
- Possessed; being
- Separated – body – spirit had separated from body

Mind
- Abrupt
- Abusive, insulting
- Ailments from – embarrassment
- Anxiety – conscience; of
- Ardent
- Censorious
- Confusion of mind – time; as to
- Courageous
- Cruelty
- Cut, mutilate, slit; desire to
- Death – thoughts of
- Deception
- Destructiveness
- Detached
- *Eccentricity*
- Fear – dark; of
- Forsaken feeling – isolation; sensation
- Grief – silent
- Harshness, rough

- Imbecility – negativism
- *Indifference, apathy – welfare of others, to*
- Indifference – joyless
- Industrious
- Loquacity – changing quickly from one subject to another
- Music; desires – playing; piano
- *Mocking – sarcasm*
- Offended, easily
- Optimistic
- Pessimist
- Rage
- Remorse, repentance
- Reproaching oneself
- Sadness – injustice; from
- Selfishness, egoism
- Sensitive – noise; to
- Sentimental – past; about
- Sighing
- *Strange – crank*
- Thoughts – persistent; morbid
- Thoughts – sexual

Dreams

Boat / Busy; being / *Climbing – falling; and* / Country – foreign / *Criminals*; of / *Dead* bodies / Death – relatives; of / Desserts – detail; in great / Driving – car; a / Earthquake / Face / *Face – two faces – only sees one; there are two faces but he* / Father / Fights / Flying / Food / Food – preparing food – desserts / Forgotten something; one has / Friends – old / *Guns* / Light; of – candle light / Music / Parties / People – crowds of / Plants – growing – fast / *Robbers* / Sexual / Singing / Snakes – leaping out at her / Swimming / Unsuccessful efforts – climbing – sand dune / Urinating – public; in / Vegetables / Walking – dark; in / Watching – helicopter / Water

"Loxosceles is derived from 'loxos' from Greek for oblique and 'sceles' from Latin 'scelus', 'scelestus' for impious, wicked, villanous, roguish, infamous, accursed, heinous." Bonnet[17]

Provers speaking as one

"**Bewitched – under a spell.** Problems interacting with patients; they are too attached to me . . . Very quick speech. Sarcastic . . . Usually big energy, but now I'm feeling **condensed**. Never felt like this before . . . Want to **crouch** into a tiny space, like a little animal. Want to take the littlest amount of space and not be visible. . . . **Contracture** – amel. sitting down legs crossed, hunched over crouched, in a small space. Even my personality is smaller; ie. at a party I didn't try to be the chatelaine, as usual. Like I'm occupying a smaller space. . . . Strong sense of **time**: wasting my days. Never thought of **dying** before when **leaving**. Death thoughts – gift of knowledge of near mortality; **how precious time is wasted on trivial stuff**. . . . Thinking about time wasting . . . Timing off – Lost my watch. Arrived at the workshop one day late. . . . Another hit of depression. **Suicidal** thoughts. Felt, what's the use . . . a desire to **escape** my life here as it is. . . . Supervisor could sense the prover was getting **edginess** about her again. As if she was present and in the conversation one minute, and then answering to a strong **impulse** beckoning her to **flee, move, get out**, in the next minute. On the receiving end, it feels as if one is being 'brushed off'. . . . **Brushed off** is definitely one of the tones of this proving . . . **How old and unattractive I am**. . . . I look in the mirror now and see an ugly, old, corpse. An ugly, saggy, sallow, drooping, wrinkling face. . . . Feeling ugly, obsessing about that and about how I looked, prevented me from presenting my well thought out opinions about the subject at hand. . . . Driving home it was a real **battle between myself and my 'proving' self.** I would think, oh, I should go and meet him where he was going. Then I'd think, no! He should pay for what he said. This'll teach him – that sort of thinking. . . . Terrified to have photo taken; felt **exposed** . . . Inward Experience; Felt insulated from every other human or experience. Apathy for others. I was always alone, even when with others. Self Absorption. Observer and isolated from everything going on . . . **Cocoon.** No Interest, stay in bed, stay home . . . desire to wrap in one and be alone. Do not disturb . . . Dream: I was hiding behind these big rocks in this huge cave. . . . I was all alone and I have no idea who or what I was hiding from. Strange feeling of hiding, woke up with that feeling. . . . Under Attack / Invincible. . . . No fear I find I have no fears, like I can just go into anything. I drove home in a blinding snow storm on the highway. I never once considered I wouldn't make it. *Not careless, just not as fearful.*"[10]

Toxicological [Bonnet][17]

Convulsions, seizures / Headache, severe / Jaundice, rapid development, progressive / Vomiting, intermittent, frequent or continuous / Dark red-to-black urine / Bloody urination / Haematuria, gross / Tachypnea, rapid respiration / Dyspnea, labored breathing / Rapid pulse / Chills, continuous / High fever / Cellulitis / Cyanosis / Dusky, mottled skin lesion / Ecchymosis / Scarlatiniform rash, erythematous, generalised / Myalgia / Pain: increasing continuously / Anemia, hemolytic

Painful, necrotic, slow-healing ulcerated wounds, creating long term disabilities . . . with recurrent wound breakdown and poor healing. . . . Generally, the skin lesion presents as a rapidly expanding tiny blue area and a sudden increase in local tenderness which can evolve to severe pain. The superficial skin infarcts, and a blue macule with fixed, dull, grey centre develops. [Bonnet][17]

Natural behaviour

Shy / Innocence / Hunting / Dark corners / Cracks and crevices / Viscid silk / Maze of threads / Retreat / Hibernation / Invasion

"The brown recluse spider forms an irregular web consisting of loose threads extending in all directions with a densely central *retreat.* It is a long-lived and hardy spider capable of *surviving for six or more months without food or water.* This longevity is remarkable for such a small animal. It is nocturnal, retiring and shy. It does not attack or bite except when molested, preferring to run for cover when disturbed." [Bonnet][17]

Clinical

"His dreams are all about killing and being killed . . . tied up, beaten, starved, misled, escape when least expected, fraud, revenge, attack, ambush, hunt, poison, torture . . . mean, evil, malicious, ambush, scheming, can't hardly wait to attack, suddenly attack and kill . . . malicious woman throwing another from a cliff." [Vervarcke][7]

Mygale lasiodora (Cuban spider)

Unfortunately, the true origin of the species is difficult to discern owing to conflicting information in the Homeopathic literature.

Proving & poisoning information from: **J.G. Houard, USA (1850s).**

Keywords
Chorea / Revenge / Rapid / Twitching / Jerky / Feigning – sick; to be / Tourette's syndrome / Abused / Violent / Kill / Escape / Hurry / Suddenness

Clinical Indications: Chorea, tics, twitching, jerking of limbs and speech, violent erections. "The characteristic mental state of Mygale is abrupt speech with restlessness, the patient is worse on waking. Like Bryonia, constantly talks of business with a strong fear of death. There are two polarities of **extreme sensitivity on one end and feeling of hatred and revenge** on the other."[11]

Phatak's repertory[36]
- Automatic acts – one arm and leg, head etc
- **Chorea** – face; of / Chorea – sleep – amel.
- Eyelids – twitch – **rapid** succession; in / Eyes – open – rapid succession; in
- Face – **twitching**, trembling / Gait – dragging / Legs – **jerking** up
- Mouth – open, hangs, jaws drop – rapid succession; in
- Nausea – palpitation; with / Nausea – vision, dim; with
- Red, redness skin, discharges etc. – streaks / Skin – *stripes, streaks*; on
- Sleep – amel.; *loss of agg.*
- Speaking, talking agg. – **jerky**
- Tongue – protruded – difficulty; with

Mind
- Delirium – *business*; talks of
- Fear – death; of
- *Feigning – sick*; to be
- Gestures, makes – one arm or leg or head
- Hatred – *revenge; hatred and*
- Hysteria
- Praying
- Restlessness – night
- Sensitive – *chorea*; in
- Sensitive – *music*; to
- Speech – *jerks*; by
- *Tourette's syndrome*

Clinical
"When I saw this young man in my consulting room; restless, aggressive, fast talking about his business, the first thing that came to my mind was that he looked like a spider . . . he had the following symptoms: restlessness, aggressiveness, workaholic, extreme thirst, *eats only what is necessary to stay alive*." Woutman[25]

New rubrics for Mygale based on this cured case:

Mind
- **Ailments from – abused; after being – violence; from**
- Anger / Kill; desire to / Violent
- Cut, mutilate or slit; desire to – knife; with a sharp
  - *(The patient actually killed somebody in self-defence and was sent to jail for it)*
- **Escape**; attempts to (*from prison, and succeeded*)
- Fanaticism (*in his pursuit of learning kick-boxing*)
- Hurry – occupation; in
- Industrious
- Face – Perspiration
- Extremities – Perspiration – Feet – **offensive**
- Perspiration – Profuse

Natural behaviour
"This spider does not make a web but *kills his prey instantly*. It is one of the biggest spiders in the world, very hairy and usually lives underground. Mothers carry their young ones on their back ('fear to touch the ground'). A useful tip: the Mygale spider *stiffens* when he is *suddenly* exposed to light." Mangialavori[1]

Tarentula hispanica (Lycosa tarantula / Wolf spider)

Class: Arachnida.
Order: Araneae.
Suborder: Araneomorphae.
Family: Lycosidae.

As with other wolf spiders, the silken sac containing over 100 eggs is carried attached to the mother's spinnerets, then after they hatch the spiderlings climb on their mother's abdomen and ride around with her for some time until they are sufficiently mature to survive on their own. The Lycosidae have a very strong tendency to flee at the approach of any large animal.

Proving by: **Jose Nunez Pernia** (aka **Jose Nunez/Marquis of Nunez**), **Spain (1846).**

Keywords
Music / **Dancing** / Destructiveness / Attack / Hysteria / Hurry / Threatening / Restlessness / Cheated / Taken advantage of / Vulnerable / Treadmill / Overdrive / Accelerated / Insatiable / Industrious

Bold type mind symptoms

- **Anger – touched; when**
- Attack others; desire to
- Breaking things – *desire to break things*
- Colours – aversion to – strong colours; aversion to
- Destructiveness – clothes; of
- Hurry – everybody – must hurry
- Hysteria – *music amel.*
- Insanity – restlessness, with – lower limbs; of
- Insanity – strength; with increased
- Insanity – *threatening destruction and death*
- **Rage – chained; had to be**
- Restlessness – anxious – walking – rapidly
- Sensitive – noise; to – music amel.
- Speech – abrupt
- **Threatening**

Fundamental delusions

- Sick – being
- Assaulted; is going to be
- Legs – cut off; legs are
- Strangers – room; seem to be in the

Ailments from

- Embarrassment
- Excitement – emotional
- Love; disappointed
- Punishment
- Reproaches

SRP delusions

- Absurd, ludicrous – figures are present
- Air – cold air; he were entering
- Insulted; he is
- Persecuted – he is persecuted
- Small – body is smaller
- Unseen things; delusions of
- Black – objects and people; sees
- Visions, has – monsters, of
- Faces; sees – *diabolical faces crowd upon him*
- Fall; something would – him; on

Remedy portrait

These delusions suggest that underpinning the well-known antics, cunning & mischief of Tarentula lies a core feeling that they are being assaulted, insulted and persecuted. They feel they are small and therefore at a disadvantage – something might even fall on them. This is why they like to create webs of intrigue around them, such as feigning illness – it gives them a feeling of control over their environment, such as suffocating parents. In a developed Tarentula state, loved ones may start to seem like strangers (leading to a forsaken feeling). As this intensifies, or perhaps during a febrile illness, others may come across as absurd, monstrous or even diabolical. Yet their desire to escape these enemies is prevented by the feeling that their legs are cut off. The legs also represent support – the ability to stand on one's own two feet – which they feel is missing. The tarentula mother keeps her children under close control, bound onto her back, hence the feeling can arise of being too tightly bound with an authority figure and wanting to break free from such constraints. This explains the pent-up tension that often expresses itself as restlessness and manic energy in uncompensated states. When suppressed, it may come through in dyspraxia or sudden awkward movements, tics or cursing (as in Tourette's syndrome).

The folklore of the Tarantella dance (being a cure for Tarentula bites) fits the theme of using pent-up energy to release oneself from restrictions. "They respond compulsively to fast and rhythmic music, and are compelled to dance to it. Music alleviates the restlessness of the extremities. Sepia types also love to dance, but for different reasons: their sluggish system is ameliorated by the activity, though because of this sluggishness it may take some effort to get started. Tarentula has no choice: he is itching to get up and dance the minute the right kind of music starts."[29]

They dream of wild and poisonous animals, of being insulted, falling from a horse and jumping into water.

Clinical
Misha Norland[29] writes:

> The babies of the Tarentula hispanica are independent from birth, but the mother spider binds them up in silk to stop them wandering. Considering that the babies will grow into aggressive predators that catch their prey by running, bounding and jumping, these **silk bonds must be a maddening restriction.** . . . Tarentula types are 'foxy', **deceptive and cunning** by nature, as expected of a spider that hunts by stealth. **The alternation of violent or aggressive behaviour with cowardice is a feature of this remedy.** They fear being assaulted, injured and trapped themselves, but inflict hurts on others. Typical Tarentula behaviour in a child might be for her to creep out of her hiding place and create mischief when no one is looking, then, when someone looks, to retreat and hide, while keeping a furtive eye on the effect she is producing.

Vasillis Ghegas writes:[14]

> The picture of Tarent. Is usually provoked by the following situations: work under strong pressure and much responsibility, jobs where any detail is important, where all your attention is required, and particularly in situations with high time pressure (such as reporters, stock brokers, air traffic controllers, the secretary who has to answer three calls simultaneously etc.) It is characteristic in Tarent. that they feel as if they were obliged to do three jobs at the same time and perfectly: they are super-workaholic and industrious.

CASE 2.1 Depression, with suicidal tendencies

Patient: **Female, age 42**

Prescription: **Tarent 200c**

Spider Themes
∫ They don't recognise my strengths, they don't recognise my gifts, I am very dynamic and then I am shat on.

∫ I am not recognised for my strengths – Feel I am dying inside because of it.
∫ I scream and cry. *I have Tourette's*!
∫ Feel **judged** and silly, it is hard to shake, it creeps up.
∫ I feel **cheated, or taken advantage of** – really? This is what I am?
∫ Strong ***chest pains*** on left side w/ shortness of breath, where the *anger* and *despair* come together and are unleashed.
∫ I push my lovely daughter away.
∫ I retreat, want to be alone, run away. I just want to **hibernate and disappear.**
∫ Feel **vulnerable** and exposed.

Animal language
∫ Money gives you status and self-worth.
∫ I'm wasting my energy – jealous of my husband getting easy offers for work. ***I would kill* to have his connections.**
∫ I must worry about **feeding two young humans**.
∫ Comparing myself to brother and sister – they're very successful.

Miasmatic pace
∫ Urgency, catch a rush, insatiable, treadmill, overdrive, constant hurry, can't keep up, accelerated.

		caust.	ign.	sep.	tarent.	bell.	nux-v.	phos.	sil.
		1	2	3	4	5	6	7	8
		24	24	24	24	23	23	23	23
MENTAL QUALITIES - Low self esteem	(273) 2	2	2	4	2	2	2	2	2
MIND - AILMENTS FROM - love; disappointed	(57) 1	2	4	1	1	2	1	1	
MIND - INCONSOLABLE / WEEPING - consolation agg	(62) 1	2	3	3	2	1	2	1	3
MIND - DESPAIR / SUICIDAL DISPOSITION	(330) 3	2	3	2	2	2	2	1	1
MIND -FIGHT- wants to + disposition to contradict	(101) 4	3	1	1	2	1	3	1	1
MIND - ABUSIVE / CURSING / CONTEMPTUOUS	(170) 3	1	1	2	2	2	3	1	1
MENTAL QUALITIES - Big ego	(237) 1	2	2	2	1	3	4	4	3
MENTAL QUALITIES - Money	(236) 2	2	2	4	2	4	4	2	2
MENTAL QUALITIES - Music	(284) 1	2	4	4	4	2	4	3	2
MIND - DANCING - amel.	(15) 1	1	2	3	2				1
MIND - HURRY / INDUSTRIOUS	(306) 2	1	2	2	3	2	2	1	3
RESPIRATION - ARRESTED	(188) 1	2	2	1	1	1	1	2	2
CHEST - OPPRESSION	(387) 1	2	3	3	2	3	3	3	2
GENERALS - FOOD AND DRINKS - sweets - desire	(285) 1	1	1	2	1	1	1	2	1

Figure 2.2 Repertorisation

Tela araneae (Spider's web)

Webs of various spiders;
Araneus diadematus, Tegenaria atrica, Tegenaria domestica, **and / or**
Tegenaria medicinalis.

Spiderwebs have existed for at least 100 million years. When spiders moved from the water to the land in the Early Devonian period, they started making silk to protect their bodies and eggs. They gradually began to use silk for hunting purposes, first as guide or signal lines, then as ground or bush webs, and eventually in the form of the aerial webs that are familiar today. Also referred to as cobwebs, it is a structure spun out of silk extruded from spinnerets located at the tip of the spider's abdomen. Spiders use different glands to produce an array of silks; a trailed safety line, sticky silk for trapping prey or fine silk for wrapping and binding it. Many spiders build webs specifically to catch insects, but they don't all catch prey in the web – some are more active hunters – whilst others do not build webs at all.

*Proving of **Tela aranaeae** spider silk by:* **Christopher Sowton, Toronto (2003).**[24]

Keywords
Invaded / Lost / Disconnected / Jealousy / Fog; enveloped in / Contemptuous / **Clairsentient** / Biting – himself / Dance / Angina pectoris / Numbness / Tingling / Apocalypse / **Intruder** / Seduction / Knives

Key Delusions
* Invaded; one's space is being
* Lost; she is
* People – behind him; someone is
* Young again; she is

Mind
* Anxiety – health; about
* Biting – arms; bites his own
* Biting – hands
* Biting – himself
* Cheerful
* *Clairsentient*
* Communication – inability for
* *Consolation – desire for; touching, without*
* *Contemptuous – society, mankind, at; mediocrity, people are succumbing to*
* Dance – desires to
* Dancing – Jumping; and
* Disconnected feeling
* Dullness – fog; feels enveloped in
* Fear – bitten; of being
* Fear – dark; of
* Fear – evil; fear of
* Insightful
* Jealousy
* Offended easily – jokes; by
* Restlessness – move; must, driving from place to place
* Touched – aversion to being; *invaded* feeling

Physicals

- Head – Pain – Forehead – pressure – amel.
- Rectum – Haemorrhage from anus – stool – during – agg.
- Stool – Hard
- Respiration – Asthmatic – accompanied by – sleeplessness
- Cough – Exhausting

- Chest – **Angina Pectoris**
- Extremities – **Numbness** and **Tingling**
- Chill – Chilliness
- Skin – Eruptions – **Ringworm**
- **Generals**
  - Narcotics – opium; as if had taken
  - Periodicity

Selected Dreams

Apocalypse, end of the world / *Captured*; being / *Drugs*; of, hallucinogens; being drugged / *Glass*, of; broken / *Incestuous* / *Intruder*, intruders; he is a / *Killing*; drugs in drink; by putting / *Knives*; sharpening / *Lost*, being; place, in a strange / *Monsters*; capturing and killing people / *Seduction*; of / *Treasure*; finding

Clinical

"Tela aranea was successfully used in a case of a middle-aged woman who was diagnosed as a case of Supra Ventricular Tachycardia. Her constitutional remedy was selected as Calcarea ars. During the acute phase Digitalis, Gelsemium failed. Later Tela aranea was given on the following indications and she improved considerably: Rapid pulse rate. Weakness, want of energy. It also calmed the patient with a feeling of tranquility." Master[11]

"Tela (Cobweb of the Black Spider) furnishes us with an unusual but fragmentary remedy for **sleeplessness**. It rapidly lowers the frequency of the pulse rate and further tests make it a valuable remedy to *reduce high blood pressure*. In some people it has produced a *calm and delightful state of feeling followed by a disposition to sleep*. The most delicious tranquillity resembling the action of Op. and followed by no bad effects. Twenty grains given to an old, infirm asthmatic produced slight but pleasant delirium. Muscular energy is increased, could not be kept in bed but danced and jumped about the room all night." Grimmer[33]

Source words

Dark / Cellar / Cobwebs / Old and ancient houses / Clinging / Sticking

Theridion curassavicum (Orange widow / Cobweb weaver)

Phylum: Arthropoda.
Class: Arachnida.
Order: Araneae.
Family: Theridiidae.

This species was originally described in 1776 by the German zoologist Philipp Ludwig Statius Müller, with the scientific name of Aranea curacaviensis. The cobweb weavers make flat or irregular tangle webs in corners of rooms and on plants, consisting of a disorganised, three-dimensional mess of loose threads.

Proving by: **Constantine Hering, USA (1832).**

Keywords
Twitching / Busy fruitlessly / Estranged / Head – divided / Jumping / Meniere's / Neuralgia / Neuritis / Tetanus / **Vibration**, sound / Vertex, separated / Blood losses / Haemorrhage / Hysterical / *Knitting* / *Obsessive* / Cerebrospinal axis

Mind
- **Delusions**
  - Dying – he is
  - Head
    - § Belongs to another
    - § Divided; is
    - § Lift it off; can
    - § Separated from body; head is
    - § Strange head; his head were another
  - Jumping – things jumped upon the ground before her; all sorts of
- *Time – earlier; time seems*

- **Themes**
  - Detached – Disconnected
  - Separated – Estranged
  - Industrious – Overactive – Busy fruitlessly
  - Jealousy – Envy
  - Low self esteem
  - Tourette's Syndrome – Face – Twitching
  - Water – Generals – seaside; at the – agg.

Remedy portrait
Mainly known for its clinical use in Meniere's disease, menopause, puberty, vertigo, nausea and extreme sensitivity to noise. In the remedy picture there is hysterical anxiety with a compulsive need to keep busy, resulting in rather hurried and fruitless activity. This tends to express itself with constant wringing of the hands or playing with the fingers, which may find a creative outlet in *knitting* or playing *string instruments*.

The characteristic rubrics of Theridion reveal a marked polarity which swings between extremes of hilarity and cheerful hysteria to a state of nervous sensitivity to the smallest rustling of paper or ticking of a clock. Their nervous system becomes very highly strung indeed. They are extremely sensitive to touch, and may report sensations as of threads, or of being fanned by a draft of air. It is indicated for convulsions with tetanic rigidity, particularly lockjaw (trismus) – revealing an affinity for the trigeminal nerve.

Whilst in the up phase, their cheerfulness can be so strong that it remains even during a headache, hinting again at an unbalanced system with a tendency to go overboard, leading eventually to a state of jangled nerves and faintness. The remedy is well indicated for injuries to the nerves and is also known for the desire to smoke tobacco, perhaps for its sedative effect on the nerves. Boericke[30] suggests its usefulness when well-indicated remedies fail to act. When suffering, they are better for lying in a horizontal position. There may be desire for whisky or wine, with an aversion to all food apart from oranges and sour fruit. As with

Tarentula, there are dreams of horses – although in Theridion they are riding on horseback as opposed to falling from the saddle.

Clinical indications Julian[22]
- Myalgia, neuralgia, neuritis.
- Alcoholic polyneuritis.
- Facial neuralgia.
- Polyradicular neuritis with abnormality of cerebrospinal fluid.

Clinical Roberts[27]
Hysteria / **Tetanus** / Spinal irritation / Rickets / Anthrax of sheep / Sunstroke / Seasickness / Syphilis / Spasmodic cough / Phthisis / Angina pectoris / Infantile atrophy / Scrofulous glands / Nodosities

Pathogenetic Ward[26]
Air, mouth / Air, nose / Asunder, bones / Band, head / Benumbed, mouth / Broken, bones / Burnt, tongue / Coldness, teeth / Disjointed, head / Dryness, mucosa / Far, vision / Furred, mouth / Head, foreign / Lump, perineum / Numb, tongue / Oesophagus, pressure / Perineal, heaviness / Pressed, toe / Pressure, head / Scalded, throat / Slime, teeth / Slipping, oesophagus / Tapped, groin / Thick, head / Veil, eyes / **Vibration, sound** / Weight, head

Clinical Ward[26]
Anxiety, heart / Band, ears / Band, nose / Band, supra-orbital / Behind, eyes / Bones, asunder / Bones, broken / Breath, leaving / Broken, bone / Burned, tongue / Child, bounding / Coldness, teeth / Debility, blood losses / *Dying*, look / Fall, bones / Flickering, vision / Head, illusion / Hears, understands / Heat, head / Heaviness, perineum / *Haemorrhage*, exhaustion / Inhalation, excessive / Lift, vertex / Lump, perineum / Mouth, dry / Nose, air / Nose, dry / Ocular, headache / Pressed, toe / Pressing, ears / Pressure, oesophagus / Roaring, ears / Rushing, ears / Slipping, oesophagus / Tapped, groin / Teeth, cold / Thick, head / Veil, eyes / **Vertex, not belonging** / **Vertex, separated** / Waterfall, ears

Clinical Mangialavori[1]
This remedy is indicated in destructive patients, especially those who like to take risks in sports (mountain climbers) or in financial speculations. They are sensitive to fright and can be paralyzed by emotions. The remedy acts mainly on the lungs.

ARACHNIDA

Androctonus amoreuxii hebraus

(Israeli fat-tailed scorpion – not a spider, but very worthy of inclusion as part of the arachnid group)

Phylum: Arthropoda.
Class: Arachnida.
Order: Scorpiones.
Family: Buthidae.

The genus Androctonus contains some of the most dangerous species of scorpion in the world; the Latin name originates from Greek and means "man killer". Scorpions prey on insects, particularly grasshoppers, crickets, termites, beetles and wasps – also spiders, woodlice, and small vertebrates. Several scorpion species are sit-and-wait predators, whilst others are more active hunters. They detect their prey with mechanoreceptive and chemoreceptive hairs on their bodies. Scorpionic courtship rituals can involve complex behaviours such as a cheliceral kiss, where the male and female grasp each other's fangs, and sexual stinging, in which the male stings the female to subdue her, making her more amenable to his sexual advances and less likely to kill him.

Scorpions are powerful animals and formidable warriors. They were probably the first animals to leave the sea and live on land. Even more remarkable is the fact that, like no other species, they have remained unchanged for nearly 400 million years, indicating a remarkable success in the process of life and evolution.[8]

Proving by: **Jeremy Sherr, Malvern UK (1997).**[8]

Source words

Armour / Weapon / Vibrations / Accuracy / Dancing / Alone / Fight to the death / Cannibalism / Radiation; immunity to / Neurotoxic

Toxicology

Sharp / Burning / Spreading quickly / Headache / Chest pain / Dyspnoea / Nausea and vomiting / Sweating / Sneezing, frequent / Salivation, increased / Lachrymation / Discharge from mouth and nose, continuous fluid / Throat as if blocked with phlegm / Pupils dilate / White froth from mouth / Bronchial asthma / Difficult speech / Restlessness / Twitching; involuntary / Convulsions / Chills / Shivering / High blood pressure / Irregular heartbeat / Tachycardia / Destruction of red corpuscles / Hands and feet turn blue / Abdominal swellings / Loss of consciousness / Death / Pulmonary Oedema.

Proving themes

- Enormous surge of violent emotions; tearing, lashing out. Violent impulses.
- Immense sexual attraction *vs.* extreme hatred.
- Resentful, abused.

- "My eyes are staring and full of hate. I have no control over my emotions. Black, horrible moods which don't last long, but are frightening in their violence."
- Aggressive, strong, violent and cruel.
- "It seemed as though he was a different person, very similar to the way he had been in adolescence, but in a much more powerful manner. These emotions were so intense he wanted to rip his chest apart to let them out".
- Energy, confidence, magentic state. Efficiency, mental tunnel vision. Unflinching, no hesitation.
- Lack of guilt, unfeeling, want of moral affection. No remorse, lack of compassion.
- Sexual power and desire ++
- Separate, disconnected, detached from society.
- Pains: short, sharp, strong, stabbing, poking.

Remedy portrait

In Androctonus there is a central theme of self-power, heightened strength – even a sense of invincibility *vs.* a lack of all willpower, fear of his own impulses and desire for total solitude, free from any interruption. There can be selfish maliciousness, with indifference to the welfare of others expressed in a mocking sarcasm that can cut to the core of the other with unerring intuition. As with Tarentula, it is a remedy of extreme states – they can also be very restless, feeling compelled to walk rapidly. At full intensity, the Androctonus state becomes paranoid; with suspicion of their closest friends, delusions that everyone is insane and that everything around them seems like a terrifying mystery.

The remedy is also suited to adolescent states of rebelliousness; wanting to fight and abuse others, with indifference and impatience that everything moves too slowly. Juxtaposed to the warrior-like personality is the desire to be appreciated and to receive sympathy from others. Like Arnica, they may say they are well when very sick – reflecting their desire for others to keep away. Another rubric reflecting this need for solitude is the delusion that they view the world from a hole, that they want to crawl behind a rock and that one thought excludes all others; a very extreme (syphilitic) expression of monomania.

Androctonus is indicated in haemorrhagic states with dark clots of blood, persistent right-sided paralysis, numbness of the entire body, radiating pains, fevers accompanied by painful soreness and an evening modality of 6pm. Like other remedies in the arachnid group, there is a desire for smoking, and it is listed under the rubric – desire to be in the wind – along with Tarentula and Tuberculinum.

Jeremy Sherr writes

Astrologically, Pluto, Scorpion and Eagle resonate as a trio. Together, these three form a series of the same vibration in various evolutionary phases. The planet Pluto governs the sign of Scorpio, while the god Pluto rules over the shades of the dead in the Under-world. Scorpions are one of the few living creatures to survive in the proximity of nuclear explosions. In ancient times, the sign of Scorpio was represented by an eagle. Scorpio must emerge from under the rocks to fight the battle of life, so that the ashes of its ego can transcend into the mighty eagle. In this context, it is interesting to compare the remedies Plutonium, Androctonus and Haliaeetus. As the most intense sign of the zodiac, Scorpios are continually evolving, deeply sensitive and emotional. They cannot stay stagnant. Their feelings are pronounced with strong attractions or repulsion, deep affections, or unforgiving hate. Scorpios are powerful and may use their power for good or for evil. They are known to be tenacious, secretive, capable of deep betrayal and strongly sexual. They are also deeply spiritual. The colour of this sign is a deep dark red.[8]

Important rubrics

- **Ailments from**
  - Abused; after being – sexually
  - Fright
  - Love; disappointed
- Breaking things
- **Contemptuous / Cruelty**
- **Dancing – wild** (*tarent.*)
- Delusions
  - Adolescent; he was again an
  - Alone; being – world; alone in the
  - **Assaulted**, is going to be (*tarent.*)
  - **Outcast**; she were an
  - Strong; he is
- **Destructiveness**
- Driving – desire for driving
- Drugs – desire – psychotropic
- Duty – too much sense of duty – children; in
- Egotism
- Euphoria
- **Fight; wants to**

- **Indifference**
  - Company, society – while in
  - Pleasure; to – things usually enjoyed
  - **Welfare of others; to**
- Kill; desire to – child; the own
- Light – aversion to – shuns
- **Malicious** – injure someone; desire to
- Passionate / choleric
- Power – sensation of
- Selfishness
- Shameless
- Shrieking – must shriek; feels as though she
- **Striking** – desire – strike; to
- Suspicious – friends; of his best
- Sympathy from others – desire for
- Talking – others agg.; talk of
- Unfeeling
- Well – *says he is well – sick; when very*
- Wrong; everything seems

Dreams

Accidents / Affectionate / Amorous / Anger / Anxious / Biting / Buildings / Busy; being / **Climbing** – bus steps, ladders / Coloured – orange, red, yellow / Confused / **Cutting** / Events – past; long / Family, own / Frightful / Guilt / Head – cut off / Jealousy / Long / **Murder** / **Mutilation** / Nakedness / **Needles** / Pursued; being / Remorse – **want of remorse** / Sea / Stool / Unsuccessful efforts / Vegetables / **Violence** / Vivid / Water

Characteristic physicals

- **Vertigo**
  - Bending head; on – forward
- **Head**
  - Air – sensation of a current of air – passing through head
  - Congestion – Sides
  - Heat – chilliness – during
  - **Pain**
    - § Lying – hanging over side of bed; with head – amel.
    - § Lying – side; on – painful side – amel.
    - § Wind – cold – agg.
    - § Occiput – lancinating
    - § Occiput – extending to – Jaw
    - § Temples – touch – agg.
  - Sensitiveness – jar; to the least
- **Eye**
  - Pain – strained; as if
- **Vision**
  - Colours before the eyes – blue – points
  - Flashes – motion; sudden
- **Ear**
  - Pain – piercing pain
  - Pain – extending to – Jaw
- **Nose**
  - Odours; imaginary and real – catarrh; as of – old catarrh
- **Face**
  - Discoloration – cyanotic – Lips
  - Formication – children; in
  - Twitching – children; in
- **Mouth**
  - Pain – Gums – right – aching
  - Pain – Tongue – stitching pain – burning
  - Speech – difficult – words – single words – cannot utter a single word
- **Throat**
  - Mucus – lumps
- **Stomach**
  - Movement in; sensation of
  - Nausea – paroxysmal
- **Rectum**
  - Coldness in anus
  - Eruptions – Anus; about – vesicular
  - Pain – bending double – amel.
- **Bladder**
  - Urination – urging to urinate – lying – agg.
- **Kidneys**
  - Heaviness
- **Male**
  - Thrill, sexual – intense
- **Female**
  - Pain -Uterus – griping pain / sharp
  - Sexual desire – increased – contact of parts; by least
- **Chest**
  - Palpitation of heart – sleep – going to sleep; on – agg.
- **Back – pain**
  - Lumbar region – bending – amel.
  - Lumbosacral region – aching
  - Sacral region – standing – agg.
- **Extremities**
  - Abscess – Fingers
  - Discoloration – Fingers – Nails – purple
  - Excrescences – horny – Toes – spikes; with
  - Itching – Thighs – Inner side
  - Pain – sprained; as if
  - Pain – Bones – sore
  - Shaking – Hands
  - Suppuration – Toes
  - Swelling – Feet – Soles – sensation of
- **Generals**
  - Evening – 18 h – 18–21 h
  - Agility
  - Food and drinks – alcoholic drinks – amel.
  - Haemorrhage – blood – clots – dark
  - Paralysis – right – persistent
  - Weariness – evening – 18 h
  - Wind – desire to be in the wind

Ixodes scapularis (Deer tick)

Class: Arachnida.
Subclass: Acari.
Superorder: Parasitiformes.
Order: Ixodida.

Ixodes scapularis has a 2-year lifecycle, during which time it passes through three stages: larva, nymph, and adult. The tick must take a blood meal at each stage before maturing to the next. Deer tick females latch onto a host and drink its blood for 4–5 days. It is the main vector of Lyme disease in North America. It can also transmit other Borrelia species, including Borrelia miyamotoi. Deer, the preferred mammalian hosts, cannot transmit Borrelia spirochaetes to ticks. They acquire Lyme disease microbes by feeding on infected mice and other small rodents.

Proving by: **Jason-Aeric Huenecke, Minnesota (2014).**[37]

Keywords
Contaminated / Parasite / Exhibitionism / Cutting pain / Destruction / Anthrax / Alone / Had-it-with-humanity / Feed off of it / Suck people's life out / **Self interest**

Fundamental delusions
- Attacked; being
- *Barriers – removed between himself and others; are*
- Cancer; has a
- **Contaminated** – being contaminated; she is
- Dark – objects and figures; sees dark
- Invisible; she is
- Keep herself together only by a great effort; she can
- Metamorphic
- Paralyzed; he is
- **Parasite**; she is a
- *Possessed; being – evil forces; by*
- Strange – voice seemed strange; own
- Touched; he is

SRP
- Communicative – heart; desire to be from the
- Naked; wants to be – **exhibitionism**
- Unreal – cannot tell what is unreal and what is real
- Vomiting – **desire to vomit out all her insides**

Dreams
Aggressive / Bombs / Cancer / Competition / Disabled people / Evil; of / Falling – danger of / Girl – attention of a; trying to attract the / Nakedness – unashamed / Protecting / Secret – keep a; must / Stabbed; being / Supernatural things / Threatened; of being / Transformation

Nucleus: The proving brought out many characteristic rubrics revealing clear parasitic themes. There is an interesting delusion shared with the Aids nosode, that the barriers between the self and others are removed – a fundamental aspect of parasitic co-dependency. The remedy appears as though it will be useful in rather extreme states of self-loathing, with symptoms such as wanting to vomit out all her insides. There is confusion over what is real / unreal, delusions of possession by evil or dark forces and a feeling of being contaminated. There may be an exhibitionistic desire to be unashamedly naked (*Hyos*).

Characteristic physicals

- **Head** – Pain – Cutting pain – knife; as with a – followed by – coldness; sensation of
- **Rectum** – Urging – waking; on (*Sulph.*)
- **Female** – Menses – early; too – three days
- **Respiration** – Hot breath – sensation as if
- **Cough** – Burning; From – Throat-pit; in

- **Chest**
  - Cracking – Sternum – backward; on bending the chest
  - Palpitation of heart – leaning – backward – agg.
  - Vibration – Sensation as if – Heart
- **Extremities**
  - Formication – Knees
  - Shaking – lower limbs
- **Generals**
  - Cold – feeling – frozen; as if
  - Dead; affected parts look as if
  - Influenza – sensation as if
  - Lyme disease

Provers speaking as one[37]

∮ Like a microbe holding all this energy. Round, little round fish eggs, in a membrane, but don't underestimate how powerful it is. **It might be small, but it could destroy you**, if becomes too much. Too much of anything isn't good. **Destruction, like anthrax, so tiny, yet so, so deadly, without warning, without knowing what you are up against, it feels very dangerous.** It is not a bad thing out in the world, it's just this powerful tiny force. . . .

∮ Feeling slightly distracted and disconnected though. Overall still in similar place as past few days. Not really down, just sort of 'had-it-with-humanity' . . . I've felt to stay in today. **It feels so good to be alone, away from people and public places** . . . I stayed in my pyjamas until dinnertime. . . .

∮ Attached, parasitic. **Taking from something in order to live.** It is staying there because it is being able to **feed off of it** . . . **You suck people's life out of them.** You consume. The consumption. You need to feed off them. You are feeding off life force . . . Self-interest, "someone who only cares about themselves. . . . **Like something to which you give and give, but it is never satisfied.** Like a person who only thinks of themselves, never appreciating others or seeing how they may be imposing.

REPERTORY ADDITIONS FOR THE SPIDERS
(made to existing rubrics in Synthesis[28]):

Mind

- ACTIVITY – desires activity
- ACTIVITY – desires activity – creative activity
- ADDICTED; TENDENCY TO BECOME
- AILMENTS FROM – abused; after being
- AILMENTS FROM – domination
- AILMENTS FROM – love; disappointed
- AILMENTS FROM – position; loss of
- AMBITION – increased – competitive
- ANARCHIST
- ANGER – authority; against
- ANOREXIA NERVOSA
- ATTENTION SEEKING BEHAVVIOUR
- ATTRACTING OTHERS
- AWARENESS HEIGHTENED
- AWKWARD
- BITING
- BRUTALITY
- BULIMIA
- COLOURS
  - § black – aversion to
  - § black – desire for
  - § bright – amel.
  - § bright – desire for
  - § desire for
- COMPANY – aversion to
- COMPANY – aversion to – desire for solitude
- COMPETITIVE
- COMPLAINING
- CONCENTRATION – difficult – attention; cannot fix
- CONFUSION OF MIND – identity; as to his
- CONFUSION OF MIND – time; as to

- CONSOLATION – agg.
- CONTRADICTION – disposition to contradict
- CONTRADICTION – intolerant of contradiction
- CRUELTY
- CUNNING
- DANCING
  - § amel.
  - § wild
- DEATH – thoughts of
- DECEITFUL
- DECEPTION
- DEFIANT
- DELUSIONS
  - § abused; being
  - § appreciated; she is not
  - § betrayed; that she is
  - § caged
  - § cheated; being
  - § deceived; being
  - § dying – he is
  - § head – belongs to another
  - § insulted; he is
  - § invaded; one's space is being
  - § looked down upon; she is
  - § misunderstood; she is
  - § neglected – he or she is neglected
  - § persecuted – he is persecuted
  - § small – he is
  - § trapped; he is
  - § understand – being understood; she was not
  - § unreal – everything seems unreal
  - § wrong – suffered wrong; he has
- DEMANDING
- DEPENDENT OF OTHERS – ambivalence; for being
- DESTRUCTIVENESS
- DICTATORIAL
- DICTATORIAL – power; love of
- DOMINEERING

- EATING – refuses to eat
- EMOTIONS – strong; too
- ESCAPE; ATTEMPTS TO
- EXCITEMENT – nervous
- FEAR
    - § death; of
    - § evil; fear of
    - § insanity
    - § starving; of
- FEARLESS
- FEIGNING – sick; to be
- FIGHT; WANTS TO
- FORSAKEN FEELING – isolation; sensation of
- HATRED
- HATRED – revengeful; hatred and
- HELPLESSNESS; FEELING OF
- HIDING – himself
- HURRY
- HYPOCHONDRIASIS
- HYSTERIA
- IMPATIENCE
- IMPULSE; MORBID
- INDIFFERENCE – eating – to eating
- INDUSTRIOUS
- INTOLERANCE
- INTRIGUER
- JESTING
- LASCIVIOUS
- LIAR
- MAGNETIC STATE
- MALICIOUS
- MANIA
- MANIPULATIVE
- MISCHIEVOUS
- MISTAKES; MAKING – time; in
- MOCKING
- MOOD – changeable
- NYMPHOMANIA
- OBSTINATE
- ORIENTATION; SENSE OF – decreased
- PITIES HERSELF
- PLANS – making many plans – revengeful plans
- POSSESSIVENESS
- POWER – love of power
- POWER – sensation of
- QUARRELSOME
- QUICK TO ACT
- RAGE
- RAGE – paroxysms; in
- REBELLIOUS
- RECOGNITION; DESIRE FOR
- REVENGEFUL
- SATYRIASIS
- SECRETIVE
- SENSES – acute
- SENSITIVE
    - § emotions; to
    - § noise; to
    - § touch; to
- SLY
- STARTING
- STRIKING
- SUICIDAL DISPOSITION
- SUSPICIOUS
- TEASING
- THREATENING
- TIME – quickly, appears shorter; passes too
- TOUCHED – aversion to be
- TOURETTE'S SYNDROME
- TRICKY
- VIOLENCE
- VIOLENT
- WICKED DISPOSITION
- WILDNESS
- WILL – strong will power
- **DREAMS**
    - DECEIVED; BEING
    - FLYING
    - FRIGHTFUL
    - JOURNEYS
    - SPIDERS
    - STRANGE

Physicals

- **VERTIGO** – FALL; TENDENCY TO
- **HEAD** – CONSTRICTION – Forehead
- **HEARING** – ACUTE
- **STOMACH** – APPETITE – diminished / wanting
- **MALE GENITALIA/SEX**
  - ERECTIONS – troublesome
  - SEXUAL DESIRE – increased
- **FEMALE GENITALIA/SEX** – SEXUAL DESIRE – increased
- **RESPIRATION**
  - ACCELERATED
  - ARRESTED
- **CHEST**
  - ANGINA PECTORIS
  - ANXIETY – Heart; in region of
  - CONSTRICTION
  - HEART; COMPLAINTS OF THE
  - OPPRESSION
  - PAIN – Heart
  - PAIN – Heart – extending to – Arm – left
  - PALPITATION OF HEART
- **EXTREMITIES**
  - INCOORDINATION
  - JERKING
  - PARALYSIS
  - RESTLESSNESS
  - TINGLING
  - TOTTERING GAIT
- **CHILL** – SHAKING
- **SKIN**
  - ERUPTIONS
    § blisters
    § erythema
    § papular
    § rash
- FORMICATION
- GANGRENE
- **GENERALS**
  - CHOREA
  - COLD – agg.
  - CONVULSIONS – tetanic rigidity
  - EMACIATION
  - ENERGY – excess of energy
  - ENERGY – excess of energy – children; in
  - EXERTION; PHYSICAL – amel.
  - FOOD AND DRINKS
    § fruit – desire
    § liquid food – desire
    § milk – desire
    § solid food – aversion
  - HEAT – lack of vital heat
  - JERKING
  - KNITTING – amel.
  - LOCOMOTOR ATAXIA
  - MOTION – desire for
  - NECROSIS
  - PAIN – burning
  - PAIN – stinging
  - PARALYSIS
  - PARALYSIS AGITANS
  - PERIODICITY
  - PERIODICITY – year – every
  - PULSE – frequent
  - PULSE – slow
  - RESTLESSNESS
  - SUDDEN MANIFESTATION
  - TOBACCO – amel.
  - TREMBLING – Internally
  - WOUNDS – bites
  - WOUNDS – bites – poisonous animals; of

References

1 Mangialavori M, Zwemke H. *Bitten in the Soul, Experiences with spider remedies in Homeopathic Medicine.* Modena, Berlin: Matrix Editrice; 2004.

2 Fraser P. *Spiders – Suspended between Earth and Sky.* Bristol: Winter Press; 2008.

3 Sankaran R. *Sankaran's Schema* (2nd edn). Mumbai: Homoeopathic Medical Publishers; 2007.

4 Sankaran R. *System of Homeopathy.* Mumbai: Homoeopathic Medical Publishers; 2005.

5 Sankaran R. *Soul of Remedies.* Mumbai: Homoeopathic Medical Publishers; 1997.

6 Sankaran P. *The Elements of Homeopathy.* Mumbai: Homoeopathic Medical Publishers; 1996.

7 Vervarcke A. *Rare remedies for difficult cases.* Ghent, 2016. (Accessed in RadarOpus, Zeus Soft.)

8 Sherr J. *The Homeopathic Proving of Androctonus.* In: *Dynamic Provings* Vol. 1. Malvern: Dynamis Books; 1997.

9 Allen T. *Encyclopedia of Pure Materia Medica, Tarentula hispanica.* New York NY. (Originally published in 1874.) (Accessed in RadarOpus, Zeus Soft.)

10 Klein L. *Loxosceles Reclusa – The Brown Recluse Spider.* Vancouver BC: Luminos Provings; 1997.

11 Master F. *The Web Spinners.* Mumbai: B Jain Publishers; 1997.

12 Master F. *Clinical Observations of Children's Remedies.* Mumbai: Lutra Services BV; 2006.

13 Gray A. *A Homeopathic Proving of Lampona Cylindrata (White Tailed Spider).* Sydney, 2000. (Accessed in RadarOpus, Zeus Soft.)

14 Ghegas V. Seminar report – Tarentula hispanica. *Homeopathic Links*, Spring 1995.

15 Hardy J. Fruitless activity – Theridion. *Homeopathic Links*, Summer 1998.

16 Joshi B, Joshi S. *Quick Book of Minerals and Animals.* Mumbai: Serpentina Books; 2013.

17 Bonnet M. The toxicology of latrodectus mactans. *Homeopathic Links*, Autumn 1998.

18 Plant R. Pipes, wires and cords – Aranea ixobola. *Homeopathic Links*, Autumn 1998.

19 Shore J. *Investigations into the Psyche of the Spider.* (Accessed in RadarOpus, Zeus Soft.)

20 Reichenber-Ullmann J. Children with attention deficit disorder – Aranea ixobola. *Homeopathic Links*, Summer 1996.

21 Daly J. Revenge of the deer: a case of Androctonus. Troy, ME: *The American Homeopath*, 2000; 6.

22 Julian OA. *Materia Medica of New Homeopathic Remedies.* Beaconsfield: Beaconsfield Publishers Ltd; 1984.

23 Shah P. Gambling and striking immediately – Androctonus amoreuxii hebraeus. *Homeopathic Links*, Summer 1999.

24 Sowton C. *The Homeopathic proving of Spider Silk – Tela araneae (Spider web).* Toronto, 2003.

25 Woutman W. Killing by instinct – A case of Mygale lasiodora. *Homeopathic Links*, Autumn 1996.

26 Ward J. *Unabridged Dictionary of the Sensations "as If".* Noida UP: B Jain Publishers; 1995.

27 Roberts H. *Sensations as if – A Repertory of Subjective Symptoms*. Noida UP: B Jain Publishers; 2002.

28 Schroyens F. *Synthesis 9.1* (Treasure edn). Ghent: Homeopathic Book Publishers; 2009.

29 Norland M. *Signatures, Miasms, Aids: Spiritual Aspects of Homeopathy*. Uffculme, Devon: Yondercott Press; 2003.

30 Boericke W. *Pocket Manual of Materia Medica and Repertory*. Mumbai: B Jain Publishers 1980. (Originally published in 1901.)

31 Whitmont E.C. Polychrest and less used remedies. *The Homeopathic Herald*, 1950; 11 (4).

32 Twohig J, Marks B. *Deadly Romance, A Homeopathic proving of Latrodectus hasseltii, Red black spider*. Ethelton, South Australia: Marks Australien; 1997.

33 Grimmer A, Currim A.N. *The collected works of Arthur Hill Grimmer M.D.* Hartford CT: Hahnemann International Institute for Homeopathic Documentation; 1996.

34 Mueller K.J. *Tegenaria atrica cases*; 1998. (Accessed in RadarOpus, Zeus Soft.)

35 Anon. *Arachne*. Greek Mythology. Available online at: *https://www. greekmythology.com/Myths/Mortals/Arachne/arachne.html* (Accessed 21st April 2020.)

36 Phatak S.R. *A Concise Repertory of Homeopathic Medicines* (4th edn). Mumbai: B. Jain Publishers; 2012. (Accessed in RadarOpus.)

37 Huenecke J-A. *Proving of Ixodes dammini, Deer Tick*; 2014. (Accessed in RadarOpus.)

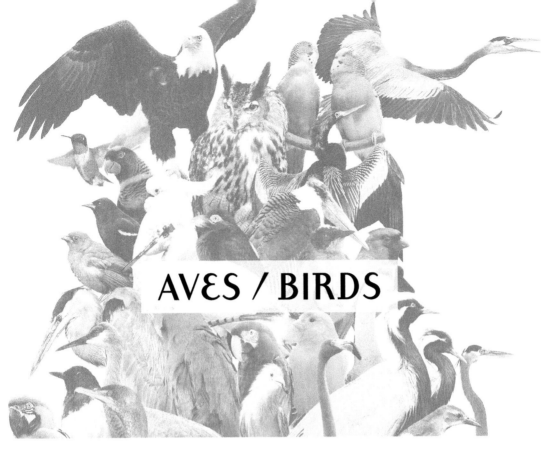

AVES / BIRDS

MYTHOLOGY

Jupiter / Zeus; Expansiveness, freedom and overview

Jupiter

Urge to connect with the spiritual realm through openness to the 'big picture'.

Spirit, Faith, Optimism, Freedom.

Joy, Vision, Expanding awareness.

Belief, Wisdom, Imagination, Exploration.

Adventurous, Scattered energy, Long journeys.

Seeing the big picture, view from the sky, over-extending oneself leading to burn-out.

Mars – Jupiter

- Fighting for liberty, freedom and expansiveness. Asserting independence.
- Desires adventure and open spaces. A passionate philosopher. Spiritual warrior.

Zeus

- *Sky god, Wisdom, Philosophical, Vision.*
- *Perceives the whole, Benevolence, Promiscuity.*
- *Excesses, Sexual, Abuse of power, Disguise.*
- *Confidence, Bravado.*
- Zeus is often depicted with an Eagle by his side.

From the point of view of those mortals whom Zeus abducts come the themes of rape and abuse which run through the bird remedies. Hera – his wife is the goddess of marriage, and whilst Zeus has many infidelities, she always maintains the sanctity of marriage (whilst employing devious means by which to get even with him). Hera's role in mythology may too have significance for patients requiring a remedy from the avian realm; individuals who have long-suffered marital abuse and yet keep the relationship going despite all they have suffered.

"According to Hyginus, Zeus was raised by a nymph named Amalthea. Since Saturn (Cronus) ruled over the Earth, the heavens and the sea, she hid him by dangling him on a rope from a tree so **he was suspended between earth, sea and sky and thus, invisible to his father.**" (Wikipedia). This has relevance to the Birds, who as Peter Fraser[4] suggests are perfectly adapted to the Sky realm, yet vulnerable when they come to Earth.

Jupiter relates to expanding one's horizons to include a world-view that encompasses more than just yourself, your job, task and place in society. You learn from different cultures, study philosophy, or travel to far-flung corners of the imagination, as opposed to staying rooted in rational thought (*Connection to Row 5 / Silver Series*).

Jupiter: Pathology / Affinities

Locomotor ataxia, sciatica, lumbago, rheumatism, hip disease, accidents to thighs. Liver, glycogen, suprarenals, arterial circulation, fibrin of blood, disposition of fats.

Hermes / Mercury

Hermes carried messages between the heavenly realm of Olympia and the hellish realm of Hades. He was the emissary of Zeus and the only god who could enter Hades and return unscathed.

Amongst many things, he was associated with:

Networks, making connections; rules the nervous system (*cf. Trees and Fungi*)

Communication, Expression and Dispersal of ideas.

Rationality, Siblings / School age, Knowledge, Understanding.

Cleverness, Duplicity, Precocity, Shape shifting, Shadow side.

Borders, Trade, Merchants, Commerce, Short journeys.

He was also an **escape** artist, turning himself into a vapour so he could escape the hermetically sealed room which housed him as an infant (*Theme – breaking free from constraints*). His very first exploit was to steal a herd of cattle from

Apollo, for which he later stood trial. He escaped punishment by inventing the Lyre which he gave to Apollo who later became the god of music.

Affinities
Nerves, bronchial tubes, pulmonary circulation, thyroid gland, right cerebral hemisphere, cerebro-spinal system, sensory nerves, vital fluid in nerves, vocal cords, ears, sight, tongue, sense perception, breath.

BIRDS IN HOMŒOPATHY

Raptors rule the Sky realm, drawing your gaze upwards towards the heavens and the light of the sun. This heavenly aspect equates to an aspiration to reach for a higher purpose in life. They do however swoop down to earth to catch prey or to nest, so they symbolically represent the relationship between heaven and earth. This theme is present in the proving of Eagle – where the two worlds (of spirit and matter, dream and reality) cannot be brought together, but are forever divided. *Raptor patients want to liberate themselves from the 'carnal cess-pits' of the material world to explore the freedom and expansiveness of the sky.*

Songbirds (especially sparrow) have a more intimate relationship with humanity. We are enthralled by the beauty and sheer creativity of their musicality. The dawn chorus is an amazing cacophony of communication. We feel that many human qualities and aspirations are shared by birds; from Sparrow as the plucky underdog, to the mightiest Eagle soaring above.

Patients often like to receive a Bird remedy; to be associated with the freedom and beauty of this kingdom is usually preferable than to be grubbing around in the dirt and disgust of the Insect world! Other Bird qualities that are evident from the provings are clear vision, or lack of it; heightened intuition or clairvoyance; chattering, communicating, wanting to speak the truth. Birds are able to break free from constraints and fly away to pastures new; travelling large distances and changing their home with the seasons.

MAPPA MUNDI

Fire / Sky realm (Spiritual, Philosophical, Divine)

Responsibility and Duty *vs.* Freedom and Independence
- The polarity between freedom and duty can be very strong in bird cases.
- When their independence is restricted (for example, by a controlling partner or difficult life circumstances) they often express a sensation of feeling **trapped, contained or tied down**.
- There is a need for freedom from the mundane and to know a higher purpose.
- Desire for meditation, alternative lifestyles, embracing spirituality and philosophy.
- Delusions – head – open and his consciousness is expanding above him; top of head is (*Falco-pe.*)

- Strong sense of **responsibility** in looking after family; a sense of honour, pride and integrity; there may be a sense of nobility in birds such as Eagle and Falcon. (*cf. Aurum*)
  Emotional clearing, my dreams have been about honouring my integrity _{arde-he.}[10]
- Need to protect, nurture and nourish very intensely. *Rescuing others less fortunate.*

Air / Underworld (Indifferent, Detached, Alone)

Caged, shackled, chained, trapped or confined to a small space
- Tethered, tortured, dominated and controlled by an oppressor.
- These aspects are equally as important as the opposite state of freedom, coupled with sensations / dreams of flying, soaring; a need for speed and breathing the fresh open air.
- Become **cold, indifferent and detached** as a result of abuse, domination and control.
- Overwhelmed from caring for the needs of others, leading to burnout.
- **Acute sense of danger**; always being alert, excessive nervous energy.
- Disorientation, getting lost, using wrong words, inability to calculate.
- Issues revolving around **pride, humiliation, shame, judgement.**
- Forsaken, isolated, repudiated.
- The falcon that was used for the proving had been held prisoner; trained to perform for their master upon whom they were dependent. The proving brought out feelings of self-condemnation for allowing oneself to be dominated and abused despite having an internal sense of power and authority, as would befit mighty birds of prey.

Key falcon rubrics pertaining to Air / Underworld
- Despair – black hole, looking into / Empty shell, sensation of being a fully functioning.

Sanguine (Open, expansive, sociable)

- Freedom of expression, desire to **travel** far and wide *without being tied down.*
- Dreams, delusions and sensations of flying and floating.
- Freedom from mundane with feeling of lightness / soaring or the opposite feeling of heaviness / containment (belonging to the closed / melancholic pole.

Melancholic (Closed, contracting, solitary)

- Grounded, down to earth, heavy, mundane, weight, burden, pressure. (*cf. Hamamelididae*)
- Falcon
  - Delusions
    - § Horses – she is a reined-in wild stallion that desires to be free
    - § Iron shield around him; has an
  - Detached – waves of detachment

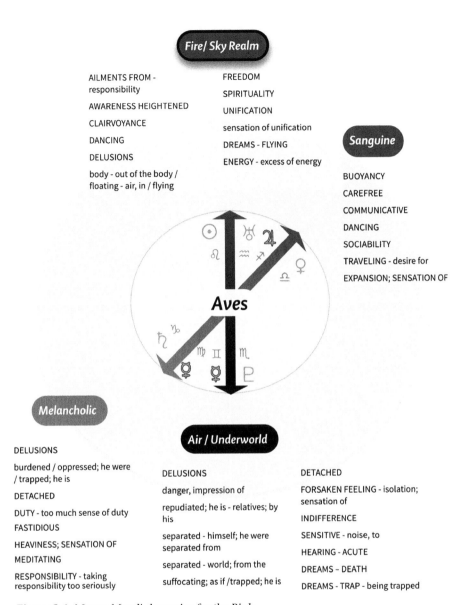

Fire/ Sky Realm

AILMENTS FROM -
responsibility

AWARENESS HEIGHTENED

CLAIRVOYANCE

DANCING

DELUSIONS

body - out of the body /
floating - air, in / flying

FREEDOM

SPIRITUALITY

UNIFICATION

sensation of unification

DREAMS - FLYING

ENERGY - excess of energy

Sanguine

BUOYANCY

CAREFREE

COMMUNICATIVE

DANCING

SOCIABILITY

TRAVELING - desire for

EXPANSION; SENSATION OF

Aves

Melancholic

DELUSIONS

burdened / oppressed; he were
/ trapped; he is

DETACHED

DUTY - too much sense of duty

FASTIDIOUS

HEAVINESS; SENSATION OF

MEDITATING

RESPONSIBILITY - taking
responsibility too seriously

Air / Underworld

DELUSIONS

danger, impression of

repudiated; he is - relatives; by
his

separated - himself; he were
separated from

separated - world; from the

suffocating; as if /trapped; he is

DETACHED

FORSAKEN FEELING - isolation;
sensation of

INDIFFERENCE

SENSITIVE - noise, to

HEARING - ACUTE

DREAMS – DEATH

DREAMS - TRAP - being trapped

Figure 3.1 Mappa Mundi dynamics for the Birds

THEMES

Freedom, independence, autonomy

The polarity between freedom and duty can be very strong in bird cases. When their independence is restricted (For example, by a controlling partner or difficult life circumstances) they often express a sensation of feeling **trapped, contained or tied down**. There is a need to liberate themselves from heavy emotional

Aves / Birds

baggage that would otherwise weigh them down. They may gravitate towards spiritual activities that enable them to explore a higher purpose.

"The intense need for freedom and space in Bird remedies and the opposite sensation of suffocation can look like Phosphorus . . . Predatory birds come close to the Lanthanides. . . . They have a desire to know more about higher consciousness . . . they question themselves, their own power, and their own strength. They have an enquiring mind." _{Joshis}[1] In both groups there is a strong accent on the need for autonomy and self-control.

> *Without freedom I wouldn't want to live. . . . I love to go back to the wilds of Scotland and go up into the mountains where I feel I can breathe. Free air, clear and pure. My husband tried to contain me, you know it is wrong but I was so young. Didn't trust my own judgment, thought of myself as stupid and had no confidence in myself. . . . He was vicious; verbally attacked and abused me 30 times a day.* _{buteo-j.} *I feel trapped. Tied down, hemmed in and un-free, constrained, limited. I am flighty, flitty, having crazy ideas, flying, flitting about, trying out new things, but find it difficult to ground myself. I don't like being tethered really. If I am feeling flighty, without a tether, I am on the verge of some stupid behaviour or addiction . . . constrained is like shackles. Just being a prisoner – having physical or mental constraints.* _{falco-pe.} *Freedom and a lack of restriction are the driving force behind their love of flight and movement.* _{Fraser}[4]

Rubrics
Freedom – desires | Independent | Space – desire for

Trapped; need to break free from constraints

One of the most fundamental themes expressed in many bird provings and cases is the core feeling of being trapped.

> *Feeling very caged, trapped and wary with partner. Terrified, not sure, how he is going to be with me. . . . I feel like that reined in wild stallion who is terrified and must fight free. I became totally detached and very angry and vengeful even though I knew these were wasted feelings.* _{falco-pe.} *Dream – People trapped below ground and I was trying to free them.* _{geoc-ca.}[5] *Intense trapped feeling . . . trapped by people and situations. People who are being weird. . . I needed to break out, a screeching feeling. I had to speak out to change the situation. I had to stop letting things slide.* _{haliae-lc.}[6]

This can be explained from the standpoint that the bird may have been held captive, as in the case with the seminal proving of Falco peregrinus. But perhaps the trapped feeling reaches even further back into the life cycle of the bird; back to the time of being contained inside the egg and feeling a great need to break free in order to make the first fledgling steps towards independence. As David Attenborough outlines:

> *Any animal that flies **must keep its weight to a minimum**. An egg kept within the body . . . while the embryo develops sufficiently to survive in the outside world, would constitute so heavy a load that flight would become seriously impeded. . . . So, all **female birds get rid of each of their eggs** just as soon as they can. . . . The egg is **ejected into the outside world** [where it is] now very **vulnerable**. Its shell cannot be impregnably*

*thick and strong for the young chick will eventually must **hammer its way out** of it (trapped sensation, need to escape to be free, flying and independent) . . . . All eggs are relatively **fragile**. Since they are also packed with nourishment, they are tempting **targets** for hungry **thieves**.*[7]

Rubrics
Delusions – caged | Delusions – prisoner; she is a | Delusions – trapped; he is

Extreme abuse

As illustrated by the relationship between Falconer and Falcon. The powerful predator is imprisoned, hooded and trained to return to the hand that feeds him. The situation is similar to Lac-c only amplified; both remedies reveal a state where the animal urges are suppressed, but the mighty falcon is lured back to a state of captivity, whereas the dog is asked to perform in order to retain their owner's love.

Misha Norland writes, "The proving of Falco would not have taken place had it not been for a patient. Her story is told in the introduction and case example to the AIDS proving:

> *There was no one to respond to my fears or illnesses. I had to learn to lock everything out. Whenever I felt bad, I would go for a run. I was into athletics. I always kept moving. It was almost like punishing myself. I still feel like this, 'I will beat this, and then I will be okay; if I keep on going I will be okay'. My father sexually abused me from as far back as I can remember. He went on doing it until I left home. My first memory is of being about three and in the bath. My father is jerking off and semen splashes on my face. When I am shocked I can feel semen on my face and I feel that others will be able to see it too. Often when I wake up, **I feel crushed, compressed**. I can only sleep if I lie with one hand over my heart and one on my throat. My mother knew what was going on. She colluded with my father. She had sex with me too. I think of her as a cardboard cutout character. I am revolted by her. I had a recurrent dream of being stuck in the birth canal with putrid pus in my nose and throat. Another recurrent dream that I have is of being a foetus, as though I have been just born and I can see the planet Earth beyond me. It is very beautiful. My umbilicus is cut and I want to tie it but I can't reach it and there is no one to ask for help. I was never given guidelines for what was right – only for what was wrong. . . .*[8]

Hints of the leprosy and AIDS miasms also come through in this shocking transcript; *"When I am shocked, I can feel semen on my face and I feel that others will be able to see it too . . . like punishing myself . . . I am revolted by her . . . being stuck in the birth canal with putrid pus."*[8] These miasms are very similar in the central theme of feeling revolting, putrid and having to make extreme efforts to be accepted by others. They feel truly outcast, that nobody can understand where they are coming from due to the horrendous acts that have been perpetrated upon them.

Ailments from – abused; after being / domination – long time; for a / humiliation / shame | Delusions – abused; being | Delusions – dominated; he is | Delusions – oppressed; he were | Humiliated; feeling

The burden of parenthood

The egg is a heavy weight; a burden on the mother's ability to fly. Once the egg is ejected into the outside world, the mating pair must work around the clock to care for their defenceless young. To come to the earth is when birds are at their most endangered, so the process of becoming a parent may be perceived by the bird patient as an incredibly arduous and dangerous task. The provings of several Bird remedies have brought out symptoms that correspond with post-natal depression.

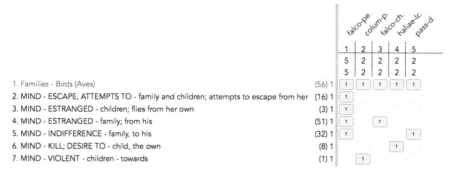

1. Families - Birds (Aves) (56) 1
2. MIND - ESCAPE, ATTEMPTS TO - family and children; attempts to escape from her (16) 1
3. MIND - ESTRANGED - children; flies from her own (3) 1
4. MIND - ESTRANGED - family; from his (51) 1
5. MIND - INDIFFERENCE - family, to his (32) 1
6. MIND - KILL; DESIRE TO - child, the own (8) 1
7. MIND - VIOLENT - children - towards (1) 1

Figure 3.2 Bird remedies in post-natal depression

Nurturing, rescuing and protecting

In birds there is a strong desire, perhaps even compulsive tendency, to nurture and protect others (often those who are more vulnerable than themselves). This may be a compensation for a history of domestic / sexual abuse in cases requiring remedies derived from captive birds (or those species with a close link to humankind).

Parents in the avian realm work incredibly hard to protect and nurture their young. In many cases, birds will form life-long monogamous partnerships as opposed to the pattern in herd mammals whereby an alpha wins breeding rights through strength in combat and then dominates a hareem. The mammal alpha male usually plays only a minimal role in rearing the young, whereas birds tend to share the responsibility for nurture more evenly.

The mammal features of play-fighting, cuddling and bonding through suckling are mostly lacking in birds. Their style of nurturing is certainly less playful than in mammals; the accent is more on how hard the parent has to work to keep their dependents well fed and protected whilst they are at the vulnerable fledgling stage. However, pigeons are an exception to this rule, and do secrete 'crop' milk on which their offspring are nurtured.

Rubrics
Duty – too much sense of duty | Love – family; for | Protecting – desire to protect | Responsibility – taking responsibility too seriously

The bringer of messages; seeking and speaking the truth

Patients responding to avian remedies may see the world through a wide-angle lens; having this 'bird's eye view' allows them to be philosophical about the meaning of life's events. They are truth-seekers, and desire to share their wisdom with others who have a more restricted worldview. Theirs is a gift of intuition, perceiving whole concepts as opposed to getting bogged down in tiresome details. The desire for openness and to speak one's own truth can be a strong feature in bird cases.

> *Themes around true communication, speaking for the real you. . . Where does the "inner, sacred you" find its voice to communicate its needs and pains and fears.* falco-pe.[8] *Communicative, expansive. . . . The "Do I tell the truth?" question flashed through my mind a few times during the day. I felt . . . much more objective, as if I was standing farther back.* sia-cr.[9] *Speaking one's truth – Unacceptable to speak one's truth.* ara-maca.[10] *I have been more communicative and chatty than usual, I am usually a quiet person who does not talk a lot.* pass-d.[11] *Communication and messages were another theme found in the proving. Much of [this] was associated with frustration or feeling blocked in [their] efforts to communicate. It is interesting to note that the bird is voiceless.* cath-a.[12]

Rubrics
Truth – telling the plain truth | Truth – desire for | Truth – tell the truth to everyone; has to

Communication, creativity, song, signals, plumage

Birds are natural communicators, heralding the dawn of each new day with a cacophony of song, or through visual messages displayed in the colouring of their feathers. In the Avian realm, a partner is usually chosen based on **creative** abilities such as song, colourful plumage, or the male's home-making skills. In all these scenarios there is an element of **performance, creativity and uniqueness** which perhaps places many birds in the Silver Series of the periodic table.

> *Although birds are safe in the air they are forced to come to earth . . . this is the time at which they are most vulnerable. . . . Birds are creatures of the air and as air is the carrier of sounds, of music and of voice, so communication and song are of great importance to birds.* Fraser[4] *(cf. Row 5, Silver Series) [Birds voices] come from a different structure [than the larynx] that lies much deeper within their body, one that is possessed by no other creatures, called the syrinx. . . .* **Birds use both sound and vision to communicate. . . .** **They issue battle cries, send warnings, summon mates, declare war and even, on occasion, tell lies.**[7]

The French composer Debussy wrote a wonderful piece of music for solo flute entitled Syrinx, whilst Messiaen spent many years studying birdsong and composing music to reflect this. As Anne Vervarcke has observed clinically, patients who respond to bird remedies may also play or prefer the sound of wind instruments. Colours and patterns of feathers are also used to communicate different messages. Pigments are commonly derived from melanin or carotenoids. Or colours can be created by microscopic bubbles in the keratin of the feathers, refracting the light.

Disturbances of appetite and thirst. Raven-ous appetite

The power of flight requires a considerable quantity of fuel and yet birds also need to remain lightweight and energetic. They like energy-rich food, eating little and often to keep their metabolism running at this high tempo. Interestingly, the proving of *Corvus corax* (Raven) brought out this raven-ous symptom in the most marked way. These patients do not want to each rich, heavy food or big portions that weigh them down; they want to feel energised and buoyant. They also dislike the feeling of being weighed down by heavy emotions (too much Water). It is far better for them to focus on communication and philosophy; they exist more naturally in the Air realm of ideas, corresponding closely to Jung's 'thinking' archetype.

Faith, optimism, expansiveness and spirituality

Astrological Jupiter brings new opportunities, adventures and an openness to discover greater meaning to one's life. Negatively, one can get caught over-promising, scattering one's energy and, as a result, letting people down. Because the natural inclination of Jupiterian types is to sense opportunities and have the faith and optimism that they will rise to any occasion, they can end up spreading themselves too thinly and burning out, as did Icarus who flew too close to the sun.

> *There has been a profound deepening of my spiritual awareness – that everything is one and everything matters, even the smallest blade of grass.* pass-d.[11] *Feel inward calm and peace; usually I am frantic, overly busy, running and wearing myself out; I am content . . . calm, cool and collected.* geoc-ca.[5] *Sensation of overwhelming love for everyone and mankind, and opening in the heart.* cygn-cy.[13] *People who . . . are dreamers, wandering from job to job, without goals or direction. But inspiration and success come if searching is continued.* dio-e.[14] *Spiritual experience in car, singing praises to god.* sia-cr.[9]

High energy

"**Flying demands so much energy** that a bird needs a very large supply of oxygen. The air sacs are an essential part of its breathing system and enable it to extract far more oxygen from each breath than a similar-sized mammal is able to get."[7]

*I feel so fizzy inside, there is too much going on in my head, and I hop from one thought to the next. . . . Want to drive my car full pelt to loud, fast heavy metal. . . . There's something inside of me that's **faster**, nastier, more raging, more berserk, it is totally wild. . . . It is fucking crazy in an instant, wildly **explosive**. The feeling of well-being is starting to spill over into mild **hyperactivity**. I am **buzzing** – excited, focused, feel I have fantastic concentration, socially too **wired**.* _{pass-d.}[11] *Tight jaw, like past experiences when doing cocaine . . . ragged breathing, feeling stoned, **twitchy**, dazed and confused . . . the cramps came on quickly and went quickly, more intense, like I was in "**hyper-drive**".* _{calyp-an.}[15]

Need for speed

MIND – DELUSIONS – railway train – she is a rushing. _{haliae-lc}[6]

I drove at high speed, I was aware of the speed but I didn't care. At one stage I spotted a police car in my mirror, fully aware that I was well over the speed limit, I carried on. . . . I was aware that if I was not more careful I would have an accident, but it didn't stop me. _{falco-pe.}[8] *Driving to the college on a dark night and had problems with another motorist. Feelings of wanting to get away, to escape, out of control, why me? To hide and then when that failed to flee. I ended up travelling much faster than I wanted to. . . . The Duel continued for about 6 miles and ended when the other vehicle swooped across in front of me. That night and the following night I had cold sweats in bed with considerable fear of the consequences of the events. I was expecting to be 'found' by the police and possibly brought to trial with the worst outcome being imprisonment.* _{pass-d.}[11] *Happy feeling when driving, especially over 60 mph. . . . Still have maniacal feeling. Still have euphoria with driving.* _{haliae-lc.}[6] *We drive home, one near-miss, partner freaked on adrenaline – my heart didn't even beat any faster. Was driving faster than usual with no fear. Scary. Usually pretty much adrenaline-pumped when I drive anywhere. Dream of driving fast up a road where the walls either side became narrower and narrower, and finally the end was blocked.* _{cygn-be.}[16]

General symptoms

- **Tension, stiffness, drawing, cramping of neck, shoulders and upper back.**
- **Stabbing, stitching pains in general** (heart, chest, abdomen, shoulders, limbs).
- Nervous restlessness, accompanied by buzzing, twitching and vibratory sensations (especially strong in the provings of Passer domesticus and Calypte anna).
- Throat symptoms. Especially in Cygnus cygnus; the proving brought out symptoms of obstruction in the throat, accompanied by grief or strong emotions.
- Vision extremely sharp or the opposite.
- Great oversensitivity.
- Diseases of nervous system affecting extremities.
- Getting lost, lack of orientation.
- Warm-blooded.
- Desire for open air.

- Refined – fine bone structure, eyes clear and intense.
- Birds have hollow bones to allow for better aero-dynamism.

The bird family includes symptoms of *"nervous energy, trembling or twitching and neuropathies; disturbances of appetite and water metabolism; sharp, stitching or tense and cramping pains; pattern rather than sequential thought; empathy, spirituality and sensitivity; detachment; perfectionism and a love of nature; a lack of understanding of time and space and perhaps most important a feeling of being trapped and a desire for freedom."* Fraser[17]

Source words

Flight, Float, Height, Gliding; effortless.
Nesting, Home-making, Fledgling, Juvenile.
Pecking order, Preening. Wind-pipe, Syrinx.
Excel, Stability, Balance, Direction, Control.
Diving, Aerial skills. Migration. Swooping, Flocking.
Order, Clarity, Vision, Strong, Speed, Competition.
Colours; iridescence, shimmering, patterns, metallic glint.
Bird's eye view. Beating of wings, Flapping, Air-brained, Flightiness.
Tuneful, Singing, Braying, Calling, Resonating, Trilling. Dawn chorus.

Differential Diagnosis

- Tubercular, Leprous / Aids and Syphilitic Miasms
- Silver Series / Lanthanides
- Lepidoptera (freedom, flying)
- Hamamelididae (flying *vs.* contained)

- Cactaceae (bound, oppressed)
- Euphorbiaceae (bound, tied)
- Violales (stabbing pains)
- Gases
- Stage 15 and 16

REMEDIES

Aves (Birds)

anas-i, anas-i-ov, ans-as, ans-as-d, aquil-ch, aquil-ht, **ara-maca**, arde-he, ardea-cn, astu-cc, bran-cn-o, bubo-v, **buteo-j**, **calyp-an**, **cath-a**, colum-ld, **colum-p**, **corv-cor**, corv-sp-o, **cygn-be**, **cygn-cy**, **cygn-ol**, dio-e, diom-ml, falco-ch, FALCO-PE, gallus-d, gallus-d-pn, gallus-em, gav-im, gav-sl, geoc-ca, guan, HALIAE-LC, ing, lars-arg, lars-hb, lars-rb, nid, oscilloc, ovi-p, ovum-g, **pass-d**, **pavo-c**, pavo-c-o, pelec-o, pharo-mc, pull-g, serin-ca, **sia-cr**, **sphen-h**, thres-a, tub-a, **tyto-a**, **vult-gr**

Ara maçāo (Scarlet Macaw)

Phylum: Chordata.
Class: Aves.
Order: Psittaciformes.
Family: Psittacidae.

The scarlet macaw is a large red, yellow, and blue Central and South American parrot. They form monogamous partnerships and are dutiful parents, expending a lot of energy in raising their young during the extended nestling and post-fledging periods. Their vocal communications are diverse; ranging from raucous honks to the mimicking of human speech. Whilst relatively docile at most times of the year, scarlet macaws can become formidably aggressive during the breeding period.

C4 Trituration Proving by: **Jonathan Shore, USA (2000).**[10]

Keywords
Defence – has none / Truth – telling the plain truth / Extravagance / Eccentricity / Humiliated / Communicative / Chronic sadness / Honoured / Appreciated / Brutality / Flayed / Vibrant

SRP delusions
- **Protection, defence; has no**
- **Separated – himself; he were separated from**
- Bubbles – blood; sensation as if bubbles in
- Double – existence; having a double
- Light – is light; he – internal organs
- Light – is light; he – skeleton
- Strike – struck; being

Nucleus: Communication is a key theme; the need to express one's truth in the social group is of paramount importance (*cf.* Milks). Learning skills may be disrupted by dyslexia which would be quite an impediment for one who places such importance on the need to express themselves. The dreams of being too passive, and of being flayed connect with the delusion that they have no defence and that they feel helpless – highlighting the Avian themes of domination, abuse and control. Other bird-like symptoms were expressed by provers – such as the feeling of being humiliated, that their skeleton and internal organs feel light and a sensation of bubbles in the blood. Another theme revolves around love; expressed in the delusion they had taken a love drug and the desire to ardently embrace everybody, especially those in their group. They may be over-the-top and extravagant, trying to make others laugh and enjoy themselves. The remedy is very Sanguine in this regard. "Worried that they are too colourful, too flagrant, too exuberant and that this will attract criticism. Worry 'Have I gone too far?' **Wanting to be honoured and appreciated for who she is (*cf. Sparrow*)."** Fraser[4]

Characteristic rubrics

- **Truth, speak one's own**
- **Truth – <u>telling the plain truth</u>**
- Speak, feels comfortable to, in a group
- <u>Extravagance</u>
- Freedom – doing what he had to do; remarkable freedom in
- Love – people in the group; for
- **Communicative**
- *Ardent – desires to be*
- Being in the present; feeling of
- *Benevolence*
- Blissful feeling
- Drugs – taken drugs; as if one had – **love-drug; a**

- Dyslexia
- **Eccentricity**
- Embraces – everyone
- Fear – accidents; of
- *Fear – failure; of*
- Helplessness; feeling of
- **Humiliated**; feeling
- *Laughing – desire to laugh*
- Love – people in the group; for
- Responsibility – taking responsibility too seriously (*Birds*)
- Sadness – **chronic sadness**
- *Sensitive – psychic environment; to*
- Speech – convincing

Dreams

Al Capone / **Brutality** / *Evil; of – power of evil; the / Rise of evil; the* / **Flayed**; people being / Flies – wall; fly on the / Friends / Good and evil / Murderer / Observer / ***Passive – change the situation; unable to*** / Prophetic / Reunion / Tropical places / Ugly / Violence / Water – clear water

Physicals

- **Stomach**
  - Appetite – ravenous (Raven)
- **Extremities**
  - Awkwardness – Hands – drops things
  - Lower limbs – *stumbling* when walking
  - Lower limbs – *trips* over things

- **Generals**
  - Allergic constitution – cats; to
  - Heat – sensation of
  - Pulsation
  - Pulse – frequent
  - Tension – Externally
  - Wavelike sensation

Natural behaviour

Vibrant, colourful plumage, raucous screeching calls, squawking, intelligence, copying.

Ardea herodias (Great blue heron)

Phylum: Chordata.
Class: Aves.
Order: Pelecaniformes.
Family: Ardeidae.

Ardea herodias is a large wading bird in the heron family. They are solitary feeders, locating their food by sight and swallowing it whole which can lead to choking on prey that is too large. They feed opportunistically on aquatic insects, small mammals, amphibians, reptiles, birds and more – based on whatever is in abundance. As large wading birds, they are capable of feeding in deeper waters, so are able to harvest from areas inaccessible to most other heron species. The most commonly employed hunting technique is wading slowly with their long legs through shallow water – quickly spearing fish or frogs with their sharp bills. They have many other fishing techniques at their disposal – standing still, hovering, diving, swimming and more. Predators of their eggs and nestlings include turkey vultures, ravens and crows.

Proving by: **Jonathan Shore, USA (2002).**[10]
Clinical additions by: **Gabriel Blass.**

Mind

- Absorbed
- Ailments from
  - Anger – suppressed
  - Criticised; from being
  - Domination – long time; for a
  - Shame
- Anger – alternating with – tranquillity
- **Benevolence**
- Buoyancy
- Change – desire for
- Colours – green – desire for
- Company – aversion to – desire for solitude
- Confidence – want of self-confidence
  - Self-depreciation
  - Support; desires
- Delusions
  - Abused; being
  - Alone; being
  - Division between himself and others

- Enlarged – body is – parts of body
- Separated – group; he is separated from the
- **Separated** – world; from the – he is separated
- **Suffocated; she will be**
- Watched; she is being
- Wrong – done wrong; he has
- **Detached**
- Emotions
  - Strong; too
  - Unclear about one's feelings
- Estranged – self; from
- Excitement – bad news; after
- Fear
  - Opinion of others; of
  - **Suffocation; of**
- Forsaken feeling – isolation; sensation of
- High-spirited
- Hindered; intolerance of being
- Independent
- Industrious

- **Introspection**
- **Intuitive**
- Irritability – driving a car
- Joy
- **Patience**
- **Pertinacity**
- Rage
  - Paroxysms; in
- Reproaching oneself

- Responsibility – taking responsibility too seriously
- Sensitive
  - Certain persons; to
  - Criticism; to
  - Emotions; to
- **Spirituality**
- Truth – telling the plain truth
- Unification – sensation of unification

Physicals
- **Head**
  - Heat
- **Eye**
  - Heat in
  - Inflammation – Lids
  - Lachrymation
  - Pain
    - § Burning
    - § Stinging
  - Tears
    - § Acrid
    - § Salty
- **Vision**
  - *Large field of vision*
- **Mouth** – taste
  - Bitter
  - Putrid
- **Teeth**
  - Grinding – sleep agg.; during
  - Moved to another location; as if teeth had
- **Throat**
  - *Choking*
  - *Constriction*
    - § Throat-pit
    - § Uvula
  - Pain – sore
- **Abdomen**
  - Constriction
  - Liver and region of liver; complaints of
- **Rectum**
  - Constipation

- **Bladder** – urination
  - Dysuria – erections; with
  - Incomplete – obliged to urinate five or six times before the bladder is empty
- **Male**
  - Erections – troublesome
  - Sexual desire – increased – easily excited
- **Chest**
  - Constriction – Sternum
- **Back**
  - Spine; complaints of
  - Stiffness – Cervical region
- **Extremities**
  - Awkwardness
  - Constriction – Lower limbs
  - Constriction – Thighs
  - Raynaud's disease
- **Sleep**
  - Short – catnaps; in
  - Waking – frequent
- **Generals**
  - Food and drinks
    - § Fish – desire
    - § Nuts – desire
    - § Oil – desire – olive
    - § Spices – desire
    - § Vegetables – aversion
  - Heat
  - Flushes of – extending to – Upward
  - Lack of vital heat

Buteo jamaicensis (Red-tailed hawk)

Phylum: Chordata.
Class: Aves.
Order: Accipitriformes.
Family: Accipitridae.

Buteo jamaicensis is an extremely territorial bird of prey. They form monogamous partnerships, and can live a long time with their versatile and opportunistic approach to hunting and foraging. Mobbing by other birds can be a daily disruption to their lives – the most aggressive and dangerous attackers are crows or other corvids. In flight, they prefer to soar with wings beating as little as possible to conserve energy. A typical sky-dance (thought to be performed to designate their territory) involves the male hawk climbing high in flight with deep, exaggerated wingbeats before diving at great speed, checking, and shooting back up or plunging less steeply and repeating the process in a rollercoaster motion across the sky.

Provings by: **Jonathan Shore & Elizabeth Schulz, Germany, USA, Finland, Scotland (1995).**[10]

Keywords
Taking – More than wanted to give / **Freedom** / **Leash, tied to** / Oneness / Knives – body / Injury, about to receive / **Neglected** / Separated / Ambition / Clawing / Power, love of / Driving – fast / **Suffocation** / Excess of energy

Central theme
Sacrificing freedom – drawn back to care-taking, giving more of herself than she wanted to. Suffocated and trapped by responsibility.

Nucleus: The remedy has a strong affinity for individuals who need independence and freedom whilst being constantly drawn back into the role of care-giver, particularly for their family or for people (or animals) who need rescuing in some way. There is a great deal of energy and a need to be active and creative although there may be others in their life who try to control and contain their free-spirit. The remedy suits people who naturally seem to have a very strong sense of responsibility, taking care of others whilst also feeling exploited, abused or insulted. The feeling of being unfairly contained or abused by others leads to an increased need for independence and freedom. However free they desire to be, they are still drawn back to their role in taking care of others less well off than themselves.

SRP Dreams
- **Leash; connected by, gloved hand to**
- **Care-taking – family member; taking care of** – paralyzed legs; with
- Disabled People

- Divorced; of getting – abusive husband; because of
- Freedom – desire for
- *Injections – receiving many*
- Oneness; feeling of
- Taking – More than wanted to give
- Zooming through stars

Delusions
- **Knives – body; shot into the**
- Injury – about to receive injury; is (*cf. **Snakes***)
- Neglected – he or she is neglected (*cf. Matridonals, Milks, Palladium, **Oxygenium**, Spiders, Stage 16*)
- Separated – group; he is separated from the (*cf. Halogens, Insects, **Milks***)

Mind
- *Affection – yearning for affection*
- **Ambition – increased**
- Anger – kill; with impulse to
- Antisocial
- Athletics; ability for – increased
- **Checking** – twice or more; must check (OCD)
- *Clarity* of mind
- Company – aversion to – alone amel.
- Concentration – difficult – *spaciness*
- Despair – *black cloud; as if in*
- Dictatorial – **power; love of**
- Driving – **desire for driving – fast**
- Duty – too much sense of duty
- Extravagance – purchases; in
- **Fear – suffocation; of** – sit up; must
- Forsaken feeling – isolation; sensation
- Gestures; makes – hands; involuntary motions of the – **clawing**
- Inactivity – unmotivated; and
- Insecurity; mental
- **Longing – good opinion of others**
- Nature – loves
- *Self-control – increased*
- Travelling – desire for
- Understood; being – desire for – friend; by

Physicals
- **Head**
  - Pain – Forehead – **Eyes – behind – right**
  - Pain – Occiput – extending to – Shoulders
- **Eye**
  - Pain – Left – **splinter**; as from a
  - *Pain – Eyeballs – pushed forward; as if*
  - *Vision – Acute – movement; for*
- **Chest**
  - Pain – boring pain
- **Extremities**
  - Pain – **cramping**
  - Restlessness – Legs – night – bed – in bed – agg.
- **Generals**
  - **Energy – excess of energy – alternating with – low energy**
  - Pain – Muscles – sore
  - *Periodicity – day – alternate day*
  - Wavelike sensation

Source words

- Broad wingspan, hooked beak, sharp talons, large eyes, fierce expression.
- Versatility and opportunism as a predator.
- Attacks with a controlled dive from an elevated height.

CASE 3.1 Rheumatoid arthritis, worn-out caregiver

Patient: **Female, age 75**

Prescription: **Buteo-j 200c, repeated weekly**

∫ Chief complaint of Rheumatoid arthritis, worse in the **neck and shoulders** (*Birds*).

∫ Great sensitivity to allopathic drugs since operation for Gallbladder removal. This was performed unnecessarily and led to the patient being announced clinically dead on the operating table. Food intolerances and drug sensitivities ever since.

∫ The doctors treated "me as if I was contaminated" (*hint of leprosy miasm*).

∫ Father: high-end Asperger's syndrome, eminent scientist, controlling.

∫ She used to volunteer in the Samaritans.

Features of the case

∫ Sensitive, and tuned-in to spiritual realm – a Reiki master.

∫ "I'm tough, never say die. Life is very full-on. I have animals around all over the place. I pick up injured animals."

∫ Creative – pyrography, stained glass, jewellery – "but husband didn't want me to work. . . . He is a controlling bully. Married me young to mould me to what he wanted. My parents put me in the marriage market".

∫ **"Without freedom I wouldn't want to live. . . . Love to go back to the wilds of Scotland and go up into the mountains where I feel I can breathe. Free air, clear and pure".**

∫ "My husband tried to contain me, you know it is wrong but I was so young. Didn't trust my own judgment, thought of myself as stupid and had no confidence in myself. . . . **He was vicious; verbally attacked and abused me 30 times a day.** Really horrible; left me without the strength to continue to practice Reiki. When practicing Reiki my hands were burning, **buzzing, vibrating.** . . . I saw a counsellor, you must try and sort it out; **I am a human being.** . . . With the RA, the pain goes into different areas and **it suddenly strikes** ++ after stress.

∫ Effect of the Rheumatoid arthritis:

∫ "Being incapacitated, unable to move. Pain so excruciating, I gave up. **Feel beaten.** I can't be me. I couldn't see any point in being alive."

Opposite

∫ **"Being free, creative, having loads of animals around. Favourite animals are my dogs, cats, horses and birds of prey.** They always appear in front of me and do something weird. A buzzard flew straight at the car, nearly a kamikaze bird! That night my husband was so foul, I decided to leave him. There was a fire in our kitchen that night. I was so incandescent with rage, I thought I must have started it. The smoke hit my vocal chords, and **now I can't sing anymore. I could only croak afterwards."**

Analysis

Buteo-j was selected as it matched the situation of being a care-giver for the one who oppresses you.

Shore: "They feel a very strong sense of responsibility to family. More than a duty, they naturally want to care for and support members of their families. . . . In one proving, a man dreamt he had cared for a disabled person for five years in complete freedom, voluntarily and happily. In another proving, the primary prover wished she could be like her sister. The sister has two disabled kids she spends all her time caring for without any complaining."

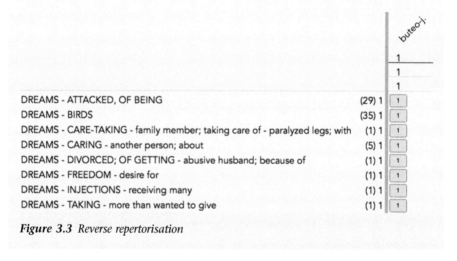

	buteo-j
	1
	1
	1
DREAMS - ATTACKED, OF BEING (29) 1	1
DREAMS - BIRDS (35) 1	1
DREAMS - CARE-TAKING - family member; taking care of - paralyzed legs; with (1) 1	1
DREAMS - CARING - another person; about (5) 1	1
DREAMS - DIVORCED; OF GETTING - abusive husband; because of (1) 1	1
DREAMS - FREEDOM - desire for (1) 1	1
DREAMS - INJECTIONS - receiving many (1) 1	1
DREAMS - TAKING - more than wanted to give (1) 1	1

Figure 3.3 *Reverse repertorisation*

Calypte anna (Hummingbird)

Phylum: Chordata.
Class: Aves.
Order: Apodiformes.
Family: Trochilidae.

Calypte anna has an iridescent bronze-green back, a pale grey chest, and green flanks. Its bill is long, straight, and slender. They feed on nectar – and occasionally tree sap – using a long extendable tongue; in so doing, they assist in plant pollination. They also eat small insects and other arthropods caught in flight. They can shake their bodies 55 times per second to shed rain or to remove pollen and dirt from feathers. During courtship rituals, the male sings with thin and squeaky tones interspersed with buzzes and chirps. Males can also be observed performing an aerial dive over their territories during the breeding season.

Proving by: **Cynthia Shephard, Canada (2003).**[15]

Keywords
Tingling / Twitchy / Pulsating / Hyper-drive / Fellowship / Care-taking / Iridescent / Buzzing / Humming / Stealth / Restlessness / Cocaine

Sensations
Tingling, burning, crawling / formication, cold, heat / burning (*Insects*)

Mind
- Air; in open – desire
- Anger – interruption; from
- Ardent (passionate)
- Brotherhood; sensation of
- Confusion of mind – talking, while
- **Decisive**
- Delusions
  - Trapped; he is
  - Young; she is again
- **Efficient**, organised
- Fear – attacked; fear of being
- Gestures; makes – tics; nervous
- Helplessness; feeling of – **overwork**; from
- **Hurried**; being
- **Industrious**
- Interruption – agg.
- Masculinity – increased sensation of
- Memory – weakness of memory – thought; for what he just has
- **Mistakes**; making
  - Speaking; in – spelling, in
  - Writing; in – omitting – letters
  - Writing; in – thoughts; from fast
- **Naive**
- **Overactive**
- **Rage**
- Secretive
- Sitting – inclination to sit – stare; and
- Space – desire for
- Thoughts
  - Intrude and crowd around each other – sexual
  - **Sexual** – tormenting

Physicals
- **Head**
  - Lightness; sensation of
- **Eye**
  - Eruptions – Lids – crusts – Margins of lids – morning
  - Pain
    - § stinging
    - § noise agg. – loud
- **Hearing**
  - Distant – sounds seem
- **Face**
  - Discoloration – red – heat – with
  - Eruptions – herpes – Lips
  - Tension – Jaws
  - Tic
- **Mouth**
  - Speech – unintelligible
- **Throat**
  - Pain – eating – amel. – sore
  - Pain – swallowing – amel.
- **Stomach**
  - Appetite – easy satiety – bites; after a few
- **Abdomen**
  - Pain – eating – after – agg. – cramping
- **Female**
  - Menses – painful – accompanied by – nausea
  - Pain – Ovaries – cramping
- **Chest**
  - Stiffness
- **Back**
  - Constriction – Cervical region
  - Pain
    - § Bending – backward – agg.
    - § Bending – forward – agg.
    - § Cervical region – looking – downward – agg.
    - § Cervical region – looking – upward – agg.
    - § Lumbar region – extending to – Legs
  - Stiffness
    - § Morning – rising agg.
    - § Morning – waking; on
  - Tight feeling
- **Extremities**
  - Pain
    - § Pulsating
    - § Shooting
    - § Bones – aching
    - § Hands – waking; on
    - § Nates – extending to – Lower limb
  - Perspiration
    - § Foot – warm
    - § Hand – heat; with
  - Shaking – Hands
  - Stiffness
    - § Morning – waking; on
    - § Motion – amel.
    - § Ankles
    - § Elbows
    - § Hips
    - § Nates
  - Walking – after – agg. – Lower limbs
- **Sleep**
  - Short – catnaps; in
- **Skin**
  - Stiffness
- **Generals**
  - Activity – increased
  - Alternating states – rapid alternation
  - Eating – small quantities – amel.
  - Electricity; sensation of static
  - Food and drinks
    - § alcoholic drinks – agg. – intoxicated; easily
    - § chocolate – agg.

Provers speaking as one

"Tight jaw, like past experiences *when doing cocaine* . . . [accompanied by] ragged breathing and feeling stoned, **twitchy**, **dazed** and confused. . . . Feel better for cold air, but then become extremely **dizzy** (NS), rising in waves and **pulsating** from my feet to my head. I have vertigo and feel like I am going to **pass out**. I'm sweating all down my back (OS) and on upper lip. My face is grey and I must sit down, and am **breathing heavily and rapidly** (NS). I must focus to keep from losing consciousness . . . **like I was in "hyper-drive"** . . . higher **sexual arousal** than prior to taking the remedy. . . . Feel excited, enlivened. . . . Even though I was very upset (in response to crisis with partner) I felt very sexually aroused; very confusing. Never felt it so extreme like this. When depressed usually not sexually aroused. . . . **Profound talk about what we care about**; acknowledged ideas and inspirations back and forth, which was quite wonderful – **enhanced my feeling of fellowship**. Great sense of enthusiasm and well-being now . . . I'm changing. *I'm more aligned with the **masculine** side of myself*, and I'm being more **assertive**. . . . I would feel better if [my sister] wouldn't try to be me. It is me wanting to be more **separate and distinct from her. I wish she wouldn't climb into my skin. . . . She isn't separating our identities enough**. . . . She used to leech on me when I was little too, but it is more particular now, boldly and defiantly stated by her. . . . I'm not looking after her, not **care-taking** my younger sister any more. It is like **I've abdicated from that role** and I'm easier. Not trying to bring her up."[15]

Source words
Bright, metallic, iridescent, buzzing, high speed, nectar, sugar.

CASE 3.2 (edited) Attention Deficit Hyperactivity Disorder

Case by: **Sally Williams**[23]
Patient: **Age 10**

"I am so incredibly happy most of the time. I can really get out of control. I have **lots and lots of energy**. I can read the same book three or four times. The thing I love best though is music. I just love being in the band. **I play clarinet**." C.B.'s mother reports that when he is not playing the clarinet he is **constantly humming**. "He hums and sings all day. He is all over the house all the time. **He cannot sit still even to eat**, but there are those times where he will be running around the house and all of a sudden he will just stop and day dream. He will just go off somewhere in his mind and he will be just kind of frozen there. Then something will bring him back and he will be off and running." He is very **smart** and **talented**, but that he is either too **distracted** or **day-dreamy** to use his abilities productively. C.B. has very little appetite and **eats "like a bird."** He **craves sugar** even though his mother strictly forbids it. He will even sneak into the kitchen to steal candy from the cupboard. C.B.'s mother calls him **"Professor Stealth,"** because he **"quietly flies into the kitchen, steals candy, and flies out."** C.B. is very **sensitive to pain** and can become **melodramatic if injured.** He is also **sensitive to ridicule by his peers** and becomes "furious" when bullied because of his **small size and restlessness."**[23]

Cathartes aura (Turkey vulture / Turkey buzzard)

Phylum: Chordata.
Class: Aves.
Order: Cathartiformes.
Family: Cathartidae.

The turkey vulture is a scavenger, feeding almost exclusively on carrion. They locate their food with keen eyesight and acute sense of smell (the latter of which is an uncommon ability in the avian realm) – flying low enough to detect the gasses emanating from the putrefying remains of animal corpses. They are lighter than other vultures, making them more buoyant in air as they effortlessly glide on thermals, preserving energy. They are gregarious, roosting in large communities and foraging independently during the day. Lacking a syrinx, the only vocalisations they can muster are grunts or low hisses. The name *vulture* is derived from the Latin word *vulturus*, meaning *tearer*, and is a reference to its feeding style. Their chicks are helpless at birth and both adults feed the young by regurgitating food, parenting for up to 10/11 weeks. Adults may flee or feign death when threatened during nesting – they have also been known to regurgitate on the intruder.

Proving by: **Todd Rowe, Phoenix AZ (1999).**[12]

Keywords
Abused / Chaotic / Invisible / **Stabbed – back; in the** / Motorcycles / Scorpions / Kidnapped / Clairvoyant / Blocked / Parasites / Desquamating / Acne / **Scavenger** / Communication / **Community** / Underground / Groups

Mind

- Ailments from – **abused**; after being
- Biting – himself
- Chaotic
- Clarity of mind
- Compulsive disorders
- Confident
- Content
- **Delusions**
  - **Appreciated; she is not**
  - Abused; being
  - Bird, birds; phoenix rising from ashes
  - Invisible; he is
  - Stabbed – back; in the
  - Transparent – he is
  - Trapped; he is
  - Vulnerable (*injury – about to receive; is*)
- Ennui
- Euphoria
- Flashbacks (*Thoughts – past; of the*)
- Flying – desire to fly
- Peace – heavenly peace; sensation of
- Hiding – himself
- Honest
- Meditating
- Order – desire for
- Rash / Temerity
- Religious affections – want of religious feeling
- Somnambulism
- Speed; desire for
- Suspicious – trick him; people are trying to
- Sympathetic – animals; towards

Dreams

Airplanes / *Balloons* / Blood / Bugs / **Buildings – big and beautiful *vs*. neglected** / Cats / Ceiling – collapsing / *Children*; about – *kidnapped*; being / *Children*; about – sick / Children; about – taking care of endangered parents / **Clairvoyant** – solving important questions of the day / **Cliff** / Crime / Danger – escaping from a danger – **fruitless efforts to escape** / Difficulties – journeys, on / Dogs / Driving – car; a / **Falling – confidence, with** / Falling – height; from a / Families / Fire – people on fire / Floating – water; on / Friends / Horses – riding / Hospitals / House – big – mansion / Island / Journeys – bus; by / *Killing* / Lascivious / Lions / Money / *Motorcycles* / Obscene / Ocean / Prisoner / Pursued; being – man; by a / Rocks / Romantic / Sailing / Scorpions / Secret / Sexual / Sick people / **Snakes** – biting him / Sneaking / Spies; about – she is a spy / Stealing / Threatened; of being / Wedding

Themes

Clairvoyance / Compassion / Dictatorial / Divided / Floating / Flying / Fragility / Hiding / Imprisoned / Nature / Organisation / Peace / Perfection / Pessimism

Clinical indications Shore[10]

Acne / Suppurating skin eruptions / Parasites / Itching.
Feelings of being stuck / blocked (*cf. Cruciferae, Anacrdiaceae, Sarcodes*).

Physical[10]

Back pain, headaches behind the eyes, itching, formication and chilliness.

- **Throat**
  - Scratching / Swelling – Tonsils
- **Larynx and Trachea**
  - *Voice – hoarseness*
- **Respiration**
  - Impeded, obstructed – swelling; from – throat; of
- **Chest**
  - Pain – Sternum – burning and stitching pains
- **Skin**
  - Eruptions – *Acne / Desquamating / Pimples – Painful / Pustules / Rash*
  - *Cicatrices – sensitive*
  - *Itching – crawling*

- **Rectum**
  - Constipation / Inactivity
- **Back**
  - *Pain – Dorsal region – Scapulae – Between* – sneezing agg.
- **Generals**
  - Complexion – black – hair
  - Complexion – dark
  - Food and drinks
    - § Alcoholic drinks – agg.
    - § Salt – desire
  - Inflammation
  - Mucous secretions – gray
  - Tumors – cystic

Provers speaking as one[12]

"A strong central feeling that arose in the proving stemmed around the idea of *catharsis* followed by feelings of *calmness* and *peace*. One prover described it as a *"little exorcism going on inside."* The vulture is a **scavenger**, one who gets rid of dead, old material. **Foraging** for food and **rummaging** through old things. . . . Scavenger bird; dreams of *dirty going to clean* . . . **vulnerability** *like an egg without a shell*. . . . The vulture is vulnerable on the ground. Several provers had dreams of the **ground being paper thin and falling through the floor**. . . . The maternal animal side came through strongly in images of **guardianship** and **care taking**. . . . Anxiety about who would play the role of caretaker was also an issue. . . . **Communication** and messages were another theme found in the proving. Much of the communication was associated with *frustration or feeling blocked in efforts at communication*. It is interesting to note that *the bird is voiceless*. . . . Theme of going back for something that one has forgotten came up frequently. The vulture when it identifies carrion, often does not approach at that time but returns to **feed with its community** on the following day. . . . Another theme was the idea of *getting away with something*. The provers often felt that rules did not apply to them or that **rules could be broken**. Much of this focuses on the feelings of **underground, secret operations**. These themes were prominent in the Raven proving as well."

"The most common cured symptoms were increased energy and feelings of calmness, peacefulness and contentment. A number of individuals pursued meditation or yoga, which they either had never done or not done for years"

Rowe[12]

Source words

Plumage dull, scavenging, well developed sense of smell, lacking tunefulness.

Columba palumbus (Woodpigeon / Ring dove)

Phylum: Chordata.
Class: Aves.
Order: Columbiformes.
Family: Columbidae.

An interesting & unique behaviour of the Woodpigeon is the secretion of crop milk to feed their young. Unlike mammalian milk, which is an emulsion, pigeon crop milk consists of a suspension of protein-rich and fat-rich cells that proliferate and detach from the lining of the crop. Their flight is quick, performed by regular beats, with an occasional & characteristic flick of the wings. In their nuptial display, they walk along a horizontal branch with swelled neck, lowered wings, and fanned tail. The call is a characteristic cooing. Most of its diet is vegetable, round and fleshy leaves from Caryophyllaceae, Asteraceae and Cruciferaceae.

C4 Trituration Proving by: **Jonathan Shore and Elizabeth Schulz, Germany (1999).**[10]

Keywords
Ugly / Criticised / Neglected / Abused / Domination / Affectionate / Remorse / Freedom / Yielding / Shameful / Naive

Nucleus: Ailments from abuse and domination for a long time with feelings of low self-worth, guilt and shame. Feels judged and criticised and compensates by wanting to serve the community (*Lac-d*). They serve others selflessly to the point of becoming a door-mat (*phlegmatic temperament*).

SRP delusions
- Body – **ugly**; body looks (*Birds, Milks, Insects, Leprosy miasm, Latex*)
- Crime – **committed a crime**; he had (*cf. Iron Series, Kalis, Talp-eu., anac., plb., verat.*)
- **Criticised**; she is (*cf. Lac-lup., Stage 2., Carc., Lyss.*)
- **Neglected – duty**; he has neglected his (*cf. Gold series, Stage 11, Lyc., cyc., staph.*)
- Reproach; he has neglected his duty and deserves (*cf. Aur., Germ-met.*)
- Wrong – done wrong; he has (*cf. Aur., Snakes., Iron Series., Lil-t., Ign.*)

Ailments from
- <u>Abused</u>; after being (*cf. Birds, Milks, Animals, Cancer miasm, Carcinosin*)
- Anger – suppressed (*cf. Staph, Plut-n, Stage 11, Carcinosin, Nat-m*)
- Domination – long time; for a (*cf. Folliculinum, Lac-leo, Ign, Mag-m*)
- Mortification (*cf. Ambr, Ign, Lyssin, Heroin, Palladium, Staph*)

Mind

- Abusive – children
- Affectionate
- Anxiety – conscience; anxiety of
- Blissful feeling
- Dependent of others – children; in
- Fastidious
- Fear – high places; of
- Freedom
- Grief – silent
- Hatred
- Heaviness; sensation of
- Light – aversion to – shuns
- Naive
- Pleasing – desire to please others
- Remorse
- **Reproaching oneself**
- Resignation
- Sensitive – cruelties; when hearing of
- Shameful – sexuality; about
- Travelling – desire for
- Violent – children – towards
- Will – *control over his will; does not know what to do; has no*
- Yielding disposition

Source behaviour

Monogamous relationship, feed milk to their young (*cf. Mammals*), young growing rapidly.

The remedy is similar to columba livia (*Rock pigeon / Homing pigeon*)

The rock dove has an innate homing ability, meaning that it will generally return to its nest – (it is believed) using magnetoreception.

Extracts from the proving by Priti Shah[21]

- Being at the bottom of the pile and having to live with the consequences.
- Being treated as someone of no consequence.
- No value – deserving no consideration.
- Being ordinary.
- Response – wanting things to be extraordinary.
- Need to progress continually – to make efforts to be of greater worth.

Corvus corax (Raven)

Phylum: Chordata.
Class: Aves.
Order: Passeriformes.
Family: Corvidae.

The common raven is the biggest member of the crow family. The bird is black with a large bill, and long wings. In flight, it shows a diamond-shaped tail. Ravens breed mainly in the west and north although they are currently expanding their range eastwards. Most birds are residents, though some birds – especially non-breeders and young birds – wander from their breeding areas but do not travel far.

In his book entitled *Raven*, David Lilley makes the following observation,

A bird as black as the night, indicating its chthonic and lunar connotations, yet, when caught in the light of the sun, displaying glorious, iridescent plumage, announcing its solar affinity: a bird for all dimensions, able to soar to the sublime heights of transcendence and descend into the infernal darkness of the abyss![18]

Proving by: **Greg Bedayn, USA (1998).**[24]

Keywords
Invaded / Invincible / **Revengeful** / Humiliated / Shameful / Destructiveness / Floating / Higher dimension / Poisoned / Hunger / Quicksand – sinking into / Tortured / **Ravenous** / Croaking / **Betrayals** / Un-woundable / Proud / **Queen-like** / Plundering / Conspiracies / Regal

Themes
Defenceless, unprotected and invaded *vs.* Invincible and regal.
Vengeful when humiliated or deceived.
Between worlds.

Fundamental delusions
- *Protection, defence; has no*
- **Invaded**; one's space is being
- **Invincible**; he is
- **Queen**; she is a
- Worlds; *she is in the divide between two worlds* (**cf.** *Eagle*)
- **Delusions**
  - *Beaten; he is being*
  - *Danger; impression of*

- Defenceless; feels she is; with panic and anxiety
- Enlarged – body is – parts of body
- Floating in a higher dimension
- Head – separated from body
- Smell; of
- Torture – tortured; he is
- Worthless; he is

- **Mind**
  - Absorbed – ***concentrate on inner world; wants to***
  - Ailments from – abused; after being – sexually
  - Anxiety – anger – during
  - Clairvoyance
  - Death – thoughts of
  - Despair – world; for the
  - **Destructiveness**
  - Detached
  - Fear – poisoned – being poisoned; fear of
  - Fear – terror
  - Hatred – ***revengeful; and***

  - Haughty
  - Helplessness; feeling of
  - <u>**Humiliated; feeling – deception; from**</u>
  - Indignation
  - Injustice; cannot support
  - Power – sensation of
  - Rage – cursing; with
  - **Sensual**
  - **Shameful**
  - Spaced-out feeling
  - Sympathetic – animals; towards
  - Unreal – everything seems
  - Violent

Dreams
Conspiracies / Crime – committing a crime / Death – friend; of a / Dogs – bitten by dogs; being / Eating / Fire – danger; of / **Food** / *Helping – people* / **Humiliation** / **Hunger** / Locked up / Oil rigs – destruction / Plundering / Society and community / Stealing / Suicide / Teaching / **Tortured**; of being / War / Water – waterfall / Waves – tidal wave / *Quicksand – sinking into; a woman is*

Physicals
- **Head** – Pain – pressing pain – downward
- **Vision** – Blurred
- **Nose**
  - Odours; imaginary and real – animals
  - Smell – acute
- **Stomach** – <u>Appetite – ravenous</u>
- **Larynx** and trachea
  - **Voice – hoarseness**

- **Respiration** – Anxious
- **Chest**
  - Inflammation – Lungs
  - Phthisis pulmonalis
- **Extremities**
  - Pain – Hands – rheumatic
  - Pain – Shoulders – *cutting pain*
  - Pain – Upper arms – *cutting pain*
- **Generals** – Strength; sensation of

Source words
Hackles, croaking, communicative, scavenger, omnivorous, hopping and soaring.

Proving
- **Themes**
  - Breakdowns of life and organisations
  - Betrayals, not being treated fairly
  - *Deceit of and lack of integrity in others*
  - *Hyper acute senses and delusions*

- **Symptoms**
  - External throat and neck sore
  - Blackness, suicidal. Blacking out, darkening of room
  - Not really here – detached
  - Everything is falling apart

Queen-like; powerful, proud and beautiful
"My chest in the breast area feels enlarged tremendously, like the ribs are bowing out. . . . Feeling very good, clean, **strong, proud, un-woundable**, like "shoulders back, chest out. . . . Generally feeling really good energy, feeling strong, proud, queen-like. . . . The last few days I was **incredibly hungry**. Grazing through the refrigerator, looking for anything edible. I am hungry all the time. I must cook immediately, big meals, good meals, and I enjoy it tremendously. I prepare a lot. I eat everything, even the crumbs."[18]

Clinical
"Raven is not valued by others so there is a fierce need to protect the core self at all times. This is the primary motivation for all their behaviour. They are not recognised, validated or respected for what they say or do or who they are. Their reality and truth are denied by the outside world. There is nothing of their own that is private and it makes them MAD! They are not quiet about this **invasion**". Shore[10]

Cygnus bewicki (Bewick swan / Tundra swan)

Phylum: Chordata.
Class: Aves.
Order: Anseriformes.
Family: Anatidae.

Bewick swans are the smaller subspecies of *Cygnus columbianus*. In adult birds, the plumage is entirely white, with black feet and a bill that is mostly black. They are similar in appearance to *Cygnus cygnus*, but smaller, shorter-necked and with a more rounded head shape. Tundra swans have high-pitched honking calls and are migratory – at which time they can fly at altitudes of 8 km. They pair monogamously until one partner dies. Should one partner die long before the other, the surviving bird will tend not to mate again for some years, or even for its entire life.

Proving by: **Penny Stirling, UK (2003).**[16]

Keywords

Underworld / Web / Banished / Conspiracies / Relentless hatred / Blackness / Lucifer / **Hideously ugly** / Wretched / Sexual thoughts / Despised / **Dirty** / **Ostracised** / Exalted love / Dancing / Sadistic / Homosexuality / Infertility / Obese / **Leper** / Taboos / Tobacco / Glamorous / Shabby / Unattractive / Bulimia

Polarity

Hideous, ugly, inadequate and unattractive vs. *Gorgeous, glamorous, attractive and able.*

A strong underworld dynamic was carried in the proving as conveyed by the rubrics listed below. The film *Black Swan* is brought to mind, in which the main protagonist – Nina, a ballerina whose passion for dance dominates every aspect of her being, is given the opportunity to take the lead role in Swan Lake. The sadistic director puts her in direct competition with newcomer Lily (*Lilium tigrinum?*). While Nina is perfect for the role of the White Swan, Lily naturally personifies the Black Swan. Yet, as rivalry between the two dancers transforms into a twisted friendship, the tables begin to turn as Nina's dark shadow world emerges, causing her to lose her tenuous grip on reality and descend into madness.

Fundamental delusions
- **Trapped; he is – underworld; in the / spider's web; in a**
- Banished; she is
- Conspiracies – against him; there are conspiracies (*cf. Plb., Kali-br., Lach., Puls*)
- Hatred; her centre is full of relentless hatred and blackness
- Devil – chuckling; she hears Lucifer (*Underworld themes*)

SRP delusions

- **Body – ugly; body looks – hideously ugly**
  (*cf. thuj., leprosy miasm, loxo-recl., falco-pe., haliae-lc.*)
- **Wretched; she looks – looking in a mirror; when** – beautiful; but for a split
  second she looks (*cf. Nat-m.* ++)
- **Thoughts – sexual – person he sees; sexual thoughts at every**
  (*cf. ust., fl-ac., nux-v., sel., kali-br.*)
- Beaten; he is being
- Blanket; under a thick
- **Despised** (*cf. Leprosy miasm, arg-n., milks, orig.*)
- Dirty – he is – cruel and unworthy
- Fail; everything will
- Friendless; he is
- Hunter; he is a
- *Ostracised; she is* (*cf. Lacs, Leprosy*)
- *Outsider; being an* (*cf. Milks*)

Mind

- Anger – himself; with
- Awkward – strikes against things
- Bulimia
- Company – desire for – *group together; desire to keep*
- Confidence – want of self-confidence
- Confusion of mind – identity – boundaries
- *Contemptuous*
- Content
- Cursing
- *Dancing*
- *Defiant*
- Dress – ridiculously; wants to dress
- *Estranged – society; from*
- Fearless – danger; in spite of
- Forsaken feeling – isolation; sensation
- Frivolous
- Haughty
- *Love – exalted love*
- Rage – biting; with
- Remorse
- Thoughts – circles; move in
- Unfeeling – family; with his
- Wandering – desire to wander
- Weeping – remorse; with
- Wildness
- Wretched – body; unhappy with her

Dreams

Amorous – dark and sadistic / Children; about – **dirty** / Doors – closing / Food – insufficient / Friends – meeting friends / High places / **Homosexuality** / Inadequate; of feeling **/ Infertility treatment**; IVF / Knives / **Leper**; being a / **Obese**; being / **Outsider** – being an outsider / Sexual – **perversity / Sexual – taboos being broken** / *Shameful* / Snakes / Stabbed; being / Trap – being trapped / Urinating – desire for / Women – energy, life and power; full of

Physicals

- **Mouth**
  - Flabby tongue
  - Ulcers – painful
  - Ulcers – Tongue
- **Throat**
  - Mucus – sensation of
  - Pain – extending to – Ear – sore
  - Swallowing – difficult
  - External Throat – Pulsation – Glands
- **Stomach**
  - Appetite – ravenous
  - Vomiting – eating – after – agg.
  - Abdomen – Pain – wavelike
- **Rectum**
  - Urging – sudden

- **Female**
  - Pain – Ovaries – right
  - Pain – menses would come on; as if
- **Extremities**
  - Eruptions – Legs – rash
  - Itching – Nates
  - Itching – Thighs – outer side
- **Sleep**
  - Need of sleep – little
- **Chill**
  - Internal – coldness – Bones; as if in
- **Skin**
  - Itching – morning – waking; on
- **Generals**
  - Tobacco – desire for tobacco

Provers speaking as one

"Feeling very unattractive in my body since I have put on probably almost two stone over the past year. . . . Went to a 'do' on bus, wrapped up over my 'best' dress. Got there feeling OK – not particularly **glamorous** but **not** as fat as I felt when I left the house. Everyone had really, really dressed up and looked **gorgeous** – I felt pretty **shabby** again. Found it quite hard to mingle. Usually I would go out of my way to be friendly/outrageous, etc. but was so outnumbered by the glamorous girls, **felt totally inadequate**. They are all very gorgeous, very loud and also very drunk – **no competition** . . . felt really very **unattractive**, especially while eating and too drunk to appreciate food. . . . Went to loos with the girls – full of full-length mirrors; and to my shock and surprise in my drunkenness I actually look fine. I don't look too fat. I look OK. For one split second, when I saw myself in that mirror, I was attractive – just as glamorous as the other girls. I can still remember that feeling, now that the alcohol has worn off, and it feels like a dream. In the reflection I was normal, not **hideously ugly**, quite slim and attractive, even! I looked OK. If only this were true! It was an incredible experience. . . . Felt quite attractive, grounded and able."[16]

Source behaviour

Enormous flocks, gregarious, hierarchy (*cf. Mammals*), babbling and bugling.

Cygnus Cygnus (Whooper Swan)

Phylum: Chordata.
Class: Aves.
Order: Anseriformes.
Family: Anatidae.

The *Whooper swan is* a large and long-necked swan with a deep honking call. Despite their size, they are powerful fliers. They require large areas of water to live in, especially whilst still growing, as their body weight cannot be supported by their legs for long periods of time. They spend much of their time on the water, eating mostly aquatic plants. They form lifelong monogamous relationships, working as a pair to care for their cygnets who stay with them all winter. When the flock prepares for flight, they use a variety of signalling movements to communicate whether the flight will take place and who will take the lead. The courtship routine consists of bobbing their heads up and down as a greeting – then whilst facing each other, they turn their necks from left to right as they beat their wings fervently. Pre-copulation displays are short and include head dipping and thrusting of the neck and chest into the water.

Proving by: **Jeremy Sherr, UK (2001).**[13]

Keywords
Love; disappointed / **Grief** / Loss / Bereavement / Sighing / **Hollow** / Abused / **Partner** / Abandonment / Hole – chest / **Neck; lump** sensation / Vulnerable / Overwhelming love

Key Themes
- *Grief – ailments from loss of loved ones.*
- Sighing – grief; with.
- Hollow, empty / full.
- Dreams – grief, abused sexually; being, flying.
- Weeping – events, thinking of past.
- Despair – finding a life partner.
- Sadness – euphoria in heart; with.
- Supplementary themes – *Abandonment, isolation, loneliness, distant / detached.*
- **Throat; lump sensation; swallowing; amel.; does not.**
- *cf.* Nat-m., Ignatia., Staph.

SRP Delusions
- Hole – chest; in his
- Hollow; body, whole
- Neck; large; too
- *Insignificant*; he is
- Polluted; he gets
- Vulnerable
- World; parallel world; she is in a

Mind symptoms

- **Ailments from**
  - Abused; after being – sexually – rape
  - Death of loved ones
  - Discords – parents; between one's
  - Love; disappointed
- Anger – love; from disappointed
- Company – aversion to
- Despair – future; about
- Farewell – **separation is difficult**

- Forsaken feeling – beloved by his parents, wife, friends; feeling of not being
- Grief – silent
- Indifference – joyless
- Playing – desire to play – water – in water
- Sadness
  - Death of mother
  - Disappointment; from

Physicals

- **Vertigo**
  - Turning; as if – he turns in a circle – left; to
- **Vision**
  - Dim – water; as if full of
- **Neck**
  - *Swelling – sensation of*
- **Respiration**
  - *Impeded, obstructed*
- **Throat**
  - Constriction – swallowing; difficult

  - Lump; sensation of a
  - Narrow – sensation
  - Suffocative sensation
- **Chest**
  - Constriction – breathing – deep – agg.
  - Narrow – sensation as if too

Generals

- Emptiness – sensation of
- Weakness – accompanied by respiration – impeded

Provers speaking as one

"Felt sensation of **overwhelming love for everyone** and mankind, and opening in the heart. This is so in contrast with feelings of last week. Feel colour re-emerge into life instead of the utterly black/white severity. . . . Our common mission is to **find love**. For someone who **finds it hard to love** or to show love, then if he finds love anyway, he has succeeded. If he has given **genuine love**, he has succeeded. . . . To look at a person as a whole – with all their faults, with whatever they lacked, and to see their Soul and love them still and see the good in that person – is a pure thing. . . . Sad for the **lack of loving affection** in my life. Feel as if I have never achieved a loving and fulfilling connection with another person yet it is everything I yearn for. . . . Desperate desire for affection. . . . Feeling emotional with grief and with an **accompanying lump in my throat**. . . . Sadness, grief, depression, exhaustion, no energy at all . . . **unbelievable sorrow/grief** . . . shivering, shaking, jerking, crying . . . **Empty, hollow** and disconnected feeling . . . I just couldn't hold back my feelings anymore. I burst into tears, violent, shaking. And suddenly it was over again. . . . Feel a deep aloneness, which has been building up all week. It is as if I will never see anyone again. There is a slight **death wish**, which I find alarming. . . . Want everyone to realise what I'm suffering – to notice and be sorry – but without me telling them. . . . Feel very sorry for myself today. Lonely. Dreaming of my soul mate. . . .

Felt very vulnerable . . . and feeling out of the group. This feeling of exclusion was accompanied by immobility and stiffness of right side of face."[13]

CASE 3.3 Grief from separation

Patient: **Female, age 52**

Prescription: **Cygnus cygnus 10M**

Animal language
∫ Like competitive things. I want to win. Why would I enter competition if I don't want to win it?
∫ I can't be bottom, can't get the worst score. People will think I am shit at it.
∫ It finished me off, I was on the floor.
∫ He kept threatening to kill me . . . came back and beat the shit out of me in the shop.
∫ Would not have survived without her.

Cygnus themes
∫ Like **bereavement**, like I've been dumped, like a divorce but worse because you can't replace. Cried more than I ever have in my whole life. The separation – it just feels like pain.
∫ When you're a teenager and you really fall in love – your whole being is all about that person.
∫ When it ends, it is awful. Your whole world ends. I am not going to be in that place anymore.
∫ Not going to be taken over by anyone else. It is like you can't exist or breathe or anything anymore.
∫ Just taken over by this other person. Completely taken over, enveloped, like sucked into a black hole.
∫ I had fallen in love with him so I was 'all-in'. Scared the shit out of me. Then my being is in someone else's hands. My birth mother, didn't have me in her hands. She was supposed to. If you're not going to then who else will?!
∫ It feels like a physical knot right in the Solar plexus. Like the moment before you burp.
∫ Something stuck, radiating out, like something wants to get out but it can't.

Bird themes
∫ When body is working well, when fit and strong – it just *frees* up my whole system. My mind can *travel* to wherever it wants to. Like to be *running* outside, often with the dog running with me. Just a sense of *space*, and the music being a part of it. Running is a very peaceful space for my brain.

Aves / Birds

Spacious. No demands on me. I get into a *meditative* state when running. No longer notice what my body is doing.

∫ Feeling *trapped* in that car, going backwards and forwards.
∫ It is important to be present and communicating well.
∫ Don't want to be clinging onto kids. I would have hated that.

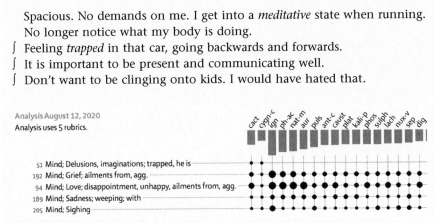

Analysis August 12, 2020
Analysis uses 5 rubrics.

51 Mind; Delusions, imaginations; trapped, he is
192 Mind; Grief; ailments from, agg.
94 Mind; Love; disappointment, unhappy, ailments from, agg.
189 Mind; Sadness; weeping; with
205 Mind; Sighing

Figure 3.4 *Repertorisation*

Cygnus olor (Mute Swan)

Phylum: Chordata.
Class: Aves.
Order: Anseriformes.
Family: Anatidae.

The mute swan is one of the heaviest flying birds. They are monogamous and often reuse the same nest each year, restoring or rebuilding it as needed. They can show marked aggression in defence of their nests and are fiercely protective of their mate and offspring – hissing at competitors or intruders trying to enter their territory. They are less vocal than the noisy whooper and bewick swans; but they do make a variety of grunting, hoarse whistling, and snorting noises – especially in communicating with their cygnets. Mute swans do not mate for life, but tend to maintain a bond for one breeding season. It is a common misconception that mute swans pair for life and that a bird will pine to death when its partner dies.

C2-C4 Trituration Proving by: **Elizabeth Schulz, Germany (1997).**[24]

Keywords
Betrayed / **Love; disappointed** / Wandering / **Grief** / Swaying / Intruders / Threatened / Vulnerability / Unicorn / Inspiration / Nurturing / Dreamers / **Soul mate** / Tenderness / Rhythm

Mind

- Ailments from – *love; disappointed*
- Clairvoyance
- Confusion of mind – loses his way in well-known streets
- Delusions – hole – chest; in his
- Grief
- Wandering – *desire to wander*
- *Weeping – violent*

Physicals

- **Vertigo**
  - Swaying; with
- **Throat**
  - Constriction
  - Lump; sensation of a
- **Neck**
  - Tension
- **Stomach**
  - Fear – sensation of
- **Respiration**
  - Impeded, obstructed
- **Chest**
  - Constriction – breathing – deep – agg.
- **Back**
  - Tension – Cervical region

Dreams

- Breathing under water
- *Betrayed*; having been
- Childbirth
- Clairvoyant
- Death – dying
- Fights – rights; for her
- Journeys
- Money – counterfeit

- **Extremities**
  - Awkwardness –
  - Hands – drops things
- **Skin**
  - Eruptions – discharging – honey; like
  - Eruptions – eczema – accompanied by – redness; intense
  - Eruptions – eczema – scales; with hard horny
  - Eruptions – papular
- **Generals**
  - Heat – lack of vital heat
  - Influenza
  - Mucous membranes;
  - complaints of – dryness
  - Pain – rheumatic – Muscles
  - Weakness – accompanied by – respiration – impeded

Proving extracts

"Misunderstood sexuality of women"

"One participant who was brutally abused by her husband and now lives alone said with deep longing in her voice: 'I want to meet my soul mate and to be with him the way I am and to be loved like that.' **The search for the soul mate** was only one part of the theme. The other was the sexual relationship. **The refusal or rejection of sexuality by the male** life partner or spouse was also present. Rough sexual treatment by men, sexual abuse of children, and child pornography were themes difficult to confront during this trituration."[22]

"Swans are loyal to each other. Their mating season starts in winter. Their **love making is characterised by great tenderness**. With their radiating white feathers ruffled up, they sway in a dance of love. The female swan decides when she is ready for mating. The male swan is then allowed during the long tender foreplay to cross his neck over hers. This loving coming closer together and then having to wait again is an attractive spectacle. **The male swan's consideration** of the female swan's rhythm and sexual excitement becomes obvious. The one-year-old brown males have difficulties in finding a mate. The female swans react very much to visual characteristics. **When choosing a partner, the male's impressive postures with lifted wings and neck feathers play a central role.**"[22]

Diomedea exulans (Wandering albatross)

Phylum: Chordata.
Class: Aves.
Order: Procellariiformes.
Family: Diomedeidae.

Diomedea exulans is the largest albatross with a wingspan up to 12 feet. It is almost completely white; with only a few dark spots on back and wings. They have webbed feet and require a long run to achieve take-off. The albatross is an excellent glider, gaining height against the wind and gathering speed by turning around in a downward plunge to the sea where they fish by ducking their curved beak into the water. When the wind is strong, the wings are bent backwards in the wrist joint. They eat sea animals, squid or refuse from ships.

Proving by: **Jan Scholten, Netherlands (2000).**

Extracts from Wad Stories vol 1 – Diomedea exulans Scholten[14]
- **The group is threatened by intruders. Taking one's stand. Saying no to intruders.**
- *Intrusion by phallus. Feeling of vulnerability in the group.*
- *The roles of men and women were not strictly divided.*
- Delusions
  - Body parts – sensation as if two sides of the body do not fit; torsion, as if
  - Oblique lines, like a reed swaying in the wind
  - Animals – unicorn – **unicorn as symbol of androgyny.**
- Restlessness – eyes, closing – amel.

"As it takes seven years for the bird to mature sexually, the albatross stands for a cycle of seven years in which groundwork and education can prepare one for the coming years. The albatross can live to be seventy years of age, reflecting the success after proper maturity. The albatross is a bird of sea, the **ancient archetype of creativity, inspiration, mothering and nurturing energies. Patience** is another symbol of the bird. People who have an albatross as totem are **dreamers, wandering** from job to job, without goals or direction. But inspiration and success come if searching is continued. It is all about conserving and using one's energy in the most beneficial manner. Without some commitment one will never succeed."[14]

Mind

- Abstraction of mind
- Closing eyes – amel.
- Concentration – difficult
- Confusion of mind
  - Identity; as to his – boundaries; and personal
  - Loses his way in well-known streets
- Delusions
  - Body – state of his body; to the erroneous
  - Danger; impression of
  - Divided – two parts; into
  - Flying
  - Trapped; he is
- Dream; as if in a
- Farewell – separation is difficult

- Fear
  - Abdomen – arising from abdomen
  - Life; of embracing
  - Tremulous
- Forsaken feeling
- Freedom
- Homesickness
- Independent
- Insecurity; mental
- Peace – heavenly peace; sensation of
- Restlessness
- Sighing
- Time – timelessness; sensation of
- Tranquillity
- Unreal – everything seems
- Unsympathetic
- Yawning

Physicals

- **Vertigo**
  - Swaying – to and fro
- **Head**
  - Heaviness – Forehead – right
  - Lightness; sensation of
  - Pain
    § Forehead
      ▪ right – stitching pain
      ▪ Eyes – Above
      ▪ Eyes – Behind
    § Occiput
      ▪ pressing pain – inward
      ▪ extending to – Vertex
- **Ear**
  - Pain – Mastoid
- **Face**
  - Air – blew upon face; as if cold
- **Face**
  - Twitching – Cheeks – left
- **Throat**
  - Lump; sensation of a
- **Stomach**
  - Eructations
  - Nausea – vomit; sensation as if about to
  - Tension

- **Rectum**
  - Constipation
  - Flatus – evening
- **Chest**
  - Open; sensation as if
  - Oppression
  - Pain – Sternum – pressing pain
- **Extremities**
  - Awkwardness – Hands – drops things
  - Coldness
  - Hands – one hand – colder than the other
  - Hands – right
  - Eruptions
    § Feet – papules
    § Hands – papular
  - Heat – Legs
  - Heaviness – Legs
  - Injuries – Foot – Heel
  - Pain
    § Legs – Spots; in
    § Lower limbs – right
    § Wrists – left
    § Wrists – Ulnar side
  - Perspiration – Fingers – Tips

- Tingling – Legs
- **Skin**
  - Eruptions
    - § Discharging – honey; like
    - § Papular
- **Generals**
  - Heat – lack of vital heat
  - Quivering
  - Shivering
  - Trembling – Externally – coldness – with

Erithacus rubecula (European robin)

Phylum: Chordata.
Class: Aves.
Order: Passeriformes.
Family: Muscicapidae.

The European robin, known also as the robin redbreast in Britain, is a small insectivorous passerine bird that belongs to the chat subfamily of the Old World flycatcher family. Male robins are renowned for their highly aggressive territorial behaviour to other birds of the same species, fiercely attacking other males and competitors that stray into their territories. In contrast, they are well-acquainted with and friendly with humans, especially gardeners, whose endeavours with the spade turn up the soil bringing to the surface earthworms and other juicy morsels.

Proving by: **Liz Fisher, Manchester, UK (2005).**[4]

Mind

- Accident-prone
- Ailments from
  - anticipation
  - embarrassment
- Anticipation
- Anxiety – anticipation; from
- *Aversion – family; to members of – others; but talks pleasantly to*
- Awareness heightened
- Caring
- **Childish**
- Children – beget and to have children; desire to
- Company
  - aversion to
    - § desire for solitude
    - § fear of being alone; yet
  - desire for
- Confident
- Curious
- Delusions
  - small – he is
  - tall – he or she is tall
- Emotions – strong; too
- *Excitement – anticipating events, when*
- Fear – happen; something will
- Forsaken feeling
- **Giggling**
- Impatience
- Impulsive
- Jealousy
- Laughing
- Loathing – oneself
- **Mischievous**
- Mood – changeable
  - quickly
  - sudden

- **Naïve** (innocence)
- Observer – being an
- **Protecting – desire to protect**
- Sensitive
  - criticism; to

Physicals
- **Stomach**
  - Appetite – changeable
- **Rectum**
  - Urging – sudden
- **Bladder**
  - Urination – urging to urinate – sudden
- **Male & Female**
  - Sexual desire – diminished / increased
- **Back**
  - Pain – Cervical region
  - Stiffness – Cervical region
- **Extremities**
  - Awkwardness
- **Skin**
  - Dry
  - Eruptions – herpetic

- reprimands; to
- Sociability
- Unification – sensation of unification
- Work – impossible

- Itching
- Numbness
- **Generals**
  - Air; in open – amel.
  - Desire for open air
  - Alternating states
  - Change – symptoms; change of – rapid
  - Dryness of usually moist internal parts
  - Heat – lack of vital heat
  - Numbness
  - Pain – shooting pain
  - Pulsation
  - Stiffness – Joints
  - Sudden manifestation
  - Tension – Joints; of
  - Trembling – Externally

Note: There appears to be a similarity between the themes of the passerines and the lepidoptera – both groups seem to align strongly with the Sanguine temperament, with naivety, giggling and childlike innocence along with sudden changeability.

Falco peregrinus disciplinatus (Trained peregrine falcon)

Phylum: Chordata.
Class: Aves.
Order: Falconiformes.
Family: Falconidae.

The Peregrine Falcon is one of 38 species of the genus Falco, the true falcons, which includes the Kestrel and the Merlin. However, such is the representative importance of the bird that it gave its name to the Falconiformes the whole order of diurnal raptors that includes eagles, hawks, vultures and buzzards. There are several features that distinguish the falcons from other raptors. They do not build nests but lay their eggs in "scrapes", depressions made on cliff ledges, in holes in trees or even on the ground. They have proportionally longer and narrower wings than the eagles and hawks which makes them stronger and faster in the air but less manoeuvrable close to the ground. They have a "tomial tooth" a projection on the upper beak with a corresponding notch on the lower one. This serration allows them to kill their prey immediately with a bite to the back of the neck and they do not generally have to contend with a struggling victim as the hawks do.[8]

Proving by: **Misha Norland and Peter Fraser, Devon UK (1997).**[8]

Keywords
Humiliation / Detached / **Wild stallion** / Freedom / Prostitute / Disintegrating / Danger / **Reckless** / Estranged / Abused / Coition – forced / Whipped / **Tethered** / **Shackles** / Escape / Force to be reckoned with / Powerful

A portrait of abuse. Standing up to the oppressor
The homeopathic remedy made from this powerful bird who is hooded, tethered and trained to return to the hand of the oppressor has proven itself to be a remarkable remedy for individuals who have suffered abuse. Along with Haliaee-tus leucocephalus (bald eagle, proven by Sherr), Falcon has become a modern polychrest and a type-remedy for other birds of prey with smaller provings. These SRP rubrics reveal the inner state of the provers who took the dose:

- *Ailments from – sexual humiliation*
- Anger – cold and detached
- **Delusions**
  - Danger; impression of – fear; but without
  - Disintegrating; the world is
  - *Horses – she is a reined in wild stallion that desires to be free*
  - *Prostitute; is a*
  - Separated – world; from the – he is separated – detached from it; being in the present yet
  - Unsupported
- Detached – daily activity; from
- *Driving – desire for driving – fast – reckless and indifferent to consequences*
- Estranged – children; flies from her own
- Reproaching oneself – stands up for himself; then

Dreams
- **Abused; being**
- Asserting herself
- Carefree
- Childbirth – worthlessness; with feeling of
- **Coition – forced**
- Eating – meat – raw
- Eating – human flesh
- **Whipped; getting**

Characteristic physicals
- Head
  - Pain – extending to – eyes
    - § Sides – alternating sides
    - § Temples – pulsating pain
    - § Temples – extending to –
      Temple to temple; from
- Vertigo
  - *Intoxicated; as if – waking; on*
- Vision
  - Acute
  - Bright – objects seem brighter
  - Colours before the eyes – swirling
  - Nearer; objects seem
  - Spirals
- Ear
  - Water; sensation of – in ear
- Nose
  - Odours; imaginary and real –
    nauseating
  - Smell – acute – unpleasant odours
- Face
  - Expression – cold, distant
- Mouth
  - Soft – Tongue – sensation as if
- Throat
  - Foreign body; sensation of a –
    swallowing – amel. – while; for a
  - Mucus – swallow – neither be
    swallowed nor hawked up; can
- Stomach
  - Alive in; sensation as if something
  - Appetite – ravenous – noon
  - Enlarged – sensation of
    enlargement
  - Trembling
- Abdomen
  - Pain – menses would appear; as if
  - Pain – twisting pain
- Stool
  - Forcible, sudden, gushing –
    explosion; like an

- Male
  - Coition – enjoyment – increased
  - Sexual desire – diminished –
    apathy; with
- Female
  - Coition – aversion to – clawing
    and biting to avoid
  - Coition – enjoyment – absent
  - Excrescences
  - Leukorrhea – offensive – fish-
    brine, like
  - Menses – copious – short
    duration; and
  - Ovulation – early
  - Pain – Vagina – coition – during –
    sore
  - Sexual desire – diminished –
    indifference; with
- Chest
  - Ceases to beat; as if heart – had
    ceased
  - Eruptions – Mammae – painful –
    touch; to
  - Pain – Mammae – Nipples –
    stitching pain
  - Palpitation of heart – tumultuous,
    violent, vehement – chest; as if
    heart beat throughout the
- Back
  - Heaviness, weight – Cervical
    region
- Extremities
  - Enlargement – sensation of – Legs
  - Eruptions
    - § Burning
    - § Dry
    - § Elbows – psoriasis, patches
  - Nails; complaints of – growth of
    nails – rapid – Fingernails
  - Separated sensation – Legs – body;
    as if separated from his
- Generals
  - Wavelike sensations

CASE 3.4 Gallstones

Patient: Female, age 40

Prescription: Falco-pe 200c

∫ "Feeling **hemmed in and un-free, constrained, limited.** I am **flighty,** flitty, having crazy ideas, flying, flitting about, trying out new things, but find it **difficult to ground myself. I don't like being tethered really.** If I am feeling flighty, without a tether, I am on the verge of some stupid behaviour or addiction . . . [*Tethered?*] I was thinking of horses. Used to love horse riding. **Having wild horses tethered to the inside, seems a bit mean.** For their survival, they also need food and shelter and looking after, and the hooves looked after. That ensures that they can go off onto the fields and the moors."

∫ "Tethered isn't as bad as hemmed in or constrained – if a horse really wanted to get away it could chew through – *it is only a bit of rope* . . . Hemmed in, constrained is like **shackles. Just being a prisoner** – having physical or mental constraints. I always keep something back – **don't ever want to completely trust anything** or anyone. That to me is weakness. I respect it in other people. I wouldn't be able to leave myself that **vulnerable or exposed.** . . . People is what I have always done – helping and supporting them and **making them fly.** But I am also mega critical of people too – they piss me off to the max. I am a critical person. I give a running psychological breakdown of every person I meet. I am good at reading people, and reading myself. . . . When alone with my thoughts it sparks an idea. Innovative ideas, solutions to problems and I get excited about that. That can happen with the right person, but there's not many of the right people out there that I can **bounce and buzz** off. . . . I would like to reach a stage **where intimacy, touching and sex are not a chore, a problem, an evil thing, a guilty thing, a bad thing.** . . . Find myself difficult to manage – I **feel overwhelmed by life and people, to have people in my personal space, or ask me in-depth questions.** . . . Being cutoff is about feeling cutoff from my body – **of feeling so hateful about myself, better to just cut it off.** I can experience pain quite easily – I can get into a zone where I **can be in pain and it not hurt.**" (Air / Underworld)

∫ "My mind is just **planning escape routes** – there's always a backup plan. That's where it comes from – If I am totally honest, it is a **fear of intimacy. It is survival, escape route,** not giving myself fully to one thing. Someone else might leave, or I might leave, or this building could set on fire. I'm never totally there . . . **I am a force to be reckoned with** – its powerful – **I feel powerful.** Its like harnessing an energy – feel in the pit of my stomach – I know that you would feel that and **you would back off** and that I wouldn't need to come near you to feel that. . . . **Not keen on animals – especially mice – hate the fact that you must kill them.** Don't like the unexpectedness of them. . . ."

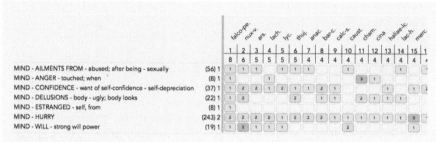

		falco-pe.	nux-v.	ars.	lach.	lyc.	thuj.	anac.	barc.	calc-s.	caust.	cham.	cina	haliae-lc.	lach.	merc.
		1	2	3	4	5	6	7	8	9	10	11	12	13	14	15	1
		8	6	5	5	5	5	4	4	4	4	4	4	4	4	4	4
MIND - AILMENTS FROM - abused; after being - sexually	(56) 1	1	1	1		1	1	1				1			1		
MIND - ANGER - touched; when	(8) 1	1			1								3	1			
MIND - CONFIDENCE - want of self-confidence - self-deprecation	(37) 1	1	2	2	1	2	1	1	2	1			1		1	2	
MIND - DELUSIONS - body - ugly; body looks	(22) 1	1	2			2		1	1		2	1	1			
MIND - ESTRANGED - self, from	(8) 1	1															
MIND - HURRY	(243) 2	2	2	2	1	1	2	2	2	1	1	1	1	1	3		
MIND - WILL - strong will power	(19) 1	1	3	1	1	1				2				1		

Figure 3.5 *Repertorisation*

MIND – Delusion – horses – she is a reined in wild stallion that desires to be free: (1) falco-pe.

Geococcyx californianus (Greater roadrunner)

Phylum: Chordata.
Class: Aves.
Order: Cuculiformes.
Family: Cuculidae.

The *Greater roadrunner* is a long-legged bird in the cuckoo family – a diverse family, well known for the parasitic breeding habits of many members, in which they lay eggs in another species' nest and leave the young to be reared by the hosts. In contrast to most others of the cuckoo family, the *Greater roadrunner* usually builds their own nest. They can maintain a speed of 30 km per hour over long distances, placing their head and tail parallel to the ground, and using their tail as a rudder to help shift direction. They kill prey by holding the victim in their bill and slamming it repeatedly against the ground. The roadrunner survives in a desert environment by a number of physiological and behavioural adaptations: they reabsorb water from their faeces prior to excretion and their nasal gland eliminates excess salt, instead of using the urinary tract like most birds.

Proving by: **Todd Rowe, AZ, USA (2004).**[5]

Keywords
Armour / **Heaviness** / Paroxysms / Benevolence / **Dirty** / Invincible / Adulterous / Old / Violent / Dancing / Deceived / Escaping / Ravenous / Bloated / Nesting / Insolent / Frantic / Sexy / Flirting

Keynote
Generals – heaviness – armour; as if wearing a suit of; external

Mind

- **Delusions**
  - ○ *Body* – *heavy* and thick; body has become
  - ○ Dirty – everything is
  - ○ *Dirty* – he is
  - ○ *Invincible*; he is
  - ○ Separated – body and mind are separated
- **Anxiety**
  - ○ Causeless
  - ○ Conscience; anxiety of
  - ○ Paroxysms; in
  - ○ Sudden
- Abrupt
- Absentminded – dreamy
- Activity – desires activity
- *Adulterous*
- Ailments from – anticipation
- Amorous
- Benevolence
- Checking – twice or more; must check
- Clairvoyance
- *Coquettish – too much*

- Defiant
- Detached
- Ecstasy
- *Escape*; attempts to
- Exhilaration
- Fancies – *lascivious*
- Fastidious
- Fear – old; of getting
- Fear – riding in a carriage; when
- Freedom
- ***Heaviness; sensation of***
- Home – desires to go
- Impatience
- Insolence
- Irritability – trifles; from
- Jealousy
- Jesting
- Laughing
- Laziness
- Orientation; sense of – increased
- Thoughts – Rapid / Sexual / Violent
- Time – quickly, appears shorter; passes too
- Tranquillity – morning – waking; on

Dreams

Animals / Caring – another person; about / Childbirth / Clairvoyant / Dancing / Deceived; being / Dirty / Escaping / Pregnant – being / Spiders / Trap – being trapped

Characteristic physicals

- **Stomach**
  - ○ Appetite – ravenous – morning – waking; on
- **Female**
  - ○ Pain – uterus – menses – during
- **Skin**
  - ○ Eruptions – menses – during
- **Extremities**
  - ○ Pain
    - § Upper limbs – night
    - § Buttocks, nates
    - § Pressing – hips
    - § Pulsating, throbbing

- **Generals**
  - ○ Coldness – bed; in
  - ○ Heat – Flushes of – morning
  - ○ Lassitude – Night
  - ○ Pain – Tearing – menses – during
  - ○ Swelling
    - § Menses – during
    - § Glands, liver, spleen etc. – menses, during
  - ○ Weariness – Night
  - ○ Weather
    - § Damp, rainy, wet – amel.
    - § Warm, wet, sultry – amel.

Proving

- Extreme jaw and teeth pain; worse in evening; "like someone has hold of your jaw and is squeezing it as hard as they can; very sharp pain".
- Lachrymation, tired sensation and blurred vision.
- Severe excruciating pain in the abdomen; "so severe that I can hardly stand it; cramping and digging; around the umbilicus".
- Cramping in the uterus during the menses.
- Ravenous appetite and thirst; "no matter how much I eat, I want more; felt like I was starving and hadn't eaten in weeks; stomach feels empty; felt dehydrated like I needed to drink a lot".
- Dryness in the lips, face, mouth, cough, nose, throat, stool and extremities.
- Peculiar sensation of tension in the skin.
- SRP – Intense craving for swimming in cold water.

Provers speaking as one

"The fatigue felt like I was wearing a suit of **armour** . . . Feeling of **heaviness**; felt like **cement** was solidifying in my veins. . . . Feel big, **swollen** and oedematous like a sausage; feel **fat** and **bloated**; feel heavy; feel like I have gained 10 pounds. . . . I am less co-dependent overall; I no longer feel like a **martyr**; I was always doing for others and not considering myself in the past. . . . Feeling doubts about my life and that I **wasted my life**. . . . I feel extremely **dirty**, even after I clean; my hair especially feels dirty even after I washed it; must wash my hair every day and still not clean; feel dirty when I am cleaning. . . . Feeling jealous; felt left out by others . . . depressed and lethargic . . . **calmness** and **focus**; won at my golf tournament; *much less nervous than usual*. . . . **Anxiety attacks** when driving; I cannot turn my head; *flesh tingles; feel I could pass out any moment*. . . . **Nesting**; just want to be a mom; the messiness of my house is bothering me. . . . I seem to be joking more and poking jokes to create an atmosphere of **friendship** and **laughter**. . . . Played a joke on somebody in the parking lot and usually I would not do that; I popped the trunk and scared them; feeling more playful; giggling. . . . **Insolent; Sullen; Abrupt; Defiant** . . . the remedy **released me from my guilt** which had been carried through all my life from my catholic upbringing . . . I feel **strong, powerful** and **knowing**; I no longer let anyone push me around . . . I feel **invincible**; strong convictions that I can do anything . . . Feel **inward calm and peace**; usually I am **frantic**, overly busy, **running** and wearing myself out; I am content to be doing nothing productive; I feel calm, cool and collected . . . **flirting** with a stranger in the presence of my husband fully aware of what I was doing and also quite **proud** of my **appearance**; I felt young, **attractive** and **sexy**. . . . Dream themes: Groups; Shunned; Panic, frantic and hurried; Rescue; Confrontation; Target Stores; Leadership role. . . ."[5]

Note

It is interesting to see themes of dirtiness coming through in an earth-bound bird. These qualities are more commonly associated with the insects, *whose transformative direction is away from the grubbiness of the earth, to the freedom of the sky.* [Fraser][4]

Haliaeetus leucocephalus (Bald eagle)

Phylum: Chordata.
Class: Aves.
Order: Accipitriformes.
Family: Accipitridae.

The bald eagle is a powerful flier, soaring on thermal convection currents to reach gliding speeds of 56–70 km/h. Its dive speed is between 120–160 km/h. They typically require mature coniferous or hardwood trees for perching, roosting and nesting. They are opportunistic carnivores with the capacity to consume a great variety of prey; swooping, turning and thrusting with razor-sharp talons and large hooked beak. Primarily a scavenger, they hunt only when there is no more easily available source of food. Though often solitary, bald eagles congregate at communal roosts and feeding sites, particularly in winter. These groups can be boisterous, with birds jostling for position and bickering over prey. They have a fast metabolism and must eat a tremendous amount to survive. It is the national bird of the United States of America.

Provings by: **Jeremy Sherr, UK and Israel (1995)[6] and Hans Eberle, Germany (1996–7).**[19]

Keywords
Danger / Betrayed / Outcast / Prisoner / Hell / Flight from reality / Egotism / Fragmentation of will / **Abyss** / Shameful / Ambition / Energised / Wild beast / Chaotic / World peace / Riots / Rape / Speeding / Father / Diplopia / **Vision** / **Conflict** / **Crack** / **Crevice** / Crazy / Frenzy / Control / Self-destructive / Belligerent / Sarcastic / Disintegrate

Nucleus
- ***Being in the present* vs. *flight from reality.***
- Symmetry, light and integration *vs.* Fragmentation, pulled into the abyss / chasm / crack. . . .
- Feeling outcast, imprisoned and betrayed . . . Frenzied, maniacal energy. . . .
- Aurum-like ambition followed by disintegration and suicidal tendencies.
- "They move between two worlds: *the world of daily life and the world of the dream.* The one informs the other and the ability to participate freely in both is essential to their well-being. Excessive difficulty in either of these worlds hinders this process and they feel stuck and trapped".[10]

Fundamental delusions[6]
- *Crack in his soul, or in the universe*
- *Pulled – he was – two directions; in*
- Danger; impression of (*cf. Animals, Lac-del, Lac-lup, Falcon, Stramonium*)
- Laughed at and mocked at; being (*cf. Baryta*)
- Legs – shorter; her legs are (*cf. Baryta*)

Aves / Birds   **143**

SRP delusions[6]

- *Betrayed*; that she is
- *Outcast*; she were an
- *Prisoner*; she is a
- *Hell* – in; is
- House – burning down; her house is
- Looking – down; he were looking

- Enlarged – body is – *fat; feeling –* pale and ugly
- Visions; has – suns; of two
- Eyes – further round side of head
- Awareness heightened – body; of – *centred in body; feels*

Mind[19]

- Ailments from – *egotism*
- Ambition – increased – *means employed; every possible*
- Confusion of mind – lost feeling
- Contemptuous – self; of
- Dancing – wild
- Decisive
- Delusions – *better than others; he is*
- Despair – *social position; of*
- Discontented – himself, with – whatever he did; about
- Energised feeling
- Fear – attacked; fear of being

- Haughty – *clothes – best clothes; likes to wear his*
- High places – desire
- Litigious
- Pedant
- Sensual
- *Shameful*
- Unification – sensation of unification universe; with the
- Violence – aversion to
- Whistling – jolly
- Wretched

Dreams[6]

Animals – attacked by a **wild beast**; of being / Blindness / **Chaotic** / Criminals, of / *Death – shadow of death; about the* / *Detective*; she is a / Fragmented / **Genealogy**; of / Ghosts / Leg – she has no legs / Lizards / Machines – **perpetual motion** or seismic activity monitor / Maps – old / Observing – participating in her dreams; rather than / *Parallel lines* / Prisoner – being taken a / Rape / Riots / Sun – being in the / **Unicorn** / *Watching – herself from above* / Waves – tidal wave / **World peace**; of

Dreams[19]

Abyss – **steep** / Accidents – fatal accident / Death – relatives; of – father; of his / Falling – danger of – height; from a / **Father** / Feasting / Forsaken; being / Helping – people – distress; in / House – old – dirty; and / Jumping – leaps; great / **Speeding** / Terror

Characteristic physicals

- **Eye**
  - Hyperesthesia – Retina
  - Open lids – sensation as if open – wide open
  - Pain – Cornea
  - Thickening – Cornea; of
- **Vision**
  - Accommodation – defective
  - Acute
  - Diplopia – below the other; one image seen
  - Diplopia – vertical
- **Nose**
  - Odours; imaginary and real – burnt – wood
- **Face**
  - Cracking in articulation of jaw

- **Female**
  - Masturbation; disposition to
  - Uterus – extending to – Hips – stitching pain
  - Larynx and trachea – Voice – deep
- **Chest**
  - Swelling – Axillae – Glands – painful
- **Perspiration**
  - Clammy – right side of body
- **Skin**
  - Heat – fever; without
- **Generals**
  - Air; open – desire for open air – mountain air
  - Menses – during – beginning of menses – amel.
  - Tension – Muscles; of
  - Weariness – eating – after – agg.

Provers speaking as one[6]

"It is like there's a **conflict**, a **chasm**, inside and my symptoms are just the surface rumblings. . . Want to antidote the remedy, but I've set out on this course and I don't think it is possible. I need to follow where it goes. It feels like a process you can't stop. A **crevice**, a **crack** that gets longer and deeper. As long as I keep busy, I'm okay . . . Like being on the edge of an **abyss**, a **crevice** that's **cracking** more deeply all the time. A crack that gets deeper and longer . . . Like there's this deep, deep, deep crack that's getting deeper and deeper. The crack is in the universe or me. It is very deep, my soul . . . Head feels **crazy**. Friends noted that I was very funny and had lots of **energy**, but sort of crazy. Everybody noticed I was in a very strange place. Hilarity – uncontrolled giggling alternating with seriousness. An **overblown reaction** to the situation . . . I can't stand it any longer. **Spiralled** and spiralled and spiralled. Feel like I'm going **mad**, like there's no **escaping** out of this. Pull, pull, **like a hypoglycaemic who hasn't eaten** and just wants to scream and yell. While I was in the shower I just wanted to kill. Feel like **I'm going to lose it**. Going stir crazy; everything is aggravated. Looking for something to antidote the remedy with and I couldn't find it. . . . In a total **frenzy** (*cf. Schistocerca americana*), like steaming **horses** that had **escaped**, running down the road (*cf. Falcon*). Very **hard to keep any control**, to be patient in traffic or the grocery store. Couldn't handle it any longer . . . I felt I had to antidote, or I thought I **might commit suicide**. I was on the edge. I thought I would **go over the edge** . . . From noon on through 11 pm, when I went to bed, felt almost **maniacal**. This feeling seems to come from my brain without much **anxiety feeling in my solar plexus**. . . . I spanked the kids for the first time in years because they had been fighting and I wanted to make a point. The strange thing was that **I did not feel remorse**, as usual, for spanking them. . . . I am deeply in touch with a **self-destructive** sense inside, the part of me that wants to **disintegrate** and **die** (*Miasm – syphilitic*). Dis-integrate, the opposite of integral **oneness**, the opposite direction. I'll have another **egg** to ground me. . . . I became **sarcastic** and very **belligerent** . . . I was in a depressed state, lost my good feeling and was angry at being asked to explain the depression. She asked me, "What do you mean?" and I said, "F*** off. If you don't understand that, too bad. Do you understand that? Do you know the English language? . . . I considered committing suicide. Feeling that life has passed me by. Thinking about my mortality. **Terrified of dying. My time has run out.**" He absolutely did not want to speak to anyone during this period. "I felt completely unable to communicate during this period." He was especially averse to any kind of phone calls and would not answer the phone or would hang up. (*Miasm – syphilitic*) . . . I kept seeing deep purple light – amazingly deep. Watched the sun rise over the house – I had a desire for **symmetry in the sky**. I felt there should be two suns. Strange because it has been so hot. An image of **light radiating towards me** – white light/full spectrum. . . . My eyes feel wide open when they are not. Unusual that I'm feeling the width and depth of the **wide openness**. I feel as if my eyes are taking in a lot of light. Repositories of light. . . . The remedy worked very directly on my will. **Fragmentation is the denial of will. Integration is the use of will.** All separate states under a unified country. . . . On chasing an escaped rabbit, wondering how it would taste. . . . I'm high up and there is water below me, and I have an image of a few of my breast feathers floating on the water. Between the breast feathers, the reflection of a very pink dawn. Noticed all birds in pairs. Thoughts of flying – Icarus![6]

Passer domesticus (House sparrow)

Phylum: Chordata.
Class: Aves.
Order: Passeriformes.
Family: Passeridae.

The house sparrow is strongly associated with human habitation, living alongside humans in urban and rural settings. Because of their numbers, ubiquity, and association with human settlements, the house sparrow is extensively – and usually unsuccessfully – persecuted as an agricultural pest. "Sparrows are one of the most sociable birds. They like to nest close together and do not like nesting sites where only one nest can be constructed. They also congregate together and play together. In the winter they form large gangs that will go off to maraud newly harvested or seeded fields. Not only do they like the company of their own kind but they seem to really like the company of humans. They like their nests to be as close as possible to human habitations, even though this does not seem to be necessary to their feeding habits. It is possible that they feel some sort of protection from the presence of humans, that many of their predators are afraid of man and so it is safer to be near human habitation."[11] Passerines generally have elliptical or short, rounded wings, designed for fast take-off speeds, sprinting ability and great manoeuvrability. They tend to have 30–70% higher metabolic rates than either non-passerines or mammals.

Proving by: **Misha Norland and Peter Fraser, Devon, UK (2004).**[11]

Keywords
Noble / Accused / Criminal / Crushed / Martyr / Starved / Wild / **Pugnacious** / Defiant / **Buzzing** / Fizzing / Ballistic / Standing up to bullies / Berserk / Mischievous / **Insulted** / Reckless / *Respect* – desires / Coquettish

Polarity
Nobility and greatness *vs.* sinned, crushed, accused and punished. Defiant, pugnacious and fizzing.

Fundamental delusions
- Great person; is a – reverenced by all around her; she ought to be (*cf. Hamamelis*)
- Looking – down; he was looking – high place; from a (*cf. Platina*)
- Noble; being (*cf. Platina*)
- Above it all; she is

SRP delusions
- Accused; she is (*cf. Zinc*)
- Criminal; he is a (*cf. Ferrum Series*)
- Crushed – she is (*cf. Insecta*)
- Hunter; he is a
- Martyr; of being a
- Old – looks old; he
- Prisoner; she is a
- Sinned; one has
- Starve – being starved (*cf. Iodatums, naja*)
- Swelling; he is gradually
- Wild; he would go
- Wrong – done wrong; he has – punished; and is about to be (*cf. Opium*)

Nucleus Norland[11]
"**Pugnacious** sums up the energy of Sparrow, which is coupled with a **buzzing, fizzing restless activity** and watchfulness. Like a teenager, it has an argumentative and defiant energy . . . [combined with] a powerful animal sexuality, connecting earth with spirit – the thrust to find the right partner and the right home. Top of the list, though, is their **sensitivity to being dishonoured** (*Staphisagria*). For sparrows, this feels unjustified; though drab to look at, and not being the possessor of a beautiful song, they feel themselves to be just dandy – a beautiful bird! *In Sparrow, the feeling of being under attack is as strong as is the violent reaction. 'I can stand up for myself and shall not be bullied!'. . .*" (Misha Norland). Dominant theme: disrespected, dishonoured and hounded out, singled out and killed – in imminent danger of extermination. Opposite: victory over injustice (*Causticum*) leading to feeling accepted and honoured"[11]

Mind

- Attracting others
- Busy – fruitlessly
- Confident – natural; feels safe to be
- Contact; desire for
- Coquettish – too much
- *Delusions – great person – reverenced by all around her; she ought to be*
- *Delusions – insulted; he is*
- Desires – full of desires – fast things
- Disposing of old things
- Driving – desire for driving – fast – reckless and indifferent to consequences
- Femininity – increased sensation of
- Fleeing away
- Forsaken feeling – beloved by his family and friends; feeling of not being
- *Giggling*
- *High-spirited*
- Honest
- Indifference – conscience; to the dictates
- Indifference – welfare of others; to
- Industrious
- Irritability – talk of others; from – loud
- Maternal instinct; exaggerated
- *Mischievous*
- Music – desire for
- Observer – being an – oneself; of
- **Overactive**
- Playful
- *Respected – desire to be*
- Sensitive – rudeness, to
- Speed – desire for
- *Talking – others agg.; talk of*
- *Talking – pleasure in his own talk*
- **Tough**
- Trance
- Tranquility – problems; not bothered by little
- Truth – telling the plain truth

Dreams

Amorous – orgasm; with / Animals – dangerous / Animals – killing / **Animals – protecting; he is** / Children; about – danger; in – water / Children; about – looking after / Children; about – wildness of / Coition – presence of others; in the / Dead bodies – smell of dead bodies / Death – fear of death; losing the / Driving – car; a – fast / Driving – car; a – recklessly / **Fire – house on fire; setting a** / Horses – running / House – old-fashioned / House – people in her house / Losing – family; his / Maggots / Remorse – want of remorse / Shooting; is / Snakes – fear, without / Soldier – being a / Teeth – becoming loose / Wasteland / Waves – huge wave approaching / Wolves

Physicals

- **Vertigo**
  - Room – entering a room; on
- **Head**
  - Pain – Lying down – agg.
  - Pain – Forehead – Eyes – above – left – lancinating
  - Prickling – Vertex
- **Eye**
  - Foreign body; as from a – hair; as from
- **Vision**
  - Accommodation – action too great
- **Hearing**
  - Acute – noise; to – slightest noise
- **Throat**
  - Bubbling in esophagus
  - Choking – sleep – during
  - External Throat – cold air agg.

- **Neck**
  - Spasms
  - Stiffness – one side
- **Abdomen**
  - Pain – breathing – hindering breathing
  - Pulsation – Ilium; crest of
  - Trembling – sensation of
- **Female**
  - Pain – Ovaries – extending downward
- **Chest**
  - Clothing agg. – bra feels tight
  - Pain – Clavicles – stitching pain – intermittent
  - Pain – Mammae – right – cutting pain
  - Prickling – Mammae
  - Stretching – amel.

- **Back – Pain**
  - Cervical region – looking – upward – agg.
  - Cervical region – motion – agg. – sore
  - Dorsal region – Scapulae – right – extending to – left
- **Extemities**
  - Jerking – sleep – going to Sleep; on – agg.
  - Numbness – Fingers – Third Finger – right
  - Pain
  - Blow; pain as from a
  - Feet – left – cramping
  - Shoulders – blow; pain as from a
  - Stiffness – Hips – motion agg.; beginning

Generals

- Buzzing
- Energy – sensation of
- Heat – sensation of – walking agg.
- Injuries – blunt instruments; from
- Injuries – contusion – bruises; and
- Weather – rainy – amel.

Provers speaking as one

"Physical fight with my daughter. I am a single mother – hit her on her head and wanted to do it more often, I walked behind her and did it again sometimes I do it as a reflex in certain situations – and feel *guilty because I did not control myself.* I felt tearful and angry afterwards, but **without regret, I wanted to show her that I am the boss; the adult, the mother!** I felt *unsupported* and somehow helpless for a few minutes. Don't want to live anymore! Want peace instead of quarrels. I felt exhausted. **I felt like throwing her out of the house so that I can live in peace. I am full of hate and I feel no regret. I want to have it done my way.** . . . . I could be one of the lads out on the town. We could get pissed, start a fight and have a right laugh. The fighting part of this comment is not an old symptom. **Go ballistic. Yes. Fight.** . . . . There seem to be issues for people around me about **standing up to bullies** and also about armed robbery. No one can bully you unless you let them. I don't think anyone would bully me at the moment! . . . . There has been a profound **deepening of my spiritual awareness** – that everything is one and that although everything matters, even the smallest blade of grass . . . A feeling that **I am the King of all I survey**. . . . During the proving I felt I wanted to be **honoured** and be honourable. I also felt accused, attacked . . . I feel totally able to **stand my ground** and state my case without becoming confused or embarrassed, or intimidated when he starts to raise his voice and it becomes emotionally charged. . . . **Want to drive my car full pelt to loud fast heavy metal.** Thank god the roads are wet so I can't go wild on my bike. There's something inside of me that's **faster, nastier, more raging, more berserk, it is totally wild.** The depth of this feeling has an extra edge that I don't recognise. It is fucking **crazy in an instant, wildly explosive.** It seems to be intensifying as the full moon comes. Something's going to get broken at this rate. Propensity to excitement growing with full moon. . . . The feeling of well-being is starting to spill over into mild hyperactivity. I am **buzzing – excited, focused**, feel I have fantastic concentration, socially too wired and not as empathetic as I would like . . . I feel so **fizzy** inside, there is too much going on in my head, and **I hop from one thought to the next.**"[11]

Pavo cristatus (Blue peafowl / Peacock)

Phylum: Chordata.
Class: Aves.
Order: Galliformes.
Family: Phasianidae.

"The peafowl is a member of the order of Galliformes which includes pheasants and turkeys. The Latin name Pavo derives from the Sanskrit epithet Pavana meaning Purity. The most notable feature of the Peacock is the magnificent tail. The iridescent nature of the feathers is caused by light interference in the nano-structure of the barbules of the feather. The peacock is one of the most extreme examples of the idea of sexual selection. In this aspect of evolution, a feature not necessarily of value in survival is selected for as an indication of overall fitness and general good health. The importance of this feature in mating rituals means it becomes more important and more overblown until it can become a liability and yet is still selected for. It is usually the male that displays these features indicating that the power of choice in sexual selection lies with the female."[17]

Proving by: **Peter Fraser, Nepal and UK (2006).**[17]

Keywords
Failure / Neglected / Trapped / Spirituality / Meditating / Feasting / Flying / Underground / Formication / Twitching / Pulsating

Mind

- *Anxiety – money matters; about*
- Cheerful
- Company – aversion to – desire for solitude
- Company – desire for – friend; of a
- Confidence – want of self-confidence – *failure*, feels himself a
- Dancing
- Delusions
  - *Neglected* – he or she is neglected
  - *Succeed; he does everything wrong; he cannot*
  - Trapped; he is
- Discouraged
- Emotions – spontaneous and natural
- Fear
  - Mice
  - Rats
- Fear – social position; about his
- High places – desire
- Indifference
- Indignation

- **Irritability**
  - Family; to her
  - Friend; to her
  - Husband; towards
  - Talking – while
- Laziness
- Love – friends; for
- *Meditating*
- *Observer – being an*
- Plans – making many plans
- Restlessness – drives him from place to place
- Sadness
  - Morning
  - Alone – when
- Sociability
- *Spirituality*
- Sympathetic
- Taciturn
- *Tranquillity – settled, centred and grounded*
- Wildness

Dreams

Amorous – fallen in love; has / Animals – wild / Army / Blood / **Bridge** / Celebrations / Children; about – lost / Classroom / Coloured – red / Dancing / Driving – car; a / **Eating – human flesh** / Elephants / *Escaping* / Examinations – failing an exam / Eyes / Failures / **Failures – examination** / Fear / **Feasting** / **Feeding** / **Flying** / Food / *Food – preparing food* / Forest / Friends – old / **God**; of / Grandparents; of / House / Ignored; she is / Insects / *Jungle* / **Killing** / Metal; about / Model; famous / **Mountains** / People – crowds of / *Photographs*, taking / **Praying** / Refrigerator / **Religious** / Revenge / River / School / Seeing again an old schoolmate / Shoes / Shopping / Snakes / Snow / Statue / Swimming / Thirsty, being / Tigers / **Underground** / *Water – dirty | muddy* / Work

Characteristic physicals

- **Vertigo**
  - Rising – sitting; from – agg.
- **Head**
  - Pain
    - § sleep – amel.
    - § sleep – preventing
    - § Sides – alternating sides – stitching pain
    - § Sides – right – then left

- **Eye**
  - Heaviness
  - Pain
    - § Opening the eyes – agg.
    - § *Pulsating* pain
    - § Reading – agg. – burning
    - § Extending to – Head
  - *Twitching* – Lids

- **Ear**
  - *Air – Sensation of air – In ear*
  - Boring fingers in – amel.
- **Face**
  - Pain – Opening the mouth agg.
- **Mouth**
  - Aphthae
- **Throat**
  - Pain – *sharp*; as from something
- **Chest**
  - Pain
    - § Inspiration – agg.
    - § Heart – Region of
    - § Heart – Region of – stitching pain
    - § Sides – left – *expiration agg.*
    - § Sides – left – *inspiration agg.*
    - § Twitching – Heart; region
- **Stomach**
  - Nausea – riding – carriage; in a – agg.
  - Pain – raw; as if
- **Abdomen**
  - *Formication*
  - *Twitching and jerking* – Sides
- **Back**
  - Coldness – ice; as from
  - Pain – Cervical region – extending to – Head

- **Extremities**
  - Emaciation – Legs
  - Eruptions – Upper limbs – vesicles – itching
  - Lightness; sensation of – Lower limbs – Legs
  - Pain
    - § Elbows – left – stitching pain
    - § Feet – Soles – bed – in bed – agg. – burning
    - § Feet – Spots; in
    - § Legs – paroxysmal
    - § Nates – cutting pain
  - Paralysis
    - § Feet – sensation of
    - § Hands – sensation of
  - Trembling – Hands – holding objects on
- **Sleep**
  - Position – stomach; on
- **Skin**
  - Eruptions
    - § *Suppurating*
    - § *Vesicular* – itching
- **Generals**
  - Numbness
  - Spots – symptom occurring in

Spheniscus humboldti (Humboldt penguin)

Phylum: Chordata.
Class: Aves.
Order: Sphenisciformes.
Family: Spheniscidae.

Penguins are flightless birds with a much heavier and more robust skeleton than birds that fly, as the lightness of bone would give them no evolutionary advantage. Their feathers are waterproof and they are incredibly natural swimmers, whilst moving clumsily on land. Each feather has small muscles allowing them to be held tightly against the body whilst swimming. When on land, the same muscles hold the feathers erect, trapping a thick layer of warm air to provide effective insulation against bitterly cold winds. In 2009 at the Bremerhaven Zoo in Germany, two adult male Humboldt penguins adopted an egg that had been abandoned by its biological parents. After the egg hatched, the two penguins raised, protected, cared for, and fed the chick in the same manner that heterosexual penguin couples raise their own offspring.

Proving by: **Peter Mohr, Germany (YEAR).**
Published by: **Jonathan Shore.**[10]

Keywords
Repudiated / Persecuted / Revengeful / Haughty / Repulsive / Secretive / Swimming / Outsider

Delusions
- **Repudiated; he is – society; by / Outsider; being an** (*cf. Hydrogen, Leprosy miasm, Latex*)
- **Persecuted – he is persecuted** (*cf. China., Kali-br., Drosera., Spiders, Snakes*)
- Loved by parents; she is not
- Right – doing nothing right; he is
- Wrong – doing something wrong; he is

Mind
- Absentminded – dreamy – amorous
- Activity – desires activity – alternating with – indifference
- Amorous – fits of amorousness
- **Anger – causeless** (smouldering)
- Animals – love for animals – dogs
- Duty – too much sense of duty
- Estranged
- Fear – failure; of
- Forsaken feeling – beloved by his parents, wife, friends; feeling of not being
- Forsaken feeling – **isolation;** sensation
- Hatred – **revengeful; hateful and**
- **Haughty**
- **Humiliated**; feeling
- Impertinence
- Injustice; cannot support Jealousy
- Laughing – loudly
- **Litigious** (*Nit-ac.*)
- **Loathing – life** (loathing – oneself) (dd. *Lac-c*)
- Mocking – **sarcasm**
- Mood – **repulsive**
- Presumptuous
- Reserved
- Responsibility – taking responsibility too seriously
- Seaside – loves
- **Secretive**
- Sensitive – noise, to – slightest noise; to the
- **Suspicious** (Paranoid)
- Swimming – desires
- Thoughts – persistent
- Timidity

Dreams – Excrements

Phsyicals

- **Head**
  - Coldness, chilliness, etc.
  - Tired Feeling
- **Nose**
  - Coldness
- **Neck**
  - Stiffness
- **Male and female**
  - Sexual desire – excessive
- **Respiration**
  - Deep – *desire to breathe*
- **Chest**
  - Oppression
- **Sleep**
  - Waking – noise – *slight noise*, from

- **Perspiration**
  - Coldness – during
- **Extremities**
  - Coldness – Feet and Hands
  - Heat – Feet
  - Heaviness
  - Pain – Toes – First
  - Trembling
- **Generals**
  - Coldness – Affected parts
  - Food and drinks
    - § Bread – desire – butter, and
    - § Fat – desire
    - § Meat – desire
    - § Rich food – desire

Tyto alba (Barn owl feather)

Phylum: Chordata.
Class: Aves.
Order: Strigiformes.
Family: Tytonidae.

The barn owl is nocturnal, relying on its acute sense of hearing when hunting in complete darkness. They specialise in catching animals on the ground – nearly all of their food consists of small mammals. They usually mate for life unless one of the pair is killed, when a new pair bond may be formed. Barn owls are cavity nesters, seeking out holes in trees, fissures in cliff faces, old buildings such as farm sheds and church towers. They are not particularly territorial but have a home range inside which they forage. They prefer to hunt along the edges of woods or in rough grass strips adjoining pasture and have an effortless wavering flight as they quarter the ground, alert to the sounds made by potential prey. They fly silently; tiny serrations on the leading edges of the flight feathers and a hairlike fringe to the trailing edges help to break up the flow of air over the wings – reducing turbulence and the accompanying noise. During nesting, the female draws in the dry furry material of her regurgitated pellets to form a carpet of shredded pellets with which to protect her chicks.

Proving by: **Liz Stone, Wales (2003).**[20]

Keywords
Invaded / **Trapped** / **Neglected** / Suddenness / Suffocation / Destroy / Sighing / Ruins / Stiffness / Clenching teeth / Cough – tickling / Stabbing pain / **Losing space** / Accidents / **Protecting children**

SRP Delusions

- **Invaded**; one's space is being (*cf. Fungi, Corvus corax*)
- Home – away from home; he is – must get there
- Neglected – duty; he has neglected his
- Pregnant; she is
- Trapped; he is

Mind

- Accident-prone
- *Anger – destroy things; with tendency to*
- Anxiety – conscience; anxiety of (guilt)
- Change – desire for – life; in
- Detached – daily activity; from
- *Hatred – persons – offended him; hatred of persons who* (Nit-ac.)
- Hurry – always in a
- Malicious – anger, with

Fear

- Alone; of being
- Control; losing
- *Mirrors in room; of – lest he should see himself*
- Sudden
- Suffocation; of
- Wind; of

- Mistakes; making – localities; in
- Order – desire for
- Sensitive – emotions; to
- **Sighing – involuntary**
- Slowness – thought and action; delay between
- *Spaced-out feeling*
- Time – quickly, appears shorter; passes too
- Truth – telling the plain truth
- Weeping – forsaken feeling; from

Dreams

Chaotic / Face – disfigured / Family, own / Fish / Glass / House – youth; like the house of her / People – influential persons / Protecting / Rocks / Ruins

Physicals

- **Head**
  - Eruptions – Margins of hair / Scalp
  - *Pain – accompanied by – Neck – stiffness in – Nape of neck*
  - Pain – Forehead – Eyes – around
- **Eye**
  - Pain – left – *cutting pain*
  - Photophobia – light; from – bright light – agg.
- **Vision**
  - **Acute** (Birds)
- **Face**
  - Swelling – Eyes – around
- **Teeth**
  - Clenching teeth together – *desire to clench teeth together; constant*
- **Throat**
  - *Mucus – difficult to detach*
- **Cough**
  - *Tickling – Throat-pit; in*
- **Chest**
  - Mammae; complaints of
- **Back**
  - *Formication – Spine*
- **Extremities**
  - Nails; complaints of – *brittle nails*
  - Pain – Bones – aching
  - Pain – Hands – Joints – aching
  - *Tingling – Forearms*
- **Sleep**
  - Position – changed frequently
  - *Sleepiness – overpowering – afternoon*
  - *Sudden – daytime*

- **Fever**
  - Coldness – externa; with
- **Skin**
  - Burning – sun; as if burned from heat of
  - Cicatrices – itching

- **Generals**
  - Biting – teeth together; biting – agg.
  - *Energy – excess of energy*
  - Periodicity – year – every

Themes from the Proving[20]
- **Despair** and **thoughts of death** and feelings of **loss in life**.
- **Accident prone**, injuries often to extremities.
- Pain – head, extremities, chest – **stabbing**, aching, **tingling**, stiff.
- Rage and **resentment of losing space for self**.
- Weeping and despair – **Grief**.
- **Polarity** – Darkness *vs.* Light.
- Confident / Confused.
- Dreams of childhood home, of **caring and protecting children**, of journeys.
- **Sleepless and busy night time** / Sleepiness afternoon.
- Head pain – frequent, crown, frontal, varied.
- Skin eruptions / Itching.
- Respiration difficult / Cough in throat pit.
- Flushes of heat.

Vultur gryphus (Andean condor)

Phylum: Chordata.
Class: Aves.
Order: Cathartiformes.
Family: Cathartidae.

The condor is primarily a scavenger, feeding on carrion – preferring large carcasses such as those of deer or cattle. They are gregarious during the non-breeding season, feeding and roosting communally. However, they become highly territorial when nesting. It is the world's largest vulture and one of the longest-living birds, with a potential lifespan of over 70 years. In flight, they flap their wings on rising from the ground, but after attaining a moderate elevation they rely on thermals to stay aloft. Charles Darwin reportedly observed them for half an hour without witnessing a single flap of their wings. Like the turkey vulture, the Andean condor has the unusual habit of urohidrosis; emptying the cloaca onto their legs and feet to cool themselves down. Because of this habit, their legs are often streaked with a white build-up of uric acid. They prefer to roost on cliff faces, caves or small rock ledges at elevations of 3,000 to 5,000 m. The Andean condor plays an important role in the folklore and mythology of the Andean regions.

Proving by: **Elizabeth Schulz and Uli Rimmler, Germany (1997).**[3]

Aves / Birds

Keywords
Ugly / Dying / Falling / Ambition / Order / Travelling / Speed / Formication /
Metallic / Itching / Burning / Darkness / Parasite

Delusions
- Body – ugly; body looks
- Flying – Andes; over the
- High – he were high
- Parasite; she is a

Dreams
- Car – racing
- Death – dying
- Falling – pit; into a
- Prophetic
- Sexual – sexual activity

Mind
- *Addicted; tendency to become* (**cf. Birds, Mammals**)
- Ailments from – **ambition – excessive**
- Ambition – increased
- Biting nails
- Checking – twice or more; must check
- Cleanness – desire for cleaning
- *Despair – itching of the skin; from*
- Fear – narrow place; in
- Humiliated; feeling
- Humility
- **Order** – desire for
- Religious affections – too occupied with religion
- *Responsibility – taking responsibility too seriously* (*Birds, Mammals*)
- Sensitive – music; to – classical music
- Singing – amel. complaints
- **Speed** = velocity – desire for
- **Travelling** – desire for
- Violent

Characteristic physicals
- **Head**
  - Pain – Skull
- **Mouth**
  - Taste – **metallic – disgusting**
- **External Throat**
  - *Swelling – Cervical Glands*
- **Male**
  - Pain – Testes – right – **tearing** pain
- **Female**
  - Pain – Ovaries – right – **stinging**
- **Extremities**
  - Pain – Shoulders – right – **stitching**
  - Pain – Thighs – exertion – agg. – sore
- **Skin**
  - **Formication**
  - **Itching – intolerable**
- **Generals**
  - Energy – excess of energy
  - *Influenza – sensation of – beginning stage*
  - *Mononucleosis*
  - Pain – cutting pain
  - Pulsation – Externally
  - Pulsation – Internally
  - Sick feeling; vague

Themes

- Morbidity, destruction, and death
- Nourishment and food (fear of not getting enough)
- Sexuality
- Religion
- Violence, addiction, and despair
- Grief and hope

Peter Fraser[4] writes that "the role of the Vulture is to remove the dead and decaying from the world. This role is filled by bacteria, fungi and by many of the insects but the Condor is the largest of all these and represents the pinnacle of the process. Death is therefore very important in the remedy."

Provers speaking as one[3]

"Dream: I was walking through the streets and saw **dead** and living people. I was surprised and amazed that the dead ones looked like the living ones. They looked so normal and mundane, and yet I knew they were dead. To find out who was dead and who alive I asked some "Are you dead?" They replied: "What? You can see me although I am dead?" The dead people were sad and hopeless because they were no longer seen by the living and could no longer communicate with the living. The dead people walked through the streets like lost souls. They still had to do something, but they didn't know how to do it . . . I was **surrounded by darkness**. I had **fallen far** and all of a sudden there was **fire**. My body was burning; everything was **burning**. . . . *My old life was lying broken under me . . . Narrowness creates fear . . . Magic. Who ate the moon? Hades, God of the Underworld. You catch the dead soul. The light of the darkness.* . . . Many thoughts about a fast new car . . . Desire to flirt, erotic dreams. Putting things in order and away (eating carcasses, the old has to disappear)."

REPERTORY ADDITIONS FOR THE BIRDS
(made to existing rubrics in Synthesis[2])

MIND

- ADDICTED; TENDENCY TO BECOME
- AILMENTS FROM
  - § abused; after being
  - § domination
  - § **domination – long time; for a**
  - § honour; wounded
  - § **humiliation**
  - § responsibility
  - § **shame**
- AIR; IN OPEN – desire
- ATTRACTING OTHERS
- AWARENESS HEIGHTENED
- BUOYANCY
- CAREFREE
- CARING
- CLAIRVOYANCE
- COMMUNICATIVE
- CONFUSION OF MIND – **loses his way in well-known streets**
- CONFUSION OF MIND – time; as to
- CONFUSION OF MIND – time; as to – space; and
- CONNECTION; SENSE OF
- **CONSCIOUSNESS – expanded**

- DANCING
- DELUSIONS
  - § above it all; she is
  - § **abused**, being
  - § arms – **bound** to her body; arms are
  - § body – out of the body
  - § body – ugly; body looks
  - § <u>caged</u>
  - § consciousness – higher consciousness; unification with
  - § danger; impression of
  - § dominated; he is
  - § expanding
  - § floating
  - § **floating** – **air**; in
  - § **flying**
  - § life – **burdened** by
  - § light = low weight – is light; he
  - § oppressed; he were
  - § **prisoner**; she is a
  - § repudiated; he is
  - § repudiated; he is – relatives; by his
  - § separated – himself; he were separated from
  - § separated – world; from the – he is separated
  - § suffocating; as if
  - § **torture** – tortured; he is
  - § <u>trapped</u>; he is
- DETACHED
- DISTANCES – inaccurate judgement of
- DUTY
- DUTY – too much sense of duty
- ESCAPE; ATTEMPTS TO
- EXCITEMENT – nervous
- FASTIDIOUS
- FLOATING SENSATION
- FORSAKEN FEELING – isolation; sensation of
- FREEDOM
- FREEDOM – desires
- HEAVINESS; SENSATION OF
- HIGH PLACES – desire

- HONOUR – sense of honour
- HUMILIATED; FEELING
- **INDEPENDENT**
- INDIFFERENCE
- LOVE – family; for
- MEDITATING
- MISTAKES; MAKING – calculating; in
- MISTAKES; MAKING – speaking; in
- NATURE – loves
- OPEN
- ORIENTATION; SENSE OF – decreased
- PERFECTIONIST
- POWER – sensation of
- PRESSURE; EXTERNAL
- PRIDE
- PROTECTING – desire to protect
- RESPONSIBILITY – taking responsibility too seriously
- SENSITIVE – noise; to
- SHAMEFUL
- SOCIABILITY
- SPACE – desire for
- **SPEED – desire for**
- **SPIRITUALITY**
- SYMPATHETIC
- TRAVELLING – desire for
- TRUTH – telling the plain truth
- UNIFICATION – sensation of unification
- VIOLENCE
- WANDERING – desire to wander
- **VISION** – ACUTE
- **HEARING** – ACUTE
- **THROAT** – LUMP; SENSATION OF A
- **STOMACH** – APPETITE – ravenous
- **BACK**
  - <u>PAIN – Cervical region</u>
  - <u>PAIN – Dorsal region</u>
  - STIFFNESS – Cervical region
- **EXTREMITIES** – PAIN – Shoulders
- **DREAMS**
  - **CARING – another person; about**
  - DEATH

- ○ FAMILY; OWN
- ○ FLYING
- ○ TRAP – being trapped
- ○ WATCHING – herself from above
- **GENERALS**
  - ○ AIR; OPEN – desire for open air
  - ○ ENERGY – excess of energy
  - ○ EXPANSION; SENSATION OF
- ○ PAIN
  - § cramping
  - § cutting pain
  - § sharp
  - § stitching pain
- ○ **TREMBLING** – Externally
- ○ **TWITCHING**
- ○ **VIBRATION, FLUTTERING, ETC.**

References

1 Joshi B, Joshi S. *Quick Book of Minerals and Animals*. Mumbai: Serpentina Books; 2013.

2 Schroyens F. *Synthesis 9.1* (Treasure edn). Ghent: Homeopathic Book Publishers; 2009 (plus author's own additions).

3 Schulz E. *Vultur gryphus – Andean condor*. (Accessed in RadarOpus.)

4 Fraser P. *Birds – Seeking the Freedom of the Sky*. Bristol: The Winter Press; 2009.

5 Rowe T. *A proving of Roadrunner* (*Geococcyx californianus*). Phoenix AZ: AMCH Publishing; 2004.

6 Sherr J. *The Homeopathic proving of Haliaeetus leucocephalus*. In: *Dynamic Provings* Vol. 1. Malvern: Dynamis Books; 1997.

7 Attenborough D. *The Life of Birds*. London: Domino Books; 1998.

8 Norland M. *Collected Provings*. Uffculme, Devon: Yondercott Press; 1998.

9 Rowles J. *A Proving of Sialia currucoides – Mountain bluebird*. Phoenix AZ: American Medical College of Homeopathy Publishing.

10 Shore J, Schriebman J, Hogeland A. *Birds: Homeopathic Remedies from the Avian Realm*. Berkeley CA: Homeopathy West; 2004.

11 Norland M, Fraser P. *Passer domesticus – The Homeopathic Proving of Sparrow*. Devon, 2004. Available online at: *https://www.homeopathyschool.com/the-school/provings/sparrow* (Accesssed 18th September 2020.)

12 Rowe T. *Cathartes aura – A Proving of Turkey vulture*. Phoenix AZ: AMCH Publishing; 1999.

13 Sherr J. *The Homeopathic proving of Cygnus cygnus*. Malvern, 2001. Available online at: *https://homeopathyforhealthinafrica.org/product/cygnus-cygnus* (Accessed 18th September 2020.)

14 Scholten J. *Wad Stories – Homeopathic lectures from a sailing trip – Proving of Diadema exulans – The magnificent albatross*. Utrecht: Stichting Alonnissos; 2001.

15 Shephard C. *Homeopathic Proving of Calypte anna (Anna's hummingbird)*. Victoria BC; 2003. (Accessed in RadarOpus.)

16 Stirling P. *The proving of Cygnus bewickii*. Bristol, 2003. Available online at: *http://www.hominf.org/swan/swanfr.htm* (Accessed 18th September 2020.)

17 Fraser P. *Proving of Pavo cristatus*. Kathmandu, 2006. Available online at: *http://www.hominf.org/peacock/peafr.htm* (Accessed 24th September 2020.)

18 Bedayn G. *North American Raven (Corvus corax principalis (sanguis)) A new proving of the blood of a North American Raven*, 1998.

19 Eberle H, Ritzer F. *Haliaeetus leucocephalus – Bald Eagle (Blood)*. Bad Endorf, Germany, 2009.

20 Stone L. *Tyto alba – Barn Owl Feather*. Wales, 2003. Available online at: *https://welshschoolofhomeopathy.org.uk/provings/Barn_Owl_Feather.pdf* (Accessed September 20th 2020.)

21 Shah P. Drug Proving of Columbia Livia. Haren: *Homeopathic Links*; 2008.

22 Schulz E. *Cygnus olor*. (Accessed in RadarOpus.)

23 Williams S. Case of Calypte Anna: Hummingbird. *Interhomeopathy*; 2006. Available online at: *http://www.interhomeopathy.org/hummingbird* (Accessed 20th September 2020.)

24 Lilley D. *The Raven. A Flight through an Archetypal Force Field*. Glasgow: Saltire Books; 2021.

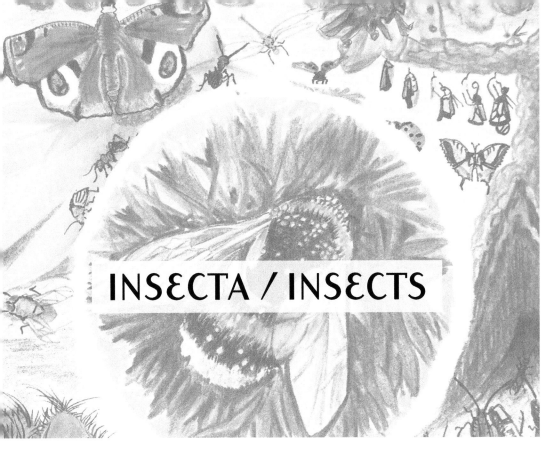

INSECTA / INSECTS

MYTHOLOGY

Uranus

Erratic, Sudden radical change, Revolution.
Metamorphosis, Unpredictability, Impatience.
Collective, New ideas, Idealism, Restlessness.
Need for excitement, Originality, Inventiveness.
Need for freedom, Purposeless rebellion.
Trapped, Independence from tradition.
Dissatisfaction, Emasculated by son.

Uranus is the first sky god who produced many offspring with Gaia. Disgusted at the sight of his own progeny (hideous beasts such as the cyclopes), he thrust them back into the womb of Gaia, banishing them to the Underworld. These aspects relate to the themes of increased sexuality and of the self-disgust found in the Insect family. The dynamic is between the Sky and the Earth which fits with Peter Fraser's concept of Insects needing to transcend the Earth to reach the freedom of the Sky.

Uranus is overthrown by his youngest son Kronus (Saturn) who plots with his mother to rid her of his father's tyranny. In this act he castrates his father, robbing him of his generative power. His genitals are cast into the ocean, and Aphrodite (Venus) is born from the sea. So, in this myth, several insect themes are present: Sexuality; prolific procreation with Uranus' disgust at his progeny. His final sexual act is to give birth to *the most* beautiful goddess in all Greek mythology. This story parallels the insect's journey from dirtiness and disgust as a grub, to metamorphosis into a beautiful and liberated winged adult.

Uranus is the planetary aspect whose sphere of influence on a person's life is associated with drastic, unpredictable and erratic change. Pluto is also concerned with transformation, but it is total annihilation and rebirth rather than metamorphosis; and thus relates more to the Actinides and Snakes. The change that Uranus governs is radical and revolutionary; suddenly reorganising the person's world around them so it is almost unrecognisable. Like the metamorphosis from Larvae to adult insect.

Uranus rules Aquarius which represents the power of the group (or hive) over the individual (Leo / Mammals). The individual is eclipsed by the society (as in the society of Bees, Termites and Ants). These individuals may compensate by busily working on self-improvement; constantly reinventing themselves and displaying a need for recognition.

Mars – Uranus

Fighting for change, transformation and the good of the collective. Revolutionary. Electrical fire. Suddenly violent. Sexual excitement.

Sensations ruled by Uranus

Dry, spasmodic, electric, explosive, convulsive, disorganizing.

Affinities

Ethers, eyes, pituitary body, gases.

INSECTS IN HOMEOPATHY

Insects have been around for much longer than we have – the nature of life is that everything lives off something else. Any organism with a blood stream is a target for the blood-sucking parasites. The host-parasite dynamic is a very deep relationship stretching far back in the collective psyche; thus, there is a very strong morphogenetic field associated with this relationship. Think of the countless millions who have suffered from malaria at the hands of the mosquito. No wonder there is such a strong feeling of loathing brought out in the homeopathic provings of parasitic insects.

Humans wage war on insects, trying our utmost to exterminate them with virulent insecticides, labelling them as pests or vermin. There are sensations of infestation and irritation; a 'get off me' feeling; 'I would tear my skin off to get rid of it'. The level of disgust felt for insects is often irrational – 'just get the damn thing out quickly'. You loathe them, they loathe you and they are loathsome. You feel dirty, invaded and foul; tearing, clutching, mutilating yourself to get rid of them (*cf.* Leprosy miasm). Parasites give a feeling of dependency; greed; laziness; taking without giving back; annoying, irritating; constantly bugging you.

Most Insects, unlike Spiders, only use their silk during the transformation from the larval stage to the adult form. The theme of metamorphosis is very strong in the natural behaviour of the Lepidoptera class, whose species undergo a massive transformation from being a small, grubby and *repulsive* larvae to becoming light, spontaneous and *beautiful* butterfly. Likewise, the Silkworm will make a cocoon within which it can turn into a pupa / chrysalis before finally metamorphosing into a Moth. The DNA is completely different from one state to the next. A less dramatic form of transformation is the process of moulting – shedding the layers that have become too restrictive (as in Beetles).

> *The insects are the things in this world for which **transformation is the most powerful and the most dramatic**. Many of them change completely in form and the transformation is from something earthbound and repulsive to something much more beautiful that is free to move through the air.* Fraser[13]

The Insect patient may also talk about the need to **reinvent** themselves, or periodically undergo **major upheavals** in their life. This may be similar to the tubercular desire to keep moving, travelling and experiencing the new. Because of the preoccupation with change and transformation, this may become a compulsive need expressing itself as purposeless rebellion or oppositional traits in children. For example, Remedies such as Culex pipiens, Cimex lectularius, Doryphora decemlineata and Musca domestica.

Uranus not only rules the process of metamorphosis, it also rules the sign Aquarius. This is the polarity point to Leo which is about expressing the creative self, being the performer and being centre stage. Aquarians acknowledge the power of groups, societies, global networks; the digital age. Ideology of the group outweighs personal power (*Leo*). They can be a spokesperson for change, renewal and progressive action in the world. Insects are vitally important to all other Animals; if they became extinct it would have disastrous ramifications for us all. Not only do they cooperate in large societies themselves, but they also contribute to the global society in their role as plant pollinators.

Termite colonies are housed in the Insect equivalent to sky-scrapers and are a true feat of engineering. These structures help to create dry islands in the flooded wetlands of the Kalahari Desert, stimulating the growth of myriad other plant and animal species whose survival depends upon these island formations. Thus there is an important and often overlooked aspect of benevolence in the insect kingdom; although the knee-jerk human response is often one of disgust or aversion, we all in fact owe a debt of gratitude to this vast and pioneering group for their ceaseless work in maintaining a healthy and diverse equilibrium in the natural world.

MAPPA MUNDI

Earth

- Materialistic; talk about work, finances and business.
- During the larval stage, the focus of the insect is on the basics; money, reproduction, sexuality, shamelessness, but especially food.
- Dirt, disgust, filthy habits and disease. Compensate by becoming OCD about cleanliness, order and a sanitised home environment.
- Fear of being crushed.

Water

- Bladder affinity. Urine infections.

Choleric

- Work, work, work.
- Hurried, hectic and fruitlessly busy.
- Need to prove their worth.
- Dry heat.
- Heavily armoured.

Sky realm (Fire)

- Escaping the mundane, exploring a deeper meaning to life.
- Finery, extravagance and fashionable clothes.
- Insects desire to transition from the Earth (material) to the Sky (spiritual).
- Sexual frenzy. Ailments from – sexual excesses | Nymphomania | Satyriasis.
- Burning pains.

Sanguine (Lepidoptera)

- In the Lepidoptera and Odonata, there may be an extended juvenile period or Peter Pan syndrome.
- Feeling like a child unprotected by adults.
- Naive. Aversion to responsibility.

THEMES

Trapped, abused, squashed vs. Recognition and admiration

Feel small, tiny, rejected and abused. Fear of being crushed, squashed or abandoned. Sankaran[18] These vital sensations can be a good indicator of the Insect kingdom, so long as the totality of characteristic themes and symptoms agree.

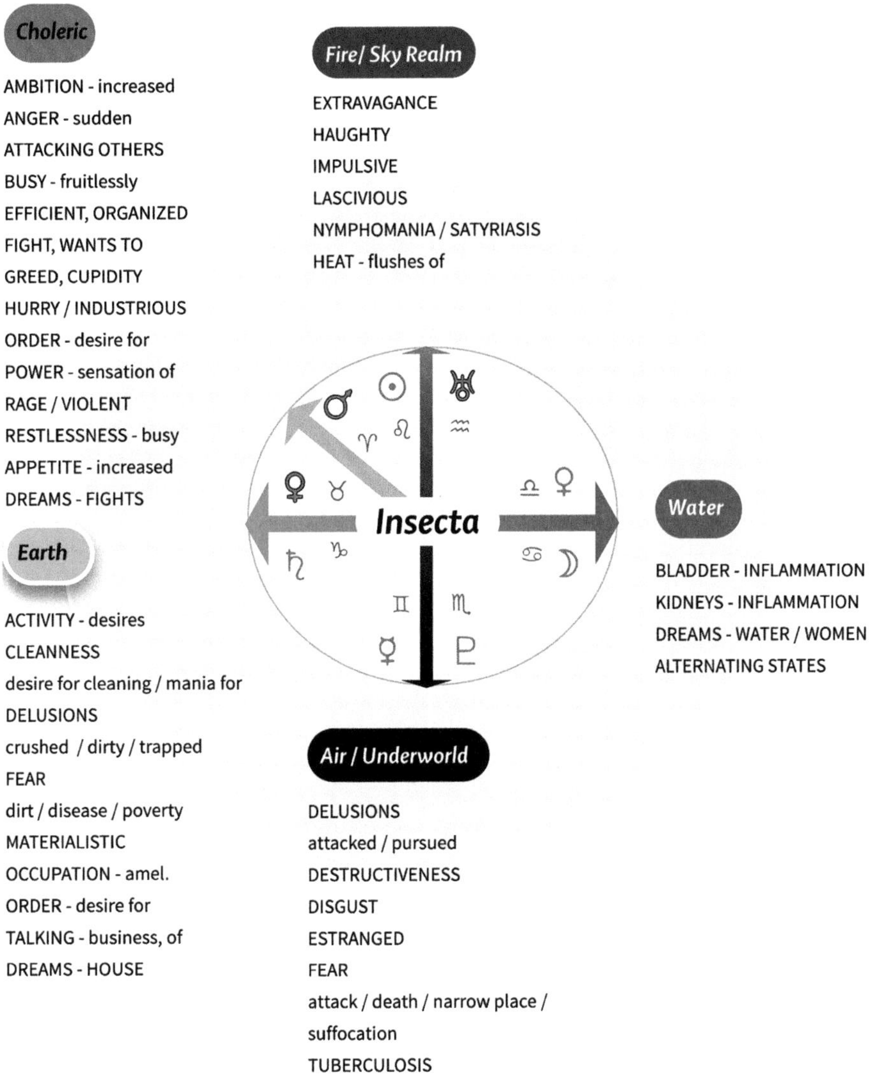

Figure 4.1 *Mappa Mundi dynamics for the Insects*

Feeling trapped, shackled, locked; irritable and evil. schist-am.[5] *feeling completely isolated . . . pities herself, forsaken feeling.* musca-d.[6] *The live animal is crushed and triturated.* blatta-o.[1] *Squashed, narrow feeling and trapped . . . crushing, throbbing pain, inward, at vertex . . . delusions – walls will crush him.* culx-per.[2] *Sensation as if crushed over the whole body, on the sides, hips, back, in short, everywhere.* apis[3] *A short excursion turns into a marathon of errands – felt trapped. Lights were driving me crazy. Finally, when we were almost done, I was accused of "whining" when I expressed my feelings.* lampro-sp.[4]

Insecta / Insects

Rubrics

Delusions – small – body is smaller | Delusions – trapped; he is | Fear – attacked; of being | Fear – death – sudden death; of | Fear – death; of – suffocation; from | Fear – escape; with desire to

Humans **wage war** on insects, trying our utmost to exterminate them with virulent insecticides, labelling them as pests or vermin. Hence there can be a strong feeling of injustice and of being unfairly treated. From the provings it is evident that there is also a contradictory sense of needing to **prove their own importance, desiring recognition and admiration.**

> *The central feeling is of very low self-worth* [with] *expressions like dirty, self-condemnation etc. due to which one needs* **recognition** . . . *appreciation, approbation and praise. Desirous of having an impressive personality and* **status**. *A strong desire to be noticed. Need to establish one's identity.* . . . *Since the proving I feel as if they are my competitors; a kind of professional jealousy.* . . . blatta-o.[7] *I need the recognition that I* **deserve**, *not that I want, but that I deserve. Only I know the hard work that I have put in to things. There is a sense of ploughing away and waiting for the harvest of my skills and talent which is a sort of recognition in the industry. If I get more recognised I will be given work more easily instead of striving to get to the next stage.* culx-per.[8]

Rubrics

Respected – desire to be | Ailments from – abused; after being | Delusions – abused, being | Delusions – appreciated, she is not

Feeling powerless, insignificant and looked down upon (low self esteem)

Delusion: people **humiliate** and **insult** them; they are **enslaved** and used.

Hive insects in particular are enslaved, controlled and dominated by their Queen. Ants are also used and abused by parasitic Wasps to rear their young. The Wasp possesses astonishingly powerful chemical weapons; these pheromones manipulate the ant's behaviour; effectively reprogramming them to take care of the Wasp larvae as if it were one of their own. Hence there can also be a feeling as though they're being **cheated, experimented on / tortured.**

> *I dreamt I was in a war – on the side of the oppressed. It involved guns and torture. Very disturbing.* culx-per.[2] *I was worried I was losing my mind; upset and questioning my life; who am I and what am I trying to do; shame, guilt, fear of failure; self-loathing.* schist-am.[5] *Feel like others put you down . . . Not an insult . . . but you should have respect. Insulted; not good enough, inferior – they are better than you are. Respect is a big thing with me.* . . . *Sometimes feels like I am a bit better than others.* . . . *Feel like I am in a worthless job – what's the point?!*[(9)] *I was worried I was losing my mind; upset and questioning my life; who am I and what am I trying to do; shame, guilt, fear of failure; self-loathing; frustration.* schist-am.[5] *I don't care to feel guilty anymore. The guilt side is the dark side – its shame originating in the body. It feels tight and burning.* lampro-sp.[4]

Delusions – insulted; he is – looked down upon | Ailments from – humiliation | Ailments from – mortification | Ailments from – shame | Delusions – wrong – suffered wrong; he has | Delusions – torture – tortured; he is

Dirt, disgust, filthy habits and disease *vs*. Finery, extravagance and fashionable clothes

Dreams of toilets, rubbish dumps and excrement, especially in *Musca domestica*. These patients can feel **ugly**, **repulsive and horrible** despite looking very well turned out, or even very beautifully dressed. The pervading feeling may be 'I'm shitty, how could anyone love me?'

Putrefaction, rotting garbage, maggots, corruption. excrement, toilets, sewers, tunnels and dirty water. musca-d.[6] *My image of myself was bad (dirty) having no control over my sexual desire. Felt like being an animal – very low, vulgar, cheap and dirty.* blatta-o.[7] *Digust – body; of – one's own . . . I'm stuck, can't get out, as if nowhere to hide. Inside me is disgusting – green brown slop. This stuff is stuck inside me, so I transmute the energy; put energy into changing it – metamorphosis.* mant-r.[10] *Feel mucky and dirty, mixing with people who have no respect. It soaks into me and I can't kick it off.* cocc-s.

They compensate very well through attention to personal appearance – **dress to attract others with bright / garish colours**. Love of shopping and wearing glamorous clothes. Inside there can be feelings of self-disgust that are often well-compensated for by dressing in expensive fashionable clothing and making a lot of effort on one's appearance.

Clothes – luxurious clothing, finery; wants. *Now I feel I must have a sober personality, you must wear decent clothes – good clothes. You must have a certain image, certain status.* blatta-o.[7] *I coloured my hair – desire to be prettier, more attractive. I put glittering makeup with pleasure. I say in front of the mirror every morning "Thank you, mum".* cocc-s.[11]

In reality, Insects want to be special, admired and successful (*especially Blatta orientalis*). Feeling 'dirty'. Compensate by becoming OCD about bacteria, dirt and germs. Desire for cleanliness, order and a sanitised home environment.

Started organising; cleaning and organizing; moving through projects. schist-am.[5] *Did a serious cleaning of my office. Remedy had an organizing influence.* enal-ca.[12] *Everything feels a mess, out of order and it is going to take a huge effort to put everything back into a new order – home, finances, work, study everything.* culx-per.[2] *For much of their down time, roaches are busy grooming themselves, licking their legs and antennae in much the same manner in which a cat washes its paws.* blatta-o.[1] *I am not a neat individual, but I groomed myself. I wore a brown belt. Haven't worn a belt in decades. Slick hair, smoothed it down.* enal-ca.[12]

Attracting others | Extravagance | Luxury; desire for | Cleanness – mania for *vs*. Delusions – body – ugly; body looks | Delusions – dirty – he is | Delusions –

repulsive fantastic | Disgust – body; of the | Fear – dirt; of | Fear – disease; of impending

Transformation / metamorphosis from larval form to adult form

Insect patients may express a sense of being trapped by their own patterns of behaviour; they can't escape the feeling of **dirtiness** / grubbiness and become **ashamed** of themselves. They would like to **transform** or revolutionise their own identity.

The language used by these patients can appear similar to mineral patients where they perceive the fault to be within themselves; who they are inside is the problem (dirty and grubby). Rather than the focus being on incompleteness or fundamental self-lack (as in minerals), the Insect patient feels as though **they must make a radical change from within in order to fulfil their true potential.**

They may feel blocked, hindered and irritated by others *dragging them down* again. Gemstones also have the theme of undergoing a transformative process. Here, the language may be more overtly spiritual; journeying from darkness / shadow into the light of consciousness. Sensations of heaviness and pressure are important expressions in Gemstone cases, compared to the squashed, stabbing, burning and crawling more intrinsic to Insect remedies.

Sensation of metamorphosis or transformation between two states. The first state was described as being in a hole or cave . . . the hole is a really transformative place; I undergo some kind of metamorphosis; it is like a deep cellular change . . . feeling I am moving into a different sense of organising my life. schist-am.[5] *All members of the muscoidea family, like the butterfly, a distant cousin, go through complete metamorphosis . . . flies, butterflies and moths become totally and magically transformed from one stage to the next: egg – maggot / caterpillar – pupa / chrysalis – fly / butterfly.* musca-d.[6] *Over the winter the larvae lie dormant in marble-sized soil chambers, and emerge as metamorphosed adults in late spring or early summer.* lampro-sp.[4]

In the Lepidoptera, there may be an extended juvenile period or Peter Pan syndrome, where the individual feels as though they will never be able to handle the duties of an adult life. Perpetual childhood – fear of, or preoccupation with, taking on responsibility.

A child feeling unprotected by adults. Naive. Aversion to responsibility. Responsibility – give up her responsibility; wanting to. Love – children; for – responsibilities; yet naive about.[14]

Rubrics
Change – desire for | Delusions – metamorphic

Safe in the luxury of a silk cocoon

A silk case protects the pupa during its time of transition from grub to imago (adult). This is quite a contrast to the way spiders use silk to encase and trap their prey, rendering them in a state of captivity whilst they await to be eaten. In the insect world, silk is used as a form of nurturing protection; to ensure the life cycle can be completed in peaceful isolation.

> In the cocoon stage *the pupas are housed in "a beautifully decorated house" of silk* . . . *Limenitis bredowii builds a silk house around itself and hangs there quietly, until its body disintegrates and magically transforms into that of the complete, adult butterfly. Silk has been obtained from the cocoon wrapping of the silkworm moth since the fifth century B.C. The princess who discovered it was given the rank of divinity for her incredible find. Silk is regarded the world over as the most elegant and sensuous fabric.* limen-b-c.[14]

For insects, a cocooned feeling may therefore symbolise protection during transitional periods, or times of upheaval; offering a means by which to escape or withdraw from the hardships of life. If a patient gets stuck or too comfortable in the safety of the pupal phase, then they will never mature to fulfil their purpose. Butterflies and moths have a strong theme of feeling unable to handle responsibility, getting stuck in an adolescent *Peter Pan* type existence; feeling unprotected and needing guidance from adults.

Collective super-societies, swarming and collaborating

Termites and Ants form super-societies in which they behave as though they are one organism; forming communities, colonies and working for the good of the collective. The hierarchy is much more basic than in Mammals. Here there is a dominant Queen and the workers. It is more like Monarchy or corrupt Communism than Democracy. Whereas Mammals have a chance to prove their worth and topple the alpha if they can beat him in combat, Insects are under strict pheromonal control. Therefore, issues of how the individual fits in with the group are also important in Insect provings and cases, especially the social ones.

> *Feeling not good enough around selection of mates; acutely aware of classes of people* . . . *sensitive to groups and group approval* . . . *polarity of wanting to be alone and then with people; frenzied desire for a mate; feeling part of a group; camaraderie; feeling of moving through time in a group together* . . . [Sensitive to not] *being good enough; rejection and rejecting; many people suffering.* schist-am.[5] *The fact that the Locust has two different forms and physically changes when it is a gregarious animal from the form it has when it leads a solitary existence is definitely characteristic.* . . . *Rejection and being on the periphery of the group and not being able to integrate* . . . *on the outside of the group and different and didn't really fit in which made me tearful.* schist-gg.[15]

Parasitic behaviour

Many types of wasps engage in parasitic behaviours to ensure their survival. This technique seems to be employed in solitary insects who do not have the security of the hive to help them raise their young. Such wasps have developed an astonishingly wide variety of skills with which to trick other organisms into caring for their young. Misha Norland conducted a proving of Knopper Oak Gall which brings out these themes very nicely. More provings are needed to gain a better understanding of how these behaviours will be expressed in humans.

*One member of the group was **ostracised**, being called a **parasite**. . . . 'They perceive me as a user of people – do things to get what I need at their expense. Felt that I hated all people and also myself. . . . Felt that I did not have the right to be with others. I feel that **I'm sucking them out**. Throwing my dirt at others.* _{galla-q-r.}[16]

Rubrics
Delusions – parasite; she is a | Delusions – sucked up; she is being / sucking people dry; she is

Industrious, fruitlessly busy and hurried

- Impulsive, instinctive, speedy, scuttling, scurrying, buzzing, flitting from one thing to another.
- Undertaking many things, persevering in nothing.
- Restlessness, nervous energy, hyperactivity. ADHD.
- Working as part of a team. Hive mentality.
- Survival depends upon constant, unrelenting efforts (*cf. Stage 8 and 12*).
- These patients can be **hurried, hectic and fruitlessly busy**.
- Lack of autonomy but a better chance of survival through working as a collective.
- *cf. Mammals*; there is a tension between the individual and the group plus an element of nurture that are both lacking in Insect cases. Mammals need to know their place within the social hierarchy, whereas Insects work as a collective to achieve their shared goals.
- **Sudden impatience** – want things done straight away. *cf. Chamomilla / Typhoid miasm.*
- The compensation for all this hectic, hurried and frenzied behaviour can also be expressed as being very organised, precise and programming everything to a strict schedule.
- Constant need for **activity and change**; these patients may do everything at an intense pace, rushing from one thing to the next. There is a predominantly tubercular miasm common to the Insect remedies. For example, Blatta orientalis has long been known as a remedy for asthma with a tormenting, harassing and violent cough. "One prover describes [the proving of *Schistocerca americana*] as 'Tuberculinum on crack'." _{Rowe}[5]

It requires focus, attention and precision to do my work; I must do a lot of work in a short space of time. If dizziness comes on then that is impossible. It is really taxing. Like got a mind of its own, this thing. It drains my energy. Another entity taking over you. _{culx-per.}[8] *The frenzy of this remedy manifested in irritability, restlessness, hurry, impatience, impetuousness, impulsivity, confrontation, violence, desire to attack others, panic and panic attacks, threatening behaviour, shrieking, hatred, mania and insanity. Sexuality was prominent even to the point of nymphomania. In this state provers described a feeling of being invincible.* _{schist-am.}[5]

Rubrics

Restlessness – busy | Industrious | Activity – desires activity | Busy – fruitlessly | Hurry – aimless | Thoughts – rush | Undertaking – many things, persevering in nothing | Occupation – amel.

Materialistic; talk about work, finances and business

During the larval stage, the focus of the insect is on the basics; *money, reproduction, sexuality, shamelessness, but especially food.* [Sankaran][18] "The larvae's main task is to eat, and they do so prodigiously. They increase their weight 10,000-fold during this period." [limen-b-c][14] "Issues of duty, task, hard work, order, systematic work. In Insect remedies there is a lot of guilt about having not completed their task. . . . Their tasks are done monotonously and instinctively. The structures are built to perfection, but these tasks are done mechanically, as part of an in-built program, with no creativity . . . everything has a specific order." [Joshis][19]

> *I have an issue with money. I don't know how to make it. I don't seem to ever have money. I realised the other day that familiar feeling of spending money. I like to shop. I feel restricted (because I don't have it). What is the block with me and money? I was able to ask. In myself are competing activities – money is good, money is bad, wrong. There's a dialogue between these two things. One says good, one says bad.* [enal-ca][12] *My sister and I have had the potential to make copious amounts of money with her business / sales skills and my artistic skill and pure magic of paint. She has denied my expertise and only treated me poorly.* [lampro-sp][4]

Rubrics

Ambition – increased | Absorbed – business matters; in | Efficient, organised | Greed, cupidity | Materialistic | Organised and methodical; desire to be | Rich; to be – desire | Talking – Business, of | Task-oriented | Simple persons | Unrefined

Escaping the mundane, exploring a deeper meaning to life

The rampant materialism which is currently at large in Western civilisation is only a superficial layer. Underneath, there can be a yearning to discover and explore spirituality or find deeper meaning in life. This is expressed very nicely in the rubric: *Mind – Conflict – higher consciousness and worldly existence; between.* [limen-b-c][14]

Spirituality is a theme common to the Birds who are at home in the sky – flying offers pure joy and freedom from an overview of the Earth. As Peter Fraser[13] explains, Insects desire to transition from the Earth (material) to the Sky (spiritual). Trapped feelings can be an expression of this desire to escape a mundane existence to explore their sense of purpose.

Insects spend most of their time busy eating as much as possible before making a winged escape from their life as a simple grub. The book / film Trainspotting is an interesting portrayal of Insect qualities. If you watch the trailer of the film, all the topics are covered. Renton (the lead character) says; "choose life . . ." and then goes onto list all the material desires that usually dominate a person's yearnings. Instead of choosing that life, he and his friends try to escape it by using heroin, which ultimately drags them further into the mire from which they are seeking to escape. There is a famous scene where he descends down the worst toilet in Scotland (going back down into the shit; see the proving of Musca Domestica).

> *I went to sit in some woods. I felt in the wrong medium. I wanted to be in another state, either planted in silence in the earth or existing in space. I wanted to be in a relative quiet state that comes in meditation, that seems to be the state that part of me is in. I didn't want to be at a mundane level.* limen-b-c.[14] *Wondrous sense of lightness, power and freedom. In a delightful mood. The inertia seems to have lifted. Singing away to myself. Seeing very clearly the pulls and tugs that family members are exerting on each other and me – all the subtle emotional manipulation. I'm watching quite delightedly. . . . When meditating, was different type of alertness. Energy became more quiet. I go "out" when meditating.* enal-ca.[12]

Rubrics
Conflict – higher consciousness and worldly existence; between | Delusions – trapped; he is | Delusions – consciousness – higher consciousness; unification with

Confusion over sexuality

There can be problems with **gender confusion / gender dysphoria**. This was especially brought out in the proving of *Musca domestica*.

> *Gender confusion: one young child who's parent's had both taken the remedy, called his mother, Daddy and his father, Mommy. Our most reliable prover had strong feelings of lurking homosexuality. He felt men were watching him, touching him and were attracted to him. He admitted to a homophobic reaction.* musca-d.[6]

Some Insects need to transform from the repulsive larval form to the beautiful adult form (from grub to Butterfly). For example, cases of gender dysphoria, where children want to undergo gender change operations. This overlaps with the theme of being experimented on. Sensation of living a double life – *Mind – Delusions – divided – two parts; into.*

Butterflies have a certain innocence and beauty that they don't know what to do with. Its as though they are still carrying the sense of being a lowly grub despite having transformed into their vivid and colourful adult form.

Rubrics
Confusion of mind – identity; as to his – sexual identity | Shameful – sexuality; about

Sexual frenzy

In some cases, Insects take to the sky for a very brief period of time relative to the time spent as a grub; 17 years for Cicadas, who then emerge as one giant population. The purpose of being airborne is often to mate. This time is very short (only 2 weeks for Cicadas) and so there is a frenzy of fornication and feeding on the Cicadas by predators. "On a more emotional level the irritability that is common to the insects builds up until it reaches a level of uncontainable anger . . . sexual excitement builds to a point of uncontrollable need that could not be denied." Fraser[13] Insect patients can feel **shameful** about their sexual habits or their animalistic instincts.

> *Suddenly began to talk vulgar things to his girlfriend, even she was surprised by my behaviour. Emphatically told girlfriend to have sex then followed by praying for forgiveness. Said "I know you will leave me and feel this man is terrible and will torture me".* . . . *Then again followed by a sudden sexual urge with a feeling as if already had sex.* blatta-o.[7] *I decided to masturbate to make me relax and to help get rid of this feeling.* . . . *Having multiple orgasms, through masturbation, not intense climax, sense of over, and over and over again, no strong emotions attached. Just do it!* schist-gg.[15] *Four of our provers had recurring sexual dreams, one more dreamt of rape, and three others had recurring dreams of gay men or homosexual issues.* musca-d.[6] *Dream: hundreds of people naked standing in rows; some were engaging in sexual activities but they were acting like animals; all mixed; very disgusting; some were crawling like snakes on the walls.* schist-am.[5]

Rubrics
Ailments from – sexual excesses | Nymphomania | Satyriasis | Love – perversity; sexual | Libertinism | Lascivious | Delirium – erotic | Obscene, lewd | Impulse; morbid – sexual | Shameless

Enslaved by Plants

Plants use insects all the time in a benign way to spread their pollen. From an Insect point of view, this could translate into a feeling of being used or enslaved by plants; they certainly must work very hard for their meal! Carnivorous plants have adopted a killing strategy so they can get the nutrients lacking in the soil in which they grow. Drosera rotundifolia deceives with an advertisement of delectable dew in order to dupe the hapless insect into becoming a slowly digested meal. In this adaptation, the plant is dependent on Insects not for pollination but for nutrition, so it deploys a technique of making itself unmistakably attractive. Yet it deceives and mercilessly devours the industrious visitor, who thinks he is coming for a meal, not that he would become one!

Supplementary themes

- **Crushed, constricting, crawling, stabbing** sensations. **Formication. Burning** pains.
- Acute violent manifestations, inflammations (especially meningitis).
- "The chief features of insects are that they fly; that they develop from juvenile forms that are often different from the adult; that they breed prolifically; and that many of them are social animals." Fraser[13]

- Skilful at cloning and improving on other people's work; because they work in an automated fashion, they lack their own creativity. Jobs like programming computer code and working in a team would be suitable for insects.
- **Organised** *vs.* **Chaotic** (*cf. Cancer miasm and Sarcodes*).
- Every insect knows its particular role in the hive society.
- Feels under attack – fear of **sudden, immediate death**.
- One sided / alternating sides – strong animal kingdom feature.
- Useful remedies in puberty especially for irritating children (ADHD). *For example, Culex-pe. Musca-d, Butterfly remedies.*
- **Hair loss.**
- Shameless sexuality. Not touchy-feely but desire sex for the physical release rather than intimacy.
- Paranoia – being throttled, or snuck up on. (Cantharis – delusion; being choked by icy cold hands.)
- Attracted to vivid colours.
- Heavily armoured but weak points in the joints – Apis, Formica rufa and Vespa.
- Need to prove their worth – especially Blatta Orientalis.

Source Words

Struggled, entangled / Pioneers / Armoured / Swarm / Cocoon / Joints weakness / Moulting – shedding layers that become restrictive (*cf. Snakes*) / Surgical precision / Genetic engineering / Broken down and reassembled / Egg, grub, chrysalis, butterfly / Probing deep into a flower / Patterns produced by tiny scales, refracting the light for an iridescent shimmer / Sexual advertisements / Drilling and sucking / Hawk moth – hovering, beating wings / Precision / Need to keep eating all the time, even during mating / Flight control / Landing upside down

Differential Diagnosis

- Tubercular, Yersinia and Malarial Miasms
- Gemstones (metamorphosis)
- Ferrum Series
- Carnivorous Plants
- Fungi (invaded)
- Geraniales (sustained effort)
- Piperaceae (desire for change)
- Berberidaceae (suddenness)
- Stages 7–9 (Collective, Industriousness)
- Araneae
- Parasites

REMEDIES

acher-at. agam-g. apeir-s. <u>APIS</u>. apisin. blatta-a. *blatta-o.* bomb-chr. bomb-pr. bombu-s. calop-sp. <u>CANTH</u>. canthin. ceto. cimx. *coc-c.* cocc-s. culx. *culx-per.* dor. enal-ca. **form**. form-ac. **galla-q-r.** galla-tu. gonep-rn. gra-sp-ch. ina-i. **lampro-sp. limen-b-c. mant-r.** mel-c-s. **musca-d.** noct-pn. papi-mc. parap-cv. ped. ped-p. pieri-b. polyom-ic. propl. pulx. pulx-c. **schist-am. schist-gg**. simul. vanes-u. vesp. vesp-xyz. vespul-germ.

DICTYOPTERA

Blatta orientalis (Oriental cockroach)

Phylum: Arthropoda.
Class: Insecta.
Order: Blattaria.
Family: Blattidae.

Cockroaches wear their skeletons on the outside. This exoskeleton is made of chitin, a durable, polysaccharide shell no thicker than the width of a human hair. To thrive, they need a place to hide – they prefer warm, damp environments such as sewer pipes, sink drains, and basements. They are incredibly strong and persistent; they can pull on average more than twenty times their own weight. When they gather in large numbers, they impart a peculiar and unpleasant odour – emanating from the roach's faeces, saliva, and waxy skin, all of which are laden with aromatic sex pheromones. Whilst relaxing, which they do for much of the day, roaches are busy grooming themselves – licking their legs and antennae in much the same manner in which a cat washes its paw. Cannibalism is common among cockroaches, particularly in laboratories, where insects are typically reared in large colonies with crowded conditions.

Provings by: **Alastair Gray, Australia (2002).**[1]
Divya Chabra, India[1] (*mentioned in Gray's proving*).[1]
Munjal Thakar, Paldi, Ahmedabad, **India. (DATE).**[7]

Keywords
Ambitious / **Appreciation** – desires / Contemptuous / Dirty / **Praise** – desires / Jealousy – venerated, to those / Repulsive / **Vulgar** / **Sophisticated** / Polished / **Finery** / Insulting / Loathsome / Triumph / Asthmatic / Emphysema

Polarity
Polished, sophisticated and ambitious *vs.* Vulgar, loathsome and dirty (*The Platina of Insects*)

SRP delusions
- Animal he is; vulgar
- Appreciated; she is not (*cf. Androctonus, Musca domestica, Palladium*)
- Dirty she is – menses; before
- Committed a crime; he had
- Talking rapidly; all around her are

Mind

- Abrupt – speak; when obliged to
- Abrupt – speaks bluntly
- *Ambition – ambitious; fame, for*
- Appreciation – desires
- Consolation – ailments from, agg.
- **Contemptuous – venerated before, to those**
- Delusions – brain; wobbling
- Delusions – dirty; he is
- Delusions – criticised; that she is
- **Despair – social position; of**
- Detached
- *Envy – venerated; to those*
- Fear – riding, when; carriage, in
- Impolite
- Indifference – music; to
- Insults – ailments from, agg.
- Irritability – alone; desires to be
- *Jealousy – venerated; to those*
- *Jesting – joke; cannot take a*
- Lewdness – obscene
- Love – approbation; for
- Praise – desires
- Responsibility – ailments from; agg.
- Rudeness
- Self-control – loss of; sexual
- Unsympathetic – unscrupulous

Themes from the proving by Divya Chabra

Feel as though:
- Cheap / Crude / Blunt / Vulgar / Low / Messy / **Repulsive** / Dirty / Stupid, dumb, no brains

Desire to be:
- **Sophisticated** / *Polished* / Status / Reputation / Cool / Systematic / Good human being / An executive / Appreciated / **Praised** / Famous / Noticed

They perceive others as:
- **Jealous** / Mean / Nasty / Deliberately laughing at them / **Insulting** and neglecting them

Dreams

Accusations / Arm – covered with vesicles / Arrested – caught; of being / **Danger** – escaping from a / Danger – *falling*; of / **Disease** – **loathsome** / Face – covered with **pustules** / Fatherland / Frightful – fear; followed by / House – big / Masks / **Pursued**; of being – man; by – **violate** her; to / **Triumph** / **Vulgar** scenes

Physicals

- **Bladder**
  - Cancer
- **Respiration**
  - *Asthmatic*
  - Accompanied by – obesity
  - Accompanied by – Bronchi – inflammation
  - Allergic
  - Exertion; from
  - Nervous
  - Old people; in
  - Difficult – accompanied by – cough
  - Wheezing
- **Expectoration**
  - Purulent
- **Chest**
  - Emphysema
  - Inflammation – Bronchi – acute
  - Pain – Sides – right

- Phthisis pulmonalis (tuberculosis)
- **Generals**
  - Allergic constitution – moulds; to
  - Ascending – agg.
  - Swelling – edematous – internal
  - Exertion; physical – agg.
- Heated, becoming
- Mucous secretions – purulent
- Obesity
- Periodicity
- Weather – cold weather – wet – agg.

Themes from the proving by M Thakar[7]
- **Dirty, self-condemnation *vs.* recognition and needs to be noticed.**
- *"This need is met through putting up a **façade of arrogance** and pride. It is also attempted through **greed for finery and social status**. The positive aspect is being ambitious and industrious [as] a way to cope with one's low self-worth."*
- **Desire for finery – good clothes.** Desire to look good.
- Jealous – comparing her possessions with those of her friends. Envious of their possessions.
- **Desire for appreciation**, approbation and praise.
- Desirous of having an impressive personality and status. A strong desire to be noticed. Need to establish one's identity, need for recognition.
- Contemptuous and envious of people generally venerated (Platina) or whom she admires.
- Competing with people whom she venerated, desire to be at par with them and be noticed or appreciated.
- **Contrary behaviour in order to be noticed.**
- Idolised and admired people of social status.
- **Sudden sexual excitement with vulgar talking** followed by sense of remorse or guilt.
- Feels one's self as being dirty and of having no control over his sexual desire.
- Felt himself like an animal – very **low and vulgar, cheap**.

Mantis religiosa (Praying mantis)

Phylum: Arthropoda.
Class: Insecta.
Order: Mantodea.
Family: Mantidae.

The name praying mantis comes from the distinctive resting posture of the first pair of legs which resembles a praying pose. Males are often found to be more active and agile, whilst females are physically more powerful. Adult females are generally too large and heavy for their wings to enable a take-off. Their deimatic display (a term for bluffing) involves wing spreading and bending of the raptorial legs to reveal two matched black eyespots with a yellow or white centre at the base of the legs, giving them a much larger and more threatening appearance to ward off attackers. Only a few days after the final moult into adults, the animals begin to show interest in the opposite sex. Owing to their inferior size and power, males are cautious in their sexual advances; after spotting a female, he usually freezes and turns his head to look directly at her, watching out for any signs he will be eaten rather than accepted as a mate. He then proceeds to approach her from behind using a stop-and-go tactic.

Proving by: **Walter Glück, Vienna, Austria (2002).**

Reference
Gluck W. Homeopathic drug proving of Mantis religiosa. B October, 2002. Abstract available online at: ***https://tinyurl.com/yyxch88q*** (accessed 29th September 2020.)

Keywords
Domination / Brutality / **Mutilation** / Violence / Sexual cannibalism / Carnivorous / **Praying** / Attacked / **Subordinating** / Agitation / Disgusting / Metamorphosis / Unfeeling

Ailments from
• Domination – long time; for a
• Excitement

Mind symptoms
• Egotism
• Euphoria
• Excitement
• Exclusive, too
• Fear – happen; something will
• Forgetful
• Harmony
• Indifference
• Mental exertion – agg.
• Mood – changeable
• Moral feeling; want of
• Morose
• Restlessness
• Sadness
• Stupefaction
• Unfeeling

Dreams
Amorous / Anger / Brutality / Children; about / Escaping / Lewd / Mutilation / Rape / Violence / Vivid / War

Natural Behaviour
Sexual cannibalism / Courtship routine / Carnivorous / Motionless / Immobile / Clasped hands / Praying / Creeping / Stalking / Caught / Attacked / Eaten

Case extracts, Pauline Wilson[10]
"My whole body and mind are scrambled. It is as though **someone comes up behind me**. . . . As if **energy grabs my whole body, overcoming my will, subordinating me**. I feel **raciness** and **agitation** – internal **quivering**. I am still and the rest of world is fast (dizziness), I feel as if in a trance, as if looking at myself from a distance . . . I'm stuck, can't get out, as if nowhere to hide. **Inside me is disgusting** – green brown slop. This stuff is stuck inside me, so **I transmute the energy**; put energy into changing it – **metamorphosis**. I take what's bad and

turn it into what's good . . . I would fall into another's energy field and the inter-action would be to my detriment. . . . I have been singing to the land and to the sea, **as if praying**. When I sang, the world would listen to me. It was a survival mechanism as if I was psychic."

ORTHOPTERA

Schistocerca Americana (American bird grasshopper)

Phylum: Arthropoda.
Class: Insecta.
Order: Orthoptera.
Family: Mantidae.

Schistocerca americana is a common pest in North America. The American Grasshopper leaps through fields and meadows and along dusty roads using their long back legs and large thighs. A grasshopper can jump 10 times higher than their body and 20 times their length. They only fly a short length at a time and land to rest and eat. The grasshopper is a serious threat to the success of agriculture. They can wipe out a crop in no time at all. The nymphs go through five or six stages before reaching adulthood. Six instars are normal, but if densities are low only five instars will be completed.

Proving by: **Todd Rowe, Phoenix, AZ USA (2007).**[5]

Keywords
Invincible / **Swarming** / Transformation / Trapped / Anxiety, paroxysmal / **Frenzy** / Industriousness / **Nymphomania** / Beside oneself / Destructiveness / **Social position** / *Tuberculinum on crack* / *Buzzing* / *Humming* / *Electrical* / End of the world / Swarm *vs* Solitary / Primitive survival / Pest

Delusions
- *Appreciated; she is not*
- Birth canal; is emerging from
- Born, newly born, overwhelmed at novelty or surroundings
- *Forced to be here against her will*
- Hole; is in a
- *Invincible*; is
- Space, bodily space, energy and dimension
- Swarming
- *Transformation or metamorphosis*
- Trapped; he is
- Watched; that she is being

Mind
- *Ancient feeling*
- Animal consciousness
- Anxiety – conscience of
- *Anxiety – paroxysmal*
- Attack others; desire to
- Aversion to herself
- *Beside oneself; being*
- Bliss
- *Busy*
- Change – desire for
- Confidence; self in
- Confrontational
- Confusion of mind – identity, as to his – *boundaries*; and personal
- Connection – feeling of
- *Destructiveness* – self destructive
- Ennui
- Fanaticism
- Flowing – sensation of
- *Frenzy*
- Handle things anymore; cannot – overwhelmed by stress
- Hurry – driving; while – wants to overtake all others
- *Impetuous*
- *Industriousness*
- *Nymphomania*
- Power – love of
- Rage
- *Social position*; concerned about
- Travel; desire to
- *Violence*

Provers speaking as one
"The core sensation for this proving was related to the sensation of **metamorphosis** or transformation between two states . . . [Solitary state] Spiralled down into this **deep hole** today; went into a hole deep in the earth . . . [Frenzy state] was very social and involved seeking a mate and various group activities. Images of flying became involved. **Sexuality** became very prominent with dreams of indiscriminate group sex and sex between children. . . . **Frenzy** (intensity) leads to the feeling of the destruction or the end of the world. There is a quality of great **destructiveness**, *restlessness, hurry, impatience, impetuousness, impulsivity, confrontation, violence, desire to attack others, panic and panic attacks, threatening behaviour, shrieking, hatred, mania and insanity.*"[5]

Themes[5]
- *Electrical, buzzing and humming* sensations.
- Panic and mania.
- Feelings of destructiveness.
- Sensation of "**the end of the world**".
- Sensitivity to noise.
- Hearing is acute; high pitched buzzing tinnitus.
- Sensation of **body vibrating all over** when going to sleep.
- Waving between dimensions of time and space or of flowing in a current.
- Chilly with hot flushes.
- Tendency towards injuries (falls), weight loss, heaviness, swelling and lassitude.
- More grounded; "I feel more connected to the ground".
- Pains: constricting, contracting, squeezing and cramping.
- Craving for meat and especially raw meat.
- Stomach; empty or hollow sensation that had to be filled, accompanied by feelings of loneliness, and anxiety.

- Torpor, confusion (of identity).
- Boundary and codependency issues.
- Swarm vs Solitary / Primitive Survival (aggression, food, sex).

Schistocerca gregaria (Plague Locust)

Phylum: Arthropoda.
Class: Insecta.
Order: Orthoptera.
Family: Acrididae.

The locust moults several times each larval stage, or instar, becoming gradually more like the adult form. Only the adult form (imago) is able to fly; the nymphs move by jumping and are called hoppers. The time taken for larvae to develop varies greatly and is much faster when in the gregarious state. When the population size increases, a serotonin-based reaction is initiated by the rubbing together of their legs – this causes a hormonal cascade and the release of pheromones – prompting the metamorphosis from solitary to gregarious form. They now reproduce much more quickly, forming the enormous and destructive swarms. Many billions of individuals will eat their own weight of vegetation every day. The largest swarms can completely devastate crops over an enormous area. Hence the place it has in biblical history as one of the plagues that afflict mankind.

Proving by: **Peter Fraser and Misha Norland, Devon UK (2007).**[15]

Keywords
Gregarious / Powerful influence / Invisible / Outsider / Persecuted / Witches / Benevolence / Boundaries / **<u>Lascivious</u>** / Vulnerable / Disgust / Narcissism / Humiliation / **Masturbation** / Sexual – disgust / Wolves / Formication / Odour / Explode / Losing control / **Over-stimulated** / *Rotten* / *Revolting* / *Repulsed* / Burrowed / Caught / Respect

Delusions
- *Appreciated; she is not*
- Body – parts – separated; are
- Divided – two parts; into
- Division between himself and others
- Forsaken; is
- *Friend – surrounded by friends; being*
- *Influence; one is under a powerful*
- Insane – become insane; one will
- Insects; sees
- Invisible; she is
- *Outsider; being an*
- *Persecuted – he is persecuted*
- Room – people; sees – bedside; at his
- Separated – group; he is separated from the
- Walking – behind him; someone walks
- Witches; believes in

Mind

- Activity – desires activity
- Anger
- Benevolence
- *Busy*
- Confusion of mind
- Confusion of mind – identity, as to his – *boundaries*; and personal
- Consolation – amel.
- Contact; desire for
- Dancing
- *Disgust*
- *Disgust – body; of the – own body; of one's*
- **Egotism (narcissism)**
- Excitement
- Fastidious
- ***Fear – attacked; fear of being***
- Fear – dark; of
- Forsaken feeling
- Grief
- Home – desires to go
- Irresolution
- Irritability
- ***Lascivious***
- Mistakes; making – time, in
- Mistakes; making – writing, in
- *Perfume – loves to use perfume*
- Rage
- Running – desire for
- Sensitive – colours; to
- Sensitive – odours; to
- Space – desire for
- Speech – hesitating
- Truth – desire for truthfulness
- ***Vulnerable***
- Weeping – amel.
- Weeping – easily

Dreams

Accidents – car; with a / Accusations – crime, wrongful of / Amorous / *Amorous – orgasm; with – multiple – masturbation, by* / Animals – wild / Arguments / Attacked; of being / Beaten; being / Beauty / Betrayed / Camping / Cats / Censorious / Chickens / Children; about – newborns / Cities / *Closet – being on – coition, during / Coition – desire for, of* / Coition – unsuccessful / Country – foreign / Dancing – circle; in a – with great agility / **Decay** / Desert / **Disgusting** / Dogs – missing / Escaping / Escaping – unable to / **Evil**; of / **Excrements – eating** / Face – *horrible face* / Fear / Fire / Fishing / Flood / Flowers / Food / Foreign language; she had to converse in a / **Forms – black** / Forsaken; being / Friends / *Ghosts* / Groups / **Hair – body hair – growing excessively** / Hair – dying her / Hiding / High places / Horrible / Horses – riding / Hotels / House / **Humiliation** / Insects / Invisible; she is / Isolated; of being / Killing / Lascivious / Lift / Lost; being / Magic / Masturbation / Meat – raw / *Meat – roasted – vegetarians; fed to* / Money / Money – problems with / Monsters / Murder / Nakedness / Nakedness – unashamed / Ocean / Orgies / Paralyzed / Poisoned; being / Rain / Rejected; being / Relatives / Robbing / Robots / Rubbish / Running / **Seduction** / *Seduction – unwanted* / Sexual / **Sexual – disgust** / Shopping / Sky / Spiders / Stones / Storms / Survival / Terrorists / Thunderstorm / Trap – being trapped / Underground / Unpleasant / Violence / Water / Waves – huge wave approaching / **Witches** / **Wolves** / Women / Worms / Wounds

Characteristic physicals

- **Vertigo**
  - Closing the eyes – agg.
- **Head**
  - Formication
  - Heaviness – Occiput – raise – difficult to
  - Pain – Pressing pain
    - § outward
    - § weight; as from a
  - Tickling in
- **Nose**
  - Odours; Imaginary and real – tobacco
  - Smell – Acute – perfumes
- **Face**
  - Eruptions – herpes – Mouth – Corners of
- **Mouth and Throat**
  - Odour – cadaverous
  - Salivation – profuse
  - Teeth – Abscess of roots
  - Pain – swollen glands; as from
- **Stomach and Gastro-intestinal**
  - Formication
  - Lump; sensation of a
  - Rectum – Flatus – offensive – cabbage
  - Stool – Fatty, Greasy
  - Stool – Forcible, sudden, gushing
- **Female**
  - Leukorrhea – bloody
  - Pain – bearing down
- **Chest**
  - Oppression – Mammae
  - Prickling
- **Extremities**
  - Itching – Thumbs – Balls
  - Nails; complaints of – brittle nails
  - Pain – stitching pain – needles; as from
  - Weakness – sensation of – Legs
- **Fever**
  - Succession of stages – heat – alternating with – chill
- **Perspiration**
  - Odour – sweetish-sour
- **Skin**
  - Itching
- **Generals**
  - Pain – appear suddenly
  - Pain – pressing pain – outward
  - Pain – stabbing pain
  - Pain – stinging
  - Touch – agg.
  - Wavelike sensations

Provers speaking as one[15]

"**I can't contain the energy and I am going to explode** . . . I can't handle this level of energy expanding within me . . . feeling pressurised in my head, like its going to explode. . . . I feel like I'm going to go mad, **sensation of losing control, loss of senses**. My mind feels **over-stimulated**, racing away with me. . . . Feel very narcissistic and talking about myself all the time! **Dancing manically** in the evening for ages, really energetically and powerfully with agility and confidence that my body could bend in strange ways and could jump and not fall. . . . A sense that I'm not in control of my actions and there is *something far bigger than me that influences me. . . .*"

Sexuality

"Had a really frustrating feeling today of being angry and not knowing what to do with myself. I decided to **masturbate to make me relax** and to help get rid of this feeling . . . afterwards I just lay on my bed and had a *huge laughing fit*, I was really **laughing loudly for no reason at all**. It was as if someone had pushed the laughing button on a doll. . . . Having **multiple orgasms**, through **masturbation**, not intense climax, sense of over, and over and over again, no strong emotions attached. **Just do it!** Matter of fact. Like a monkey. *No feelings or sensations attached, an acceptance this is how it is, reproduction, life.* A monkey just reproduces in front of anyone at any time, they will **copulate**. . . . I felt a **huge wave of sexual energy** in the pit of my stomach like a magnetic pull towards him. He was openly **flirting** with me with extremely intense eye contact. . . . Dreams of masturbation, running out of the house into a field or to some grass area to **try to get some privacy to masturbate** and my family keep chasing me or bothering me. . . . Dream: I went to some toilets and found lots of **school girls having sex with different older men in each toilet**. There was an older lady organising the session and I'd gone there to be trained for her position, so I could organise the sessions. . . . Dreams of sexual betrayal taking place in the context of shopping."

Under control
"The feeling was that **I couldn't control or alter my behaviour, it's like a hyper-awareness** where I am totally self-aware and self-conscious, aware of my eyes, where I am looking, my body language. . . . I feel as though I'm wearing an old brown (leather?) coat, which is no longer right for me, and **I need to cast it off** (moulting?) . . . . I feel like the remedy is inside me and I want to get it out. It feels like a black furry gremlin thing moving around in circles in the area of my solar plexus. **I want to get it out of my body.**"

Disgust
"I had the feeling that being in a human body disgusts me; that humans are disgusting; they hurt and kill each other and the energy feels low around some people. I feel that the inner part of a person is light and good but something about being in the body makes people behave badly. . . . Dream, woke disturbed by **horrible face** and aware of **murder**, something was horrific, a sensation of **horror**. Sensation of something **revolting, disgusting and festering, rotten and decaying**. . . . Dream: in the distance a huge wave coming and beaconed my friend to hurry put my dog lead on and we hurried to the top of a hill. The sensation was running for survival, had to be quick. . . . Dream: sense of doing something that I knew I should not be doing, sense of **dishonesty, disgust**, reaction was amazement that the person I was stealing from was not angry. . . . I dreamt that my cousins and brother were performing a sexual act on me by **pushing something into my vagina and pulling my legs apart**, it makes me cringe thinking about it! In my dream the thing they were pushing inside me was a chickens head with its long neck. . . . Dreamt that I was eating a piece of **raw chicken**. I have no recollection of putting it in my mouth in the dream, but I remember that I was chewing it and felt **disgusted** and **repulsed** by it. . . . Dreamt of black and white very thin and light centipede? Encased, **burrowed** in my skin, mostly on my abdomen, as if it were **hibernating** or being protected there! **Ugh**!; there were a few; I squeezed one out, it was **alive**; on my right thigh

I put my hand to some kind of formation that was there – hard rock-like black scab? . . . . Dreamt that I was looking after a work colleague's baby and that the **nappy fell off** when they were about to **poo** so I caught it **in my hand**! It was **disgusting** and then somehow it ended up in my **mouth** and I felt so **sick** trying to spit it out and thought I should make myself sick to get it all out of my system."

Magic / witches / ghosts

"Dreamt of lilies and wolves. The lilies had to be ground up to make a remedy along with a **magic ceremony**. There were many wolves at the place I was staying (it was a magical place). A **wolf growled** and tried to **bite** me but I managed to grab it by the back of the neck and it went away. It was ragged looking with cuts in its fur and above one eye. . . . They were a **subtle menacing presence** . . . half of it was very **magical** and **serene** yet there was this menacing presence of the wolves. When I woke up it was like the two feelings cancelled each other out. . . . Dream that I was a white witch with long red hair. . . . There has been a theme of witches coming up and I felt that maybe I needed to become a witch. . . . Dream: I could see the **ghost** and it was a black form which made me anxious. I wanted to shout at it but couldn't make any sound come out. I shot white light at the ghost and she turned white but was still coming in my direction. The ghost came right to me and started **pushing** me backwards. I was **falling** backwards with the ghost pushing me and I couldn't so anything to stop it, then I woke up suddenly with the feeling of this ghost woman's arms pressing on my chest."

Insect themes

"Dreamt that I was looking in the mirror, wearing a pretty top which had a see-through section in the cleavage area up to the throat. I saw a dark patch there and on closer inspection realised that I had an extra nipple there. It was flat, like a man's. . . . Dreamt of having **really hairy legs**, black dark hairs with wounds on my legs like gashes that had scabbed over, on my right leg and right buttock. . . . Dreams of **food**, of being in a room with many people like a canteen and being served last, and the waiter *dropped my food on the floor (bacon) and saying I should eat it anyway*, I remember saying, don't worry I will eat it, its fine. . . . Dreamt I was **dancing** for a camera like a photo shoot. My brother was dancing with me but I was the person being filmed, I was really **energetic** and spinning loads and doing really **agile** moves that meant I was really high in the air above my brothers head. It surprised me in the dream at how high I could jump. . . . Dream: We were all organised by **robots**, metal beings, looked like humans, no talking to us and anyone who didn't do their work were taken aside and either physically beaten or killed. I spent time in the dream running away from them, lots of fear in dream of being **caught** and **humiliated**. . . . Dreams where I am very **critical** of people. No sense of **respect**."

DIPTERA

Musca Domestica (Common house fly)

Phylum: Arthropoda.
Class: Insecta.
Order: Diptera.
Family: Muscidae.

The housefly is believed to have evolved in the Cenozoic Era and has spread all over the world as a close associate of humanity. Major breeding sites include garbage dumps, open privies, livestock manure, and wastes around meat, fruit and vegetable processing plants. They feed on almost all human foods as well as on carcasses, excreta, bacteria, and anything in a state of decay. They have mouthparts specifically adapted for sucking up fluid or semifluid foods. House-flies have been used in the laboratory in research into aging and sex determination. The female usually mates only once and stores the sperm for later use. She lays hundreds of eggs on decaying organic matter which soon hatch into legless white larvae, known as maggots. The adults can carry pathogens on their bodies and in their faeces, contaminate food, and contribute to the transfer of food-borne illnesses. They also play an important ecological role in breaking down and recycling organic matter.

Proving by: **Susan Sonz, USA (1999).**[6]

Possible fundamental delusion
* *Superiority, of – inferiority at the same time; and*

Keywords
Beautiful / Dirty / Corruption / **Maggots** / Vermin / Metamorphic / **Gender confusion** / Homosexual / Garbage / Decomposing / **Inferiority** / Superiority / Neglected / **Abused** / Suicidal / Watched / Eyes / **Corruption** / Flying / Floating / Crypt / Sewers / Prostitution / Disease

SRP Delusions
* *Abused; being*
* Appreciated; she is not
* *Beautiful* – things look
* Body – out of the body
* *Cancer; has a*
* *Corruption*; surrounded by
* *Decayed*; tarnished and impure; everything is
* Disease – *incurable disease*; he has an
* Die – about to die; one was – alive again; and
* *Dirty* – everything is
* Fancy; illusions of – followed by – *garbage*
* Fingers – thousand fingers – scratching the body
* Garbage – beautiful; is
* Hearing – retching
* *Maggots*; seeing

- Metamorphic
- *Neglected* – he or she is neglected
- Possessed; being
- *Pregnant*; she is
- Seeing – dead animals with insects eating out eyes
- Seeing – eggs; insect and fish
- Separated – group; he is separated from the
- Smell; of
- Superiority; of

- *Vermin*
- Visions; has – beautiful – kaleidoscopic changes; varied
- *Walking – behind him; someone walks*
- *Watched; she is being*
- *Wrong – suffered wrong; he has*
- Young; she is again
- Eyes – darting like an animal
- Eyes – hundred eyes; seeing

Mind

- Anger – easily
- Animal consciousness
- Anxiety – alone; when
- **Anxiety**
  - Conscience; anxiety of
  - Driving from place to place
  - Health; about
  - Time is set; if a
- Aversion – women; to – men; in
- Cleanness – mania for
- Company – aversion to – sight of people; avoids the
- Confidence – want of self-confidence – inferior; feels
- Confusion of mind – Identity, as to his – sexual identity
- Conscientious about trifles
- Contemptuous
- Cursing
- *Disgust*
- Elated
- Exertion – physical – amel.
- Extravagance

- Fear
  - Accidents; of – car
  - Attacked; fear of being
  - Black – men
  - Homosexuality; of
  - Neglected; of being
  - Sexual – assault
- Forgotten – something; feels constantly as if he had forgotten
- Forsaken feeling – isolation; sensation of
- Loathing – oneself
- Love – perversity; sexual
- Love – romantic love; desire for
- Mania – hands – washing face; while
- Masculinity – increased sensation of
- *Mistakes; making – gender; in*
- Pities herself
- Reproaching others
- Rest – cannot rest when things are not in the proper place
- Restlessness – pain, from
- Suicidal disposition – thoughts
- Weary of life

Dreams

Abortion / Beach / **Betrayed**; having been / **Blood** / Boat / Bombs / Buildings – glass buildings / Cats / Children; about – newborns – sick / **Cholera** – dying from / Closet – being on / Clothes – red dress / **Corruption** / Criminals, of / **Crones** / **Crypt** / Dead; of the – friends / Dead; of the – relatives / Decomposition / **Dirt** / **Disgusting** / Dogs – black / Drowning / Elevator / **Excrements** / Factory / Falling – water, into / Fire / Fish / Floating / Flood / Flying / Flying – room; from room to / Games / Ghosts / Glob – black, oily / Grass / Hair – red / **Homosexuality** /

Horses / House / Island / Italy / Landlord / Lascivious / Lascivious – orgasm; with / Obscene – orgasm; with / Looking – down from above / Money / Monsters / Murder / Nuns / Obscene / **Pedophilia** / Picking sores till bleeding / Police / Pregnant – being / **Prostitutes** / Pursued; being / Rape / **Sewers**; about / Sexual / Sexual – violence / Sharks / Skating / *Soldier – being a – Russian soldier* / Surgery / Swimming / **Threatened**; of being / **Trolls** / **Tumor** / **Tunnel** / **Violence** / War / **Water – dirty** / Water – swimming in / Wedding / Worms

Physicals

- **Vertigo**
  - Fall; tendency to – left, to
- **Head**
  - Congestion – anxiety; with
  - Dandruff
  - Pain –
    - § Caffeine; gripping like too much – dull pain
    - § Forehead – Eyes – above – pulsating pain
    - § Occiput – dull pain
    - § Temples – lying down – agg. – pressing pain
- **Eye**
  - Focus – difficult to
  - Opening the lids – shutting involuntarily; and
  - Styes – right eye
- **Vision**
  - Blurred – reading – agg.
- **Ear**
  - Eruptions – Lobes, on – moist
  - Noises In – stretched sounds
  - Pain – cutting pain
- **Nose**
  - Odours; imaginary and real
    - § Chemical
    - § Peaches
  - Smell – acute – strong odours
- **Face**
  - Eruptions
    - § Herpes – Mouth – Corners of
    - § Eyebrows – painful touch
  - Inflammation – Parotid glands – mumps – accompanied by – salivation
  - Ulcers – Lips

- **Mouth**
  - Froth, foam from mouth – waking; on
  - Odour – putrid
  - Pain – Gums – stitching pain
- **Stomach**
  - Appetite
    - § Constant
    - § Diminished – eating; when time for
    - § Disordered – cold – drinks – amel.
  - Nausea – sudden
- **Abdomen**
  - Pain
  - Hypogastrium – sharp
  - Inguinal region – walking – agg.
  - Inguinal region – walking – agg. – cracking
- **Male**
  - Flaccidity – Penis
  - Pain
    - § Testes
    - § Pinching
    - § Extending to – Thighs
- **Female**
  - Eruptions
    - § Herpetic
    - § Labia – boils
  - Masturbation; disposition to
  - Menses
    - § Intermittent
    - § Staining
  - Pain – Uterus – Cervix – sharp

- **Chest**
  - Eruptions
    - § Rash – flat
    - § Scaly
    - § Axillae – rash
  - Pain
    - § Constricting pain
    - § Mammae – Nipples – men; in
    - § Middle of chest – radiating
- **Back**
  - Eruptions – boils – Cervical region – right
  - Pain – Cervical region – dislocated; as if – separated; as if
- **Extremities**
  - Eruptions
    - § Hands – eczema
  - Insensibility – Upper limbs
  - Nodules – red – Thighs
  - Pain
    - § Hips – pulsating pain
    - § Shoulders – right – extending to – Wrist
    - § Shoulders – lying – bed; in – agg.
    - § Upper arms – aching
- **Sleep**
  - Deep – Unrefreshing
  - Position – knees – chest position; knee
  - Waking – late; too
- **Fever**
  - Intense heat
- **Skin**
  - Greasy
- **Generals**
  - Food and drinks
    - § Bacon – desire
    - § Cheese – agg.
    - § Cheese – desire
    - § Vinegar – desire
    - § Water – aversion
  - Heat – flushes of – alternating with – chills
  - Heaviness – internally – alternating with – lightness
  - Paralysis – sensation of
  - Weakness – restlessness; with
  - Weather – windy and stormy weather

Themes by *Susan Sonz*[6]

Four provers had recurring sexual dreams, one more dreamt of rape, and three others had recurring dreams of gay men or **homosexual** issues. . . . **Gender confusion**: one young child who's parent's had both taken the remedy, called his mother, Daddy and his father, Mommy. Our most reliable prover had strong feelings of lurking homosexuality. He felt men were watching him, touching him and were attracted to him. He admitted to a homophobic reaction. . . . One Sensitive Prover was drawn to garbage and the brackish water in the subway, he constantly used language like "being surrounded by **corruption and decay**", he saw garbage "moving", in fact he said he believed the remedy was about **garbage** and that the remedy was **degrading and decomposing**.

   cf. Rattus norvegicus sanguis, Yersinia miasm (Pestinum).

Culex pervigilans and Culex musca (Mosquito)

Phylum: Arthropoda.
Class: Insecta.
Order: Diptera.
Family: Culicidae.

The mosquito goes through four separate and distinct stages of its life cycle: Egg, Larva, Pupa, and Adult. They prefer polluted water with high concentrations of detritus upon which the larvae can feed. They do consume human blood but prefer the blood of bird species that are closely linked to humanity such as doves and pigeons. Females feed on blood, whilst males survive on sugary plant nectar. Once a host is bitten, the mosquito uses its proboscis to take in and digest the blood, injecting saliva instantly after the proboscis enters the host. Mosquitoes cause greater human suffering than any other organism, with over one million people dying from mosquito-borne diseases every year. In addition, mosquito bites can cause severe skin irritation through an allergic reaction to the mosquito's saliva, causing the red bump and itching. Mosquito-vectored diseases include protozoan diseases such as malaria, filarial diseases such as dog heartworm, and viruses such as dengue, encephalitis and yellow fever.

Proving by: **Alastair Gray, Australia (2002).**[2]

Keywords

Suffocating / Ugly, body / **Wrong, suffered** / Misfortune / Pursued / Antagonism / Revengeful / Cursing / *Disgust* / Ennui / Bugs / Rats / War / Wasps / *Prickling* / *Fluttering* / *Sticking* / *Stabbing* / Metallic / Sting ear / Hypersensitive / **Squashed** / Wiped out / Dizzy / **Blocked** / **Cocoon** / **Ambitious** / **Superiority** / Harassed / *Respect* / Offended / Dirty / Cockroaches

SRP delusions

- *Suffocating*; as if
- *Attack under*
- Head heavy; his own
- Misfortune
- Narrow; everything is
- *Offended; people he has*

- *Pursued*; he was
- **Walls will crush him**
- Wrong; he has done
- *Appreciated; she is not*
- *Body; ugly body looks*
- **Wrong; suffered he has**

Mind

- *Antagonism – herself, with*
- Anger – violent
- Anger – *misunderstood* when
- Alone – sensation of being
- *Checking* – twice or more; must check (OCD)

- Confusion – identity as to his – head *separated*
- **Disgust – body of one's own**
- *Disorder* – sensitive to
- *Ennui* – tedium
- *Extravagance – squandering money*
- Fastidious

- *Hatred – revengeful, and*
- *Rage – fury, cursing with*
- *Reserved*
- *Sociability*
- Shrieking – must *shriek*, feels as though she
- Thinking – complaints agg, thinking of his
- Thoughts – persistent
- Thoughts – vagueness of
- *Will – loss of will power*

Dreams

Accusations – **crime**; of wrongful / Animals, of – *biting* him / *Animals, of – wild* / *Body, body parts – cut off* / **Bugs**, insects – stung by / Busy; being / Child, children – rescuing them / Crimes – committed; he had / **Cruelty** / Driving a – car – fast / Fingers – *cutting*, cut off / **Rats** / Scientific / **Snakes** – bitten by; of being / Striving and urging, anxious / True, seem; on waking / **War** / **Wasps** / Water – swimming in

Physicals

- **Vertigo**
  - Extending from – vertex
  - Motion – agg. – head, of
  - Turning – agg. – motion of head, or
- **Head**
  - *Heat – vertex*
  - Lump sensation
  - Pain
    - § Breathing deep – amel.
    - § Darkness – amel.
    - § Sitting – amel.
    - § Stooping – agg.
    - § Touch – agg.
    - § Forehead – eyes – behind – reading agg.
    - § *Boring, digging, screwing – temples – extending to – inward*
    - § *Paroxysmal – decreasing gradually*
    - § *Tingling, prickling – Vertex*
- **Eyes**
  - Agglutination – waking; on
  - Closed – convulsive, spasmodic
  - Light – agg. – bright
  - Open, opening – hard to keep open
  - Pain
    - § Closing eyes – amel.
    - § Aching – light – bright, agg.
  - § *Burning, smarting, biting – exertion agg. – eyes, of*
  - § Pulsating, throbbing
  - Photophobia – daylight
  - Inflammation
  - Noises – agg.
- **Ears**
  - Obstruction, stopped sensation
  - Pain
    - § *Lancinating*
    - § *Piercing*
    - § *Pulsating, throbbing*
    - § Swallowing – amel.
    - § Swelling
- **Face**
  - Heat – flushes
  - Numbness, insensibility
  - Pain – *prickling*
  - Paralysis
- **Mouth**
  - *Tingling, prickling*
- **Throat**
  - *Pulsation*
- **Stomach**
  - Distension – painful
- **Rectum**
  - *Excoriation*
  - Inactivity, rectum
  - Lump sensation
  - Pain – *sticking*

- **Female**
  - *Coition – aversion to, sexual aversion*
  - Leucorrhea – *albuminous*
  - *Menses*
    - § Bright red – dark, then
    - § Clotted, coagulated – large
    - § Painful, **dysmenorrhea** – warmth amel.
    - § Profuse – gushes, in
    - § Thin, liquid – clots, with
  - Pain
  - Vagina – extending to – upward
  - Aching – vagina / *Cramping – uterus / Cutting* / Warmth amel.
- **Chest**
  - Ball sensation
  - *Fluttering* sensation
  - Pain – digging
- **Sleep**
  - Disturbed – anxiety, from / Dreams; by / Thoughts; by
  - Eruptions – red – spots
- **Skin**
  - Itching
    - § Discharges, after
    - § Violent
  - Roughness, scraped
- **Generals**
  - Pain
    - § *Boring, grinding, grating*
    - § Dragging, bearing – down
    - § *Piercing*
    - § *Pricking*
    - § *Sudden*, paroxysmal – decreasing gradually
    - § *Tearing* – cramping
  - Paralysis – lower part, paraplegia
  - Secretions of mucous membranes – Bland / transparent
  - *Separated*, parts of body feel

Pathogenetic[2]

Sting / Sting ear / Sting thigh / *Sticking* pain / *Stabbing* pain / Shaking / Business / Industriousness / Irritability / Slow mentally sluggish / Lack of concentration / Disinclination to work / No responsibilities / Desire to be alone and not talk / *Rage violence* / Dead / Shameless / Floating in air / Ungrounded / Irritation lip / *Metallic Taste* / Made things sour / Coating in mouth / **Head** symptoms / Tired and heavy the whole time / **Eyes** / Goggle / Jabbed in the chin / Bruised / As if a bee sting / Cut in leg / Cut in face / Cold hands / Shins / Tibia

Female

PMT / PMS / Menses; pain before / Clots / Late / Quick / Finished quick exit / Sudden cessation

Themes

I have added bold type to illustrate the prominent themes.

Squashed, trapped, narrow feeling

"Lying in bed; had vision on closing my eyes of being in a room **squashed against a wall**, the room was very narrow and dark. I was there for an exam. . . . I keep having this *fear / thought that I am going to* **haemorrhage** – through my mouth, ears, eyes, nose, urinary or digestive tract . . . *Impatience, willingness to quarrel, anxiety and fear of death*; poor memory and a disinclination for all work; he is so busy **scratching** to relieve the **itching** and so busy walking to relieve the **restlessness**, that any interruption makes him impatient and ready to quarrel."[2]

Mind – "Because of the sensations in head and eyes it dominated my being and all senses and was the only thing I was aware of. . . . I'm **hypersensitive** to anything – tiny amounts of noise, little niggly things. I'd say I'm happy to have my own company . . . *just not wanting to be out in public* – just cause it took so much effort. . . . I felt *over-whelmed*, confused. I just didn't have much mental capacity. I felt emotionally exhausted . . . I was just *questioning my existence . . . I am amazed at how clear my mind is. It is as if everything is brighter and clearer . . .* thoughts are more precise. . . . I had this feeling of *vagueness and detachment* as if I were watching myself from a different position while my physical self was being *observed*. Mind detached from body. Also became somewhat **dizzy** . . . Worn out. Flat. Lethargic. Reserved and focused. **Wiped out**. Even friends notice – 'seems like you are very *distant*' . . . Impossible to be left alone. Very sensitive to storms – when rain comes, I feel 'free'. Dizziness and confusion of mind . . . I cannot support *strong odours like fish* cooking, even in the street when I go shopping the fish odours coming out of the restaurants are unbearable for me. . . ."[2]

Vertigo – "Uncoordinated, knocking into things, not moving precisely . . . experiencing giddiness whilst working on the PC. It *feels like I am going to fall off my chair*. Does not last very long and is not constant but rather *intermittent*."[2]

Ear – "Very *sudden pain in my left ear, inside the ear drum*, severe. Like a tic bit my ear drum. *Throbbing and pulsating. It made my head jerk when it began.* It lasted for less than a minute. Better for swallowing. Ears feel blocked – *like I'm in a cocoon*. Not better for swallowing."[2]

Face – "Slight numb sensation coming on all over my face – like its hard to move the muscles on my face, especially my mouth. Need to ask lips to move like a delayed reaction."[2]

Provings of Culex musca by J.T. Kent and N. Shah.[20]

Mind

- **Delusions**
  - ○ *Against him; people are*
  - ○ Granted; being taken for
  - ○ *Harassed*; he is
  - ○ *Poisoned* – has been; he (Kent)
  - ○ *Raped*; is going to be
  - ○ **Superiority; of** (*Platina, Sulphur, Granite*)
  - ○ Wrong – everything is
- **Fear**
  - ○ Ghosts, spectres; of
  - ○ **Murdered**; of being
  - ○ *Panic attacks, overpowering*
  - ○ People; of, anthropophobia
  - ○ Strangers; of
  - ○ *Tunnels*; of (*Claustrophobia*)
- Abusive, insulting
- *Ambition – **ambitious** – achieve things; desire to*
- *Boaster, braggart – squanders through ostentation*
- Censorious, critical
- Colours – desires – bright
- Direct, open, blunt

- Extravagance – ostentation; by
- Fastidious
- Initiative; lack of
- Interruption – ailments from, agg.
- Irritability – trifles, about
- Mirth, hilarity, liveliness
- Offended easily
- Quick to act
- Relaxed feeling, letting go
- **Respect – desires** (*cf. Blatta orientalis*)
- Restlessness – itching – from
- Rudeness
- Sensitive, oversensitive – colours; to
- Slam the door; desire to
- Strangers; in presence of – agg.
- *Voyeurism*
- Vulnerable; emotionally

Dreams
Actors, actresses; of / Beautiful / **Bugs**, insects / *Cats* / **Cockroaches** / Competition; of / Conflict / *Crabs* / Danger / Dead; people, of; grandfather / ***Dirt, toilets, dirty*** / Dogs / Eruptions / Fights / Friends / Greenhouses / ***Hair; falling out*** / Landscapes; beautiful, of / ***Stabbing others*** / Studies; of

Physicals (Kent's proving)
- **Vertigo**
  - Forehead; In
- **Ear**
  - Fullness; sensation of – blowing the nose agg.
- **Nose**
  - Discharge – Posterior nares – crusty
  - Sneezing – ineffectual efforts
- **Mouth**
  - Salivation – sleep – during – agg.
- **Throat**
  - Swallow; constant disposition to
- **Male**
  - Pain – Penis – Glans – burning
- **Female**
  - Menses
    § Clotted – dark clots

  § Copious
  § Wash off; difficult to
- **Back**
  - Wind was blowing; as if – cool, on back
- **Sleep**
  - Waking – frequent – heat – bed; of
- **Generals**
  - Air; draft of – sensation of a draft – fanned; as if
  - Faintness – hunger; from
  - Light; from – agg.
  - Mucous secretions – ropy, tenacious
  - Pain – stitching pain
  - Pressure – hard – amel.
  - Swelling – puffy, edematous
  - Warm – wraps – amel.

Natural behaviour
Blood sucker / Irritating / Harassing

CASE 4.1 Vestibular neuritis

Patient: Female, age 34

Prescription: Culex pervigilans 30c

∫ It all starts happening in the forehead – **spinning, pressure** – this all feels a bit much but I just carry on. I end up feeling **zonked** by the experience. **Helpless, Drained, Heavy,** just want to close off to everything. It requires **focus, attention** and **precision** to do my work; I must *do a lot of work in a short space of time*. If dizziness comes on then that is impossible. It is really taxing. **Like it has got a mind of its own, this thing. It drains my energy. Another entity taking over you** (animal).

∫ Can't control how it is going to affect me. Its quite freaky!

∫ Would love to just dance – but it is stopping me . . . I am just not myself.

∫ **The thing will take over me even more** – and distract me.

∫ I just can't take it out and be like – off you go. Its like an entity.

∫ Other times I just push myself and do those things – because I am **not letting it take over me.**

∫ Don't feel like I am being myself. *It* comes on when *it* wants.

∫ It tricks me – you're ok now. Then I get dizzy.

∫ If I can't get out, I feel stuck.

∫ Best thing I can take from this is that it is life forcing me to slow down.

∫ Just want to be on my own.

∫ Not able to be more of this **adventurous** person I would like to be.

∫ **Bored** of talking about it – I don't know how I do it. . . .

∫ *Business or work* creates a pressure in the centre of my forehead.

∫ It is like a movement in my brain or my head. Not true spinning.

∫ I find that sounds can be really intense – needing to **escape**, get away from it.

∫ *Following procedures and advice of the doctors*, so I am **terrified it might never go away.**

∫ *Might be something I always must live with*. When the fuck is this going to go away? (Like the sycotic miasm, with sudden attacks when the entity takes over. Malarial miasm).

∫ **Panicky.**

∫ This is **insane**! Feel I must go slower – at a different pace to everyone else.

∫ **I need my boundaries to be respected.**

∫ Feeling that I am coming out of something that stopped me moving forwards (Delusion, hindered – malarial miasm). I just need to move forwards, but something is dragging me down so I need to *get away* from them. More than anything, I want to be moving forwards, but feel as though I am being held backwards.

∫ I need the **recognition that I deserve**, not that I want, but that I deserve. Only I know the hard work that I have put in to things. There is a sense of ploughing away and waiting for the harvest of my skills and talent which is a sort of *recognition* in the industry. If I get more recognised I will be given work more easily instead of striving to get to the next stage. . . . I feel like there is a wall – all I need to do is push through and step onto the other side. . . .

Modalities
∫ Bright lights and visual stimuli agg.
∫ Concentration agg.
∫ Sitting there – everyone talking really loudly over each other just to be heard. agg.
∫ Noise and acoustics bouncing off the walls agg.
∫ When in a calm space amel. Talking agg.
∫ Dizziness and pressure – concentrating or thinking agg. **it has got a life of its own**.
∫ Strong smells agg. Gets in nose and sinuses
∫ When the dizziness comes on – feels like when you quickly get up to stand.

SRP
∫ If I am moving my head to the side; whilst moving; the sensation follows me threefold (*as if her vision is lagging behind the actual head movement*).
∫ Disorientation – head is moving a lot – a sense of being on a boat.

Insect themes
∫ Parasite – Invaded by an entity that takes over.
∫ Work, respect and recognition important themes.
∫ Needs to work in a focused and precise way.
∫ Forced to slow down – would like to operate at a faster pace.
∫ Physical symptoms matched very well.

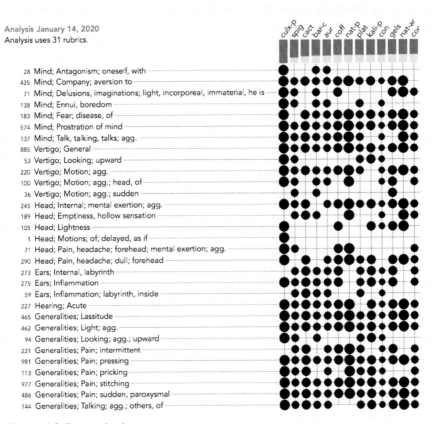

Figure 4.2 *Repertorisation*

HYMENOPTERA

Apis mellifera (Bee venom)

Phylum: Arthropoda.
Class: Insecta.
Order: Hymenoptera.
Family: Apidae.

The honeybee belongs to the Hymenoptera, an order of insects with 4 transparent wings, comprising many of the social insects. In contrast to the carnivorous dietary habits of wasps, bees gather protein from flowers as pollen. They have 4 stages in the life cycle: egg, larva, pupa, and adult. At the end of the first stage stage, the larva moults, spins a silk cocoon, and transitions to the pupa stage. Pupae undergo a complete metamorphosis taking about 7–8 days for queens, 12 days for workers, and 14–15 days for males. Once the final metamorphosis is complete, they chew their way out of the cell and they do not grow or moult after emerging. Queens drastically outlive both worker and males, living between 2–5 years. Only one bee will be the queen or mother of the whole colony. She is larger than all the others, but with a smaller brain and enormous ovaries. The queen asserts control over the worker bees by releasing a complex suite of pheromones.

Much has been written about Apis, so I will focus on highlighting the smaller rubrics rather than repeating existing materia medica.

SRP Delusions
- Bed – someone – in the bed; as if someone is – with him (*Nux-v*)
- Dying – he is
- Images, phantoms; sees
- People – beside him; people are
- **Pregnant**; she is
- Pursued; he was – fiends, by
- Tongue – wood; tongue is made of
- Walking – cannot walk, he – run or hop; must (*frantic, high tempo*)
- **Well, he is** (*Arnica, Opium, Pulsatilla*)

Themes
- Ambitious / Competitive / Driven
- Amorous / Lascivious / Libertine / Nymphomania
- Carefree / Childish / Frivolous
- Destructive – Breaking things
- Domineering / Dictatorial
- Elated / Joyful / Ardent / Ecstasy
- Floating / Flying / Light
- Foolish – Antics; playing
- Future; fear of – Forebodings
- Industrious / Overactive / Busy; fruitlessly
- Intuitive / Clairvoyant / Conscious / Prophesying
- Jealousy / Envy – Ailments from jealousy
- Persecuted / Pursued / Enemies / Victim
- Procrastinating – Undertaking many things, persevering in nothing
- Tormented / Self-punishment – Striking himself
- Yielding / Timid / Delicate

Characteristic Mind Rubrics

- Absorbed
  - business matters; in
  - family matters; in
- Affability
- Ailments from
  - celibacy
  - jealousy
  - rage, fury
- Antics; playing – children; in
- Awkward – haste, from
- Borrowing from everyone (*taking on others problems, as in a busybody*)
- Childish behaviour – delivery; after
- Coma – renal failure; with
- Death – thoughts of – fear; without
- Delirium – meningitis cerebrospinalis
- Fear
  - coughing; of – burst; lest something will
  - death; of – abortion; in
  - death; of – predicts the time (*acon.*)
  - pins; of (*sil.*)
- Hurry – awkward from hurry
- Insanity – busy
- Irritability – sends – doctor home, says he is not sick
- Mania – sexual mania – increased sexual desire; from
- Mirth – wretched; simulating hilarity while he feels
- Mischievous – children; in
- Nursed in children; being – desire – daytime only
- Obstinate – nothing the matter with him; declares there is
- Practical
- Restlessness – sleep – starting from; on
- Sensitive – steel points directed toward her
- Shrieking – piercing
- Will – control over his will, does not know what to do; has no – head; with dullness in the

Clinical _{Clarke}[26]

Abscess / Ankle – swelling of / **Apoplexy** / Asthma / Bladder – affections of / Bright's disease / Carbuncle / Chancre / **Clumsiness** / Constipation – nurslings, of / Constipation – sucklings, of / Diarrhoea / Diphtheria / Dissection wounds / **Dropsy** / Ear – erysipelas of / Erysipelas / Erythema – nodosum / Eyes – affections of / Eyes – optic neuritis / Feet – burning in / Gangrene / Glossitis / Gout / Gum-rash / **Hands – swelling of** / Heart – affections of / Heat-spots / Housemaid's knee / Hydrocephalus / Hydrothorax / **Injuries** / Intermittent fever / Irritation / Jealousy – effects of / **Joints – synovitis of** / Kidneys – Bright's disease / Labia – inflammation of / Laryngitis / Lichen / **Meningitis** / **Menstruation – disorders of** / Nettle rash / Nose – redness of / Operations, effects of / Optic neuritis / Ovaries – inflammation of / Ovaries – pain in / **Ovaries – tumours of** / Panaritium / Pannus / Peritonitis / Phlebitis / Pleurisy / Prostatitis / **Punctured wounds** / Red-gum / Rheumatism / Scarlatina / **Self-abuse** / Suppressed – eruptions; effects of / Sycosis / Syphilis / Throat – sore / Tongue – oedema of / Tongue – ulcerated / Trachea – irritation of / Tumours / Typhus fever / Urethritis / Urine – abnormal / **Vaccination** / **Varicose – veins** / Variola / Wounds

Causation – Bad – news, hearing / Eruptions checked, repelled, or suppressed / Fright / Grief / Jealousy / Mental exertion – shock / News – bad / Rage / Shock – mental / Vaccination / **Vexation**

Temperaments – Awkward persons / **Bilious** – temperament / Busy all the time, but accomplishes little / Elderly persons / **Frivolous** persons / **Jealous** / **Nervous** / Scrofulous / Thin / **Widows**

Vespa Crabro (European Hornet)

Phylum: Arthropoda.
Class: Insecta.
Order: Hymenoptera.
Family: Vespidae.

Hornets make their intricate paper-like nests out of surrounding plant materials and other fibres, preferring dark places such as hollow tree trunks as their home. They only tend to sting in response to being stepped on or grabbed, generally avoiding conflict. They are defensive of the nest and can be aggressive around food sources. They hunt large insects such as beetles, wasps, large moths, dragonflies, and mantises. Social hymenopteran species typically communicate through certain behaviours and pheromonal signals. One example is an alarm dance – this consists of persistent buzzing, darting in and out of the nest and attacking or approaching the target whose presence has triggered the alarm pheromone. European hornets have been observed to steal prey from spiders, which can be classified as an example of klepto-parasitism.

Proving:
This remedy suffers from a paucity of good Mentals, as is lacking a modern proving.

Characteristic Rubrics
- Death – **dying**; sensation as if
- Delusions – house – **fragile**; is
- Unconsciousness – periodical
- Unconsciousness – walking; while
- Extremities – Discolouration – Upper limbs – purple
- Extremities – Pain – **Joints – cutting pain**
- Extremities – Swelling – Hands – painful
- Generals – Pain – Internally – **stitching pain – needles; as from – hot needles**

Clinical
Lilienthal[8] mentions the following:
Tenderness of left ovary, with consciousness of trouble in those parts; frequent desire to urinate; indescribable pain in sacral region, sometimes extending to back; patient wants to be in a cold room.

Formica rufa (Crushed live red ants)

Phylum: Arthropoda.
Class: Insecta.
Order: Hymenoptera.
Family: Formicidae.

Formica rufa have formidable weaponry; such as their large mandibles and the formic acid which they spray from their abdomens. Formic acid was first extracted in 1671 by the English naturalist John Ray by distilling a large number of crushed ants of this species. Nuptial flights take place during the springtime and are marked by savage battles between neighbouring colonies as territorial boundaries are fought. They aggressively attack and remove other ant species from their territory. Their main foodsource is honeydew from aphids. They create part of their nest underground, piling up pine needles and twigs on top of it. Worker ants can be influenced by a chemical stimulus emitted by cocoons to practice parental nursing. They are highly polygynous, re-adopting post-nuptial queens from their own mother colony; leading to multi-gallery nests that may contain hundreds of egg-producing females.

Proving by: **Adolph Lippe, USA (1864).**

Ailments
- "The **sudden appearance** of the pains in rheumatic and gouty conditions, and their **darting from left to right** or right to left, mark the use of Formica. These pains may be more truly described as darting rather than wandering; there is more rapid change than we think of in wandering." Roberts[31]
- "This is a remedy for certain types of chronic nephritis (inflammation of the kidney), and for a tendency to develop polyps (for polyps in the nose, compare with Teucrium marum). We observe red skin with urticaria (hives), and profuse perspiration which does not provide any relief. The mental and emotional aspects of this remedy are yet to be studied." Grandgeorge[9]

Clinical Clarke[26]
Apoplexy / Brain – affections of / Bruises / Chorea / Cough / Diarrhoea / Dislocation / Dropsy / Eyes – affections of / Face – paralysis of / Feet – sweat of – checked, consequence of / Gout / Hair – falling off / Headache / Milk – deficient / Nodes / Over-lifting, complaints from / Paralysis / Rheumatism / Sight – affections of / Spine – affections of / Spleen – pain – in / Sterility / Throat – sore

Causation Clarke[26]
Foot-sweat, checked or suppressed / Sweat suppression of – feet

Mind

- Ailments from – mortification
- Ambition – increased – competitive
- Anxiety – family; about his
- Cheerful – pain – after
- Delusions – move – everything is moving – to and fro
- Dwells – past disagreeable occurrences, on
- Excitement – champagne – as after
- Eccentricity
- Fear – evening
- Forgetful – heat – during
- Forgetful – evening
- Laziness – evening
- Memory – active – past events, for
- Mental exertion – agg. – impossible – night
- Restlessness – night

Physicals

- Head
  - Bubbling sensation in – Forehead; as if a bubble was bursting in
- Ear
  - Pain – cutting pain
  - Pain – waking; on – stitching pain
- Extremities
  - Contraction of muscles and tendons – Joints
  - Discolouration – Joints – redness
  - **Heat – Joints**
  - Pain – **right – then left**
  - Pain – Joints – accompanied by – rash
  - Pain – Joints – motion – slight motion – agg.
- Generals
  - Side – left – then right side
  - Pain – **Joints – wandering pain**

COLEOPTERA (BEETLES)

Cantharis vesicatoria (Spanish fly beetle / Blister beetle)

Phylum: Arthropoda.
Class: Insecta.
Order: Coleoptera.
Family: Meloidae.

The Spanish fly (*Lytta vesicatoria*) is a slender, soft-bodied metallic and iridescent golden-green beetle. The names derive from the Greek *lytta* for martial rage, raging madness, Bacchic frenzy, or rabies – and Latin *vesica* for blister. The defensive chemical cantharidin is produced only by males; females obtain it from males during mating, as some is contained in the spermatophore. It was first isolated and named in 1810 by the French chemist Pierre Robiquet, who demonstrated that it was the principal agent responsible for the aggressively blistering properties of this insect's egg coating. The larvae are very active as soon as they hatch, climbing nearby flowering plants to await the arrival of a solitary bee. Hooking themselves on to the bee using the three claws on their legs, they are carried back to its nest, where they feed on bee larvae and their food supplies. The larvae are thus somewhere between predators and parasites.

Most of the information on Cantharis comes from self-experiments in low potencies, intoxications clinical experience and allopathic usage. Much has already been written about Cantharis, so I will keep it brief rather than repeat what is already well documented.

Important delusions
- **Choked** – ice-cold hands; by
- Injury – being injured; is

SRP Delusions
- Business – doing business / talks of money / working hard
- Hand – taking her hand; something – midnight
- Possessed; being
- **Seized**; as if

Clinical
- Principally used for **cystitis** and **burns** or burning, cutting pains
- Often there is a strong sexual drive to the remedy and a predominance of symptoms relating to the urogenital system
- Erotic mania / sexual perversity / adultery / priapism / masturbation
- Self-harm – scratching, tearing
- Hydrophobia
- Violent rage
- Roving restlessness
- Convulsive, paroxysmal, twitching
- Dysentery, yellow fever, gonorrhoea, gangrene, haemorrhage

Coccinella septempunctata (Ladybird)

Phylum: Arthropoda.
Class: Insecta.
Order: Coleoptera.
Family: Coccinellidae.

The seven-spot ladybird is the most common in Europe. Its elytra are red punctuated by a total of seven spots, hence the name. Their distinctive spots and attractive colours apparently make them unappealing to predators. When threatened, they may both play dead and secrete a fluid from their leg joints which gives them a foul taste. Adults can eat up to 100 aphids a day. Rather than using any complicated methods for eating its prey, the ladybird kills its prey outright before devouring it.

Proving by: **Eketarina Chamurliyska, Sofia, Bulgaria (2004).**[11]

Keywords
Attractive / Haughty / Clairvoyance / Beautiful / Materialistic / Vanity / Nostalgia / **Attended to; desire to be** / Gypsies / Mansions / Being taken care of / Not being protected / **Trigeminal neuralgia** / Alternating sides

Themes
The dreams brought out in this proving are noteworthy for highlighting the polarity between: **Gypsies** (representing a vagabond archetype; travellers, waifs and strays, of no fixed abode) *vs.* **Mansions**, big luxurious homes that have been renovated. The Insect remedies have a fundamental polarity between dirtiness; an inner feeling that one lacks respect *vs.* the desire to earn lots of money and make a success of oneself. Provers looked at themselves in the mirror and admired their beauty in a remarkably similar way to the provers of Firefly. Both ladybirds and fireflies are certainly less reviled than other insects; both have an innocence or magical fairy-like quality about them, which perhaps brings them closer to the butterflies. Provers of ladybird also wanted to go out and buy more materialistic things, or wanted their partners to buy them fashionable boots instead of books. There was a strong theme of wanting to be attended to; haughtily clicking one's fingers, or of spontaneously attending to the needs to others so that they can be comfortable.

Mind
- Activity – desires activity
- Animals – love for animals
- *Attended to; desire to be*
- *Attractive; desire to be*
- Benevolence
- Business – desire for
- *Cares, full of – others; about / Caring*
- Change – desire for
- *Clairvoyance*
- Company – aversion to – desire for solitude
- Company – desire for
- Confident
- Confusion of mind – time; as to
- Defiant / Inciting others
- *Delusions – beautiful – she is beautiful and wants to be*
- Delusions – light = low weight – is light; he
- Delusions – unreal – everything seems unreal
- Excitement – nervous
- Exertion – physical – desire
- Fear – disease; of impending
- Fear – water; of
- Grief
- *Haughty*
- High-spirited
- Homesickness
- Hydrophobia
- Industrious
- *Intuitive*
- Irritability
- *Materialistic*
- Memory – weakness of memory – facts; for

- Memory – weakness of memory – numbers
- Mistakes; making – calculating, in
- Quarrelsome
- *Sociability*

- *Truth – telling the plain truth*
- *Vanity*
- *Vivacious*
- *Yearning / Nostalgia*

Dreams

Accidents / Animals / Beach / Boat / *Care-taking – being taken care of* / *Caring – another person; about* / Children; about – newborns / Children; about – rescuing; of / Dead; of the – relatives / Earthquake / Father / Flood / Flood – house is in a / Forsaken; being / Friends / **Gypsies** / Helping – people / Homeopathic remedies / Horses / Horses – running / House – big – **mansion** / House – **built; houses being** / House – **collapsing** (*demolished; being*) / House – country; in the / House – **majestic** / House – moving / House – other people's; being in / Journeys / Knives / Men / Mother / People – crowds of / Pleasant / *Protected; being – not being protected from harm* / Searching – someone; for / Shooting; about / Stairs / Stairs – ascending / Walking / Women

Clinical

Neuralgia / Dentistry

Physicals

- **Vertigo**
  - Alternating with – Teeth; pain in
- **Head** – **Pain**
  - Forehead
    - § Touch – agg.
    - § Sides – right – stitching pain
- **Eye**
  - Pain – light; from – agg.
- **Face**
  - Heat
  - Pain
    - § Extending to – Ear
    - § Nerves – *Trigeminal neuralgia*
- **Ear**
  - Pain – External ears – *burning*
- **Mouth**
  - Coldness – sensation of coldness
    - § *Icy*
    - § Gums
  - Pain
    - § Neuralgic
    - § Gums – *neuralgic*
  - Swelling – Gums
- **Teeth**

- Pain
- Cold air; sensation as from – forced into teeth; were
  - § **Drawing** pain – paroxysmal
  - § **Jerking** pain – torn out; as if – teeth would be torn out; as if
- **Throat**
  - Elongated – Uvula – sensation as if
- **Stomach**
  - Appetite – insatiable
- **Kidneys**
  - Pain – radiating
- **Urine**
  - Sediment – sand – gravel
- **Female**
  - Pain – Ovaries – right
- **Chest**
  - *Formication* – Mammae
  - Fullness – Mammae – *sensation of fullness – milk in mammae; as if*
- **Extremities**
  - Pain – Shoulders – *alternating sides*

- **Sleep**
  - ○ Sleepiness – pain – after – neuralgia; after an attack of
- **Generals**
  - ○ Pain – *neuralgic*
  - ○ Side – *right – then left side*

CASE 4.2 Trigeminal neuralgia

Patient: **Female, age 49**

Prescription: **Cocc-s 30c**

Insect themes

∫ Makes you feel dirty, grubby . . . scrubbing on the ground. . . . Want to wash it all off me . . . want to get up and get out of there – like I want to go and climb up a mountain. . . .

∫ Clear my body. Get air flowing through me. (*Earth to Air*)

∫ *Feel mucky and dirty, mixing with people who have no respect.*

∫ *It soaks into me and I can't kick it off.*

∫ Feel like others put you down. . . . Not an insult . . . but you should have respect.

∫ Insulted; not good enough, inferior – they are better than you are.

∫ Respect is a big thing with me. . . . Sometimes feels like I am a bit better than others. . . .

∫ Dislike people going out drinking and flirting . . . Because I am not like it. Because I have got high standards . . . you're insulting that person you are with by eyeing someone else up.

∫ Feel like I am in a worthless job – what's the point?!

∫ Feeling like I am dying if I don't keep my mind occupied. People zap me all day.

∫ Like to be organised, like to be prepared – don't want anything to spring up on me.

∫ Impatient – quick, snappy, wanting to get on. Trying to do half dozen things at once. Panic when something wrong with me; over react and over think things.

∫ Confrontation – happens to me. Makes me feel uneasy. Out of comfort zone. (*animal*)

Symptoms

∫ **Facial neuralgia**

∫ Pain whilst moving my hair, feels tender and sore.

∫ Tingling – distracting – always there as a reminder it hasn't gone.

∫ **As if someone is gripping you.**

∫ Heat agg.

∫ Like cigarette burn on top of head. Scalding pain.

∫ Tingling cheekbones around eye. Little stabs in my ear and face.

∫ Stabbing pain in R ear / Burning on top of skull – scalp, vertex / Pain during coition – Wouldn't be able to take anymore, **just get off me.**

∫ **Pain is always lurking in the background** – always there as an irritant, not letting me enjoy myself.

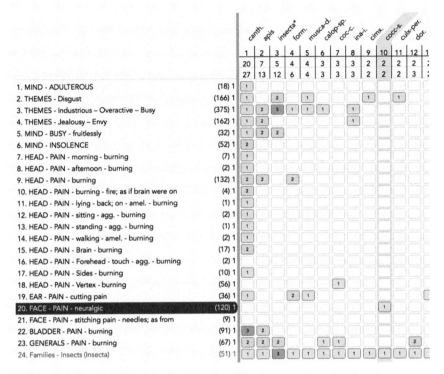

Figure 4.3 *Repertorisation* (limited to Insects)

Cantharis 30c plussed daily was my initial prescription. This failed to relieve the facial neuralgia, so I turned to the lesser-known remedy – Coccinella septempunctata – again in a 30c solution to be plussed daily. This slowly but surely relieved the complaints and allowed the patient to reduce her prescribed anti-epileptic medication.

Provers speaking as one

"I had a quarrel with a colleague. . . . I went to my boss and I told him that I will **follow the hierarchy upwards** and the problem will be solved. *I shook my finger . . . I gave my hand to my husband to kiss it* and I thought it was normal, not a kind of **haughtiness**. . . . I had a quarrel with my husband because – 'you must show consideration with me', and I shake my finger! I left a pile of dirty dishes to my husband and *I did it on purpose*. . . . I tell easier things to people, without thinking that much, more *spontaneously*. I don't think of consequences, as I usually do, I say it like something natural . . . Snapping or shaking fingers at people (haughtiness) . . . . I went to **beautician**, increased *vitality*, increased desire for work, regulated feeling of hunger, I almost don't eat now. . . . I coloured my hair – desire to be **prettier**, more **attractive**. . . . I put **glittering makeup** with pleasure. I say in front of the mirror every morning 'Thank you, mum' . . . . I wanted an *external change*, I wanted to make my entire hair on coloured tufts. . . . I want that my husband **buy me boots with high heels**, instead of books, as usual. . . . *I eat 4–5 times per day and I am still hungry*. In one week, gained 4 kg. . . . Swelling of breast, as if milk will come out, **with formication**. (*cf. Lampro-sp. The proving of which elicited a tingling sensation as if lactating. . . .*) Stiffening of deltoid muscle, *right. Goes to left*, but it is more para-vertebral (*Alternating sides – Animal feature*)."[11]

Notable dreams from the proving

- Friends are changing their residence; **I help them**. . . . Everybody makes me feel comfortable, **all the time they are doing something good for me**. Caring for me. Somebody even tells me to change my bathing suit because it is wet and I could take cold. **They take a lot of care for me.**
- I dreamed of our old house, which was demolished and now in my dream it has been rebuilt and is very beautiful. . . . Heavy earthquake. . . . I see a building, half-**demolished** and a baby inside, so I come back naturally, take the baby and start running.
- Climbing the stairs, a **gypsy** came up with me. I decided to run but he told me "Don't even think about it, and took out a gun. The next stairs another gypsy came up with me and put a knife to my back. . . . Someone rang at the door, I looked through the eyelet and I saw the same gypsy with the gun. I told my family that he was ringing, but nobody moved. . . . **I realised that I will never be able to protect myself from these gypsies**, because one of them was marrying one neighbor of mine and they would have access to our entrance at any time. Nasty dream. My sensation was that **I was alone and there is no one to protect me. I was alone among friends.** (*cf. Butterflies*)
- I look after the homeless dogs and they are all castrated, de-**vermined**, we take care of them. One of the animals sleeps in the entrance on a sofa, it is the most gentle, the best one, I take care of it for three years. There is an alcoholic, who **harasses us all**, he went back from the pub and slaughtered the animal, he virtually cut it into pieces. I called the police. . . .
- I went out for a walk and was **attacked** by dogs.
- **Pity** for everything and everybody, universal **nostalgia**.
- I dreamt that I went to the hairstylist, and I saw a woman with black shiny hair, and the lower layer was shiny blond like the hair of a Barbie doll.
- Increased intuition, whatever I think of, it happens. I like playing backgammon on the Internet and when I think of a number on the dice, it comes. I know in advance even how I will play.
- "The experiences of three of the provers are interesting in this sense – one had a dream of being threatened with knife, threatened of murder and the other

one really lost her favourite dog, which was virtually slaughtered by a sadist alcoholic. The third one was bitten by a dog. In the homes of three provers during the proving (in January) appeared . . . ladybirds!"[11]

Doryphora decemlineata (Colorado potato-bug)

Phylum: Arthropoda.
Class: Insecta.
Order: Coleoptera.
Family: Chrysomelidae.

Colorado potato beetles are orange-yellow in colour with 10 characteristic black stripes on their elytra. The specific name decemlineata, meaning 'ten-lined', comes from this feature. Around 1840, *Doryphora* adopted the cultivated potato into its host range and it rapidly became a most destructive pest of potato crops. It is today considered to be the most important insect defoliator of potatoes. The females are very prolific and are capable of laying over 500 eggs in a 4- to 5-week period.

Keywords
Solanaceae / Electric / Battery / Burning / Over-work / Stinging / Trembling / Protective outer – Vulnerable inner / Garbage / Invades / Purging / Gonorrhoea

Potatoes are the preferred host for this parasite, but it may feed and survive on a number of other plants in the Solanaceae family. Various authors have made the link between the Solanaceae and Doryphora. Both produced states of delirium in the provings, and Mangialavori has paediatric cases where the remedy has been used favourably where Solanaceae prescriptions have failed.

Pathogenetic Ward[23]
Arm galvanic (electric sensation) / Battery leg / Distress whilst sleeping / Fall, stepping / Feet, pins / Fullness, abdomen / Galvanic battery sensation / Over-work, eyes

Clinical Ward[23]
Battery extremities (sensation as if) / Blackness of eyes / **Burning of feet** / Dimness of eyes / Dimness of sight / Dreams, wild / Fall, stepping / Fatigue, eyes / Fullness, abdomen / Heaviness, abdomen / Overwork, eyes / Pins, feet / Screams, dreams / Soreness, eyes / Stinging, feet / Swelling, feet / Trembling, extremities

"In the Coleoptera family, the members have a **hard protective outer layer and a vulnerable inner body**, reflecting their duality, with emphasis on dark and light with the firefly. Taken with the theme of metamorphosis – for maturation as well as for the species as a whole within its ecosystem, we have the guideline for a beetle family prescription." Begin[21]

CASE 4.3 Extracts by Marty Begin[21]

- "Changing a toxic influence into a balance of dark and light forces."
- Being able to deal with chaos and transmute it into something productive.
- *Polarities* – Dark and light / Hard **protection** *vs.* Soft **vulnerability** (*cf. Molluscs*).
- *Themes* – Going through the dark to come into the light (*metamorphosis / moulting*). (*cf. Gemstones*)
- **Garbage** from her family **invades** her space. Feels like a **leper**.
- Beetle characteristics= amel. Sun and warmth, agg. Dark and cold / Herpes blisters / Tubercular dissatisfaction and industriousness / Empathy / Flying and escape / Need to mature or go through a metamorphosis / Intellectualism and creativity.
- **Crazy** and **addictive**. "**Purging, delete**, you're done". "**Chaotic, aggressive, insane, dark** and **demanding** energies all around her . . . these are adjectives we could use to describe the Solanaceae family . . . she also had to maintain order and stability amidst the chaos of the Solanaceae."[21]

Rubrics

- **Delusions**
  - Fall – at every step, he would
- **Eyes and vision**
  - Vision – dimness of vision were caused by film – before eyes
- **Abdomen**
  - Full – abdomen were
  - Heavy – abdomen were
- **Extremities**
  - Upper extremities – Battery – galvanic, were attached to arms
  - Lower extremities – Pins – feet were full of

- **Urinary System**
  - Urethra – Inflammation
- **Male Genitalia / Sex**
  - *Discolouration – Red – Penis – Glans*
  - *Gonorrhoea – Remedies in general*
  - Itching – Penis – Glans
  - Pain – Penis – Glans – burning
  - Swelling, genitalia – penis, glans
- **Sleep**
  - Comatose
- **Generals**
  - Sensation, of – *Burning*

Lamprohiza splendidula (Firefly / Glowworm)

Phylum: Arthropoda.
Class: Insecta.
Order: Coleoptera.
Family: Lampyridae.

These soft-bodied beetles are commonly called fireflies or glowworms for their use of bioluminescence during twilight to attract mates or prey. They produce "cold light" (with no infrared or ultraviolet frequencies) from specialised light-emitting organs on the lower abdomen. The enzyme luciferase acts on luciferin, in the presence of magnesium ions, ATP, and oxygen to produce light. Firefly luciferase is used in forensics, and the enzyme has medical uses in detecting the presence of ATP or magnesium. They hibernate over winter (during the larval stage) by burrowing underground, or under the bark of trees – emerging in the spring. After several weeks of feeding on other insects, snails, and worms, they pupate for 1–2 weeks – emerging as adults. Most fireflies are distasteful to many vertebrate predators, due in part to a group of steroid pyrones known as lucibufagins, which are similar to cardiotonic bufadienolides found in some poisonous toads.

Proving by: **Marty Begin, Canada (2004).**[4]

Polarities
Carefree, free from responsibility, no guilt *vs.* Trapped by responsibility, guilt, following the rules.

Vulnerable, raw emotionally, weeping *vs.* Fighting emotional state, detached, blocking, numb.

Present in the here and now *vs.* Disappearing, other-world, not present, outside of it.

Ungrounded, light, floating up, uplifting *vs.* Grounded, heavy, pulled down. (*cf. Hamamelididae*)

Peaceful, calm and content *vs.* Spinning, live-wire.

Homey, domestic *vs.* Get away from home, escapism.

Emptiness, openness, naked feeling *vs.* Fullness, containment. (*cf. Milks*)

Imprisoned *vs.* Breaking out of oppression.

Isolation *vs.* Sociability.

Themes
- **Vanity**, wanting attention. (*cf. Coccinella septempunctata*)
- **Foreboding**, not facing change or challenge.
- **Childlike**, children, excitement, disappointment. Growing up from / regressing to, high school.
- **Happy, excited**, dancing, singing, music, fun (*Sanguine temperament*).
- **Dark and light dynamics**: dread of approaching winter, cold, darkness, **amel. (sun)light**.
- Averse to the light, embracing the darkness. (*Mappa Mundi Fire-Air polarity*)
- **Leap of faith**, embracing change or challenge, breakthrough (*metamorphosis theme*).
- **Synchronicity**, magic, clairvoyance.
- **Confident, taking charge**; strong, calm, saying no, taking a stand.
- **Industrious, busy, active**; productive, accomplishing, handling things (*common to insects*).
- **Need to make money** (*common to insects*).
- **Division between body and mind / head, heart and intellect.**

- **Empathizing**, caring for others, helping others, **absorbing energies**.
- Re-connecting with old / distant friends, lovers, (dead) relatives, acquaintances.
- Dead, corpse, morbid, death / life.
- Jealousy, suspicion, sadness, depression, loneliness; trapped in emotions.
- Lost, losing someone / something.
- Flying, wings, free-fall, freedom, planes crashing, travelling, adventure.
- Dreams of sharks with no threat; whales, jelly fish.
- Weddings, about to commit / committing.
- Anxiety about health / Arguing / Fighting / Drugs / Sexual, sensual / Sexually invasive /
- Encounters with younger girls.

"**Polarity; vulnerability and power**, and the protection of vulnerability, which arises from being seen or **being attractive**, and from the **temptation** to give in to the **dark side. . . . She is very guarded in her relationship** with someone who is passive emotionally, active sexually, adventurous, and who perpetuates her search to be seen and loved in a committed way"[4]

Mind
- **Delusions**
  - Appreciated; she is not
  - *Beautiful* – she is beautiful
  - Betrayed; that she is
  - Body – brittle; is (*fragile*)
  - Body – *ugly*; body looks
  - Floating
  - Invaded; one's space is being
  - Light = low weight – is light; he
  - *Neglected* – he or she is neglected
  - New; everything is
  - Oppressed; he were
  - Possessed; being
  - Strong; he is
  - *Trapped; he is*
- Activity – desires activity
- *Adventurous*
- *Affection – yearning for affection*
- *Ailments from – responsibility*
- Anxiety – family; about his
- Anxiety – money matters; about
- Anxiety – work
- Ardent
- *Attracting others*
- *Benevolence*
- *Boundaries; lack of*
- Business – aversion to
- *Carefree*
- Cares, full of – others; about
- Clairvoyance
- Cleanness – desire for cleaning
- Company – aversion to – desire for solitude
- Company – desire for – alone agg.; when
- Confident
- Conflict – higher consciousness and worldly existence; between
- Content
- Dancing
- Detached – observing; as if – outside; from
- *Duty – too much sense of duty*
- *Ennui*
- Escape; attempts to
- Forebodings
- Forsaken feeling – *isolation*; sensation of
- *Freedom*
- Helplessness; feeling of
- Horrible things, sad stories affect her profoundly

- *Impulsive*
- Inactivity
- *Industrious*
- Irresolution
- Jealousy
- Laziness
- *Love – exalted love*
- *Mirth*
- Occupation – amel.
- *Optimistic*
- Peace – heavenly peace; sensation of
- Protecting
- Quarrelsome
- Reproaching oneself
- *Respected – desire to be*
- *Responsibility – give up her responsibility; wanting to*
- *Restlessness – move – must constantly*
- Running – desire for
- *Self-indulgent*
- Selfishness
- *Sensitive – emotions; to*
- Suspicious
- Thoughts – future; of the
- Thoughts – past; of the
- Timidity
- Tranquillity
- *Travelling – desire for*
- Unobserving; nonconformism
- *Vanity*

Dreams
Animals / Children; about – responsibility for / Darkness / Dirt / Friends – old / Grief / Helping – people / Hospitals / Journeys / Light; of / Long / Pets / Romantic / Stealing / Weeping; about / Women / Work

Characteristic Physicals[4]
- **Kidneys** – Twinges in my left side where kidney pains occurred pre-surgery 1999, where there is an old scar
- **Urethra** – After urinating, I felt the sensation of a bladder infection – discomfort, burning mild pain in my urethra. Lasted approximately 5 minutes.
- **Urine** – Smelly urine (kind of like asparagus) / Had this idea that I had a UTI – that I "saw blood" I my urine / Urine was very strong smelling, musty ammonium, asparagus smell / Urine still malodourous, but not as strong.
- **Mouth** – Speech – difficult – articulate, unable to
- **Throat** – Choking – sensation of
- **Abdomen** – Butterflies; sensation of / Emotions agg. / Knotted Sensation – Intestines
- **Female Genitalia / Sex** – Metrorrhagia – dark blood – clots; with / Pain – bending double – must bend double
- **Chest** – Tingling – Mammae in – lactating; as if
- **Back** – Pain – Spine – radiating
- **Extremities** – Pain – pulsating / stitching – splinters; as from / Vibration; sensation of

Case extracts *by Marty Begin*[4]
"I feel responsible for my parent's happiness . . . I'm nurturing . . . would like to be a parent . . . and I'm ambitious. . . . **When I stay busy it makes me feel attractive, strong, competent,** and connected with the world. I'm just walking along the street, just **buzzing** along – energetic, **sassy** . . . I'm a bull in a China

shop . . .what do I do?. . . In my work **I lay on the charm** . . . **People are attracted to me.** . . . When I'm travelling, the most interesting creative people are attracted to me. **I give off a kind of energy.** I'm a little firefly . . . I love **travelling** – you **leave behind all the shit** in you, you can't get out . . . **leave all the responsibilities behind you.** It cures my constipation. I feel **free, foot loose** and **fancy**, light, strong, thoughtful, clear, every historical ruin fills me . . . with a sense of **discovery** and **exploration.** . . . On the other hand things like crappy movies deplete me . . . I'm the **energy source** at my company. . . . I give out so much and **not a lot is reciprocated.** . . . My time, ideas, enthusiasm – **people feed off it.** I know it is my greatest **strength,** but it needs to be met with like-minded people . . . they're like my "be here now" hippy boyfriend. . . . I dwell in the past and future – he's totally non-committal. I'm peripheral to his decision making. . . . I **want the world to respond to me as I respond to it.** . . ."[4] "Dream – In this cave there was a beautiful woman who was pure white. . . . She was **beautiful,** but her whiteness made her **repulsive.** She was a gorgeous **dominatrix** type and her lovely spine curled into paper ribbons at her buttocks. I went to her and said I wanted to be **initiated** and that I'd do anything to be so (*embracing change / metamorphosis*). After I told her all I'd do, she said nothing, so I offered even more. She said I would have initiated you with your first offering but since you have already put forth more, you must fulfil those promises as well for your initiation."[4]

Theme of having to do more and work harder to be initiated; to undergo the rite of passage that allows a transformative process. Also, the duality of beautiful vs. repulsive is a key indication for Insect remedies.[4]

Selected Proving extracts[4]

§ "**The mundane continues to insert its presence into my esoteric realm** and demand attention to what appears to really matter above all." *cf. Limenitis bredowii californica.*

§ (Mind – conflict – higher consciousness and worldly existence; between.)

§ "Stood in front of the bedroom mirror, which is full length, mirror and **flexed my muscles.** I feel more muscular than usual. **I feel strong, tense, in shape** and as if all my muscles are flexed. I liked what I saw in the mirror, and I liked my curves and softness around my hips and thighs. This is not a usual feeling, **admiring my body.** Staring into my own eyes, with a smirk on my face, as if telling myself it was ok to admire myself!"

§ *Focus on appearance, strong sexual energy; even vanity that runs through Insect provings.*

§ "**She felt very vain:** thinking more about what to wear, thinking about style, she got bangs (that she hadn't had since elementary school). Getting the bangs was an **impulsive** move. She wanted to **make a statement,** wanting to be noticed. Wanted to show herself – very unlike her – she normally does not go out of her way to get attention: she thinks it is a sign of vanity."

§ "I feel quite apathetic to most things. . . . I really just want to **escape this life** that I am in right now although I am doing so many things that I really want to do."

§ *"It takes me away from my 'me' time that I just can't get enough of."*

§ "It is like my father's living through me – tendencies and ways of being. He's gone, but the behaviour still lives in me. My mother is a saint – don't know how she put up with us; Mother: rules are made to be followed; **Father: rules are made to be broken**."

§ "The head office people loved my work yesterday . . . **makes me feel respected for my talents and abilities**." (*cf. Blatta orientalis*)

§ "I've been very **indulgent** and there wasn't any reason not to. I have been just going for things. Last night an old girlfriend ***trapped*** me and ***seduced*** me. I was surprised I let in."

§ "Feeling overwhelmed, like taking on patients' problems. . . . Something about a patient creeped me out and **I couldn't separate his energy from mine**. Later he came back and I was totally fine."

§ "I felt the **pure energy of love**. The same emotion I felt when my twin sons were born – in my chest and in my throat. **I felt these emotions in my throat, as if I could choke**. The tears sprang from my eyes – yet – the emotion was love, pure, free-flowing love."

§ "My sister and I have had the potential to make **copious amounts of money with her business / sales skills and my artistic skill** and pure magic of paint. She has **denied my expertise** and only **treated me poorly**. . . . She views me as **competition** and vehemently refused working equally with me before. . . ."

§ "I have that same pressing feeling as if there are fingers inside my mouth pulling. At the top of my head I feel this pressure. **I'm also getting this feeling in the chest, like my breasts are tingling, as if I'm lactating.** The head pressure comes and goes all the time. I still have a domestic streak, doing laundry and putting away summer clothes."

ODONATA

Calopteryx splendens (Banded demoiselle / damselfly)

Phylum: Arthropoda.
Class: Insecta.
Order: Odonata.
Family: Calopterygidae.

The Odonata occupy completely different realms as larvae and adults – moving from water to air. In the juvenile or naiad stage, they are voracious underwater predators, hunting and eating anything they can catch. As adults, they have 2 pairs of wings, a long body and are also fierce hunters. They possess supremely good 360 vision owing to eyes that envelop the head. They are among the fastest and most impressive aerialists of the insects.

Proving by: **Jeremy Sherr, Denver CO, USA (2004).**[22]

Mind

- **Ailments from**
  - Money; from losing
  - Reproaches
  - Rudeness of others
- **Delusions**
  - *Adolescent*; he was again an
  - *Alone*, being – world; alone in the
  - *Appreciated; she is not* (Insects)
  - Body – *vibrating*
  - *Heavy*; is
  - Laughed at and mocked at; being (*Bar-c.*)
  - *Old* – feels old
  - Separated – group; he is separated from the
  - Violence; about
  - Water – under water; he is
  - Work – *accomplish her work; she cannot*
  - *Young* again; she is
  - Eyes – big; of
- **Mind**
  - Ambition – loss of
  - Anger – sudden
  - Awareness heightened – animal awareness
  - Change – desire for
  - *Cleanness* – mania for
  - *Communicative – heart; desire to communicate from the* (*Lepidoptera*)
  - *Conflict – higher consciousness and worldly existence; between* (*Lepidoptera*)
  - Content – himself; with
  - Cowardice – opinion; without courage to express own
  - Death – thoughts of – fear; without
  - Estranged – family; from his
  - *Femininity – increased* sensation
  - Hurry – movements, in – fast enough; cannot do things
  - Industrious – household affairs; in
  - Initiative; lack of
  - Meditation agg.
  - Objective, reasonable
  - Order – desire for
  - Pities herself
  - *Responsibility – give up her responsibility; wanting to* vs. *Taking responsibility too seriously* (*Lepidoptera*)
  - Sadness – heaviness – Body; with *heaviness* of
  - Secretive
  - Sombre; everything that is – aversion to
  - Struggling
  - Thoughts – monotony of
  - Violence
  - Writing – difficulty in expressing ideas in

Dreams

Adventurous / Ascending – descending; and / Betrayed: having been / Children; about – newborns / Friends – old / Losing – things / Metamorphosis; about / Numbers; of / Organizing / Penis – enormous / Please – superiors; desire to please / Secret – discovery of / Seduction / Survival / Trap – being trapped

Clinical

Acute influenza[22]

Provers speaking as one

Pain in shoulders and neck is constant and **reduces any feeling of adult power / competence to childlike vulnerability**. This feeling of childlike vulnerability is as if a catastrophe of nature or forces of nature, beyond the control of human beings, has occurred and it is humbling and *reduces adults to children* . . . throughout the proving I felt more **old and serious, full of burden and responsibility**, while my wife (also on this remedy) behaved like a care free teenager. This dichotomy was much more exaggerated than usual. I became older, she became a teenager. . . . I am aware of a **profound sense of innocence**. I am conscious of and embarrassed by my own **naiveté**. . . . Bought very young-looking hipster jeans with flares. At the hairdresser's said I wanted a 'young' cut. Ten days later someone commented on my new jeans: "Oh, you paid good money for someone to rip out the pockets." "You old fart," I thought. **Felt like I was a kid amongst adults**. . . . Everyone is complaining about how little money they're making and I am doing okay. I feel like I should be helping them more. I don't know why I feel like it is my responsibility. . . . This is the boniest remedy I've ever been on. I feel the density of my bones and the lightness of my spirit. **Suddenly I'm a skeleton**. But my spirit, the part of me that has no density, has lifted. I've been quite a bit lighter. That is the paradox of this proving for me. . . . High energy level continued throughout proving with periods of exhaustion. Used phrases: **adrenaline flow, revved up, running around like maniac**, harried, feeling wiped out, tired, needing a break from the constant work, perpetually tired, I want to be less harried and I want to have a peaceful life. . . . Seem to need an abnormally high amount of stimulus, like computer phone and TV, all at the same time. . . . Felt very **hyper-stimulated** from my core. . . . If someone snuck up behind me, I feel like I would want to spit in their face. . . . I have incredible **strength and** resolve in carrying on at functions of work, teaching and school, through adversities that would normally have emotionally debilitated me. . . . Closed eyes in sunshine and saw raw, **damaged flesh and a bloody arm** – yuck. Want to turn away. Closed eyes again and saw **malnourished, emaciated** children with damaged flesh huddled together. Then saw **blood red**. Then saw walls splattered with something – red blood – and then something silvery grey and iridescent. Then they collapsed. Also saw window splattered then shattered. Then saw green camouflage army fatigues. Saw fire red colour . . . I felt guilty, horrible, on waking. I have been very **short-fused** for several weeks, even to the point of hitting my horses. When they don't do what I want, I **hit with a violent rage**. . . . I've become obsessed with having my hair cut. I need a new cut that shows some **attitude**. I'm feeling like my exterior has to match my interior, that I have more **bite** than I look like I do. Maybe I look **soft** and **easy**. . . .

Source behaviour
From voracious water nymph to air-borne damselfly; a master of flight and speed.

Enallagma carunculatum (Tule bluet damselfly)

Phylum: Arthropoda.
Class: Insecta.
Order: Odonata.
Family: Coenagrionidae.

The tule bluet has a long slender abdomen, large eyes on the sides of the head, short antennae, and 4 heavily veined wings that are held folded together over the back. When a male locates a female, he attempts to grasp her behind the head – if receptive, she allows the male to grasp her then curls the end of her abdomen up to the base of the male's abdomen where his secondary sexual organs are located. This coupling results in the heart-shaped formation characteristic of all odonates. The nymphs are aquatic and move themselves by walking or swimming with a snake-like motion. They mature over winter and spring, undergoing several moults before they are ready to crawl up on emerging vegetation in early summer to begin their metamorphosis into adults.

Proving by: **Melanie Grimes, USA (2002).**[12]

Keywords
Two brains / Conspiracies / Hunter / Meditating / Animal consciousness / Alert / Pursued / Spiders / Electricity / Sudden / Zigzag / **Predator** / Not threatened / **Reptilian** / Conspiracy / Hibernation / Confinement / Gregarious / Frantic / **Anacardium war** / Swords / Phenomenal speed / **Groomed**

SRP Delusions
- Animals – she is an animal
- Body – centreline; of
- Brain – two brains; one within the other; has – *reptilian; as if*
- Conspiracies
- Danger; impression of – threatened
- Face – asymmetrical; features are, her
- Hibernation; about
- Hunter – predatory; he is a
- Pinball machine – sensation as of a
- Stasis; prolonged – been in; he had – liberated; from which he is
- Support – unsupported; feels
- Tentacles – back; coming from her
- Trapped; he is
- Two dimensional – three dimensional objects are

Mind
- Air; in open – desire
- *Alert*
- *Animal consciousness* – **feral feeling**
- Antagonism with herself
- Boundaries – awareness; of
- Clairvoyance
- Cleanness – desire for cleaning
- Cleanness – mania for
- Confusion of mind – Identity; as to his – *duality*, sense of
- Confusion of mind – Sides – left and right; between
- Concentration – difficult – sequential thinking; for
- Eating – after – amel.

- *Fastidious – personal appearance; about – grooming oneself*
- Forgetful – *connection of consecutive thoughts; of*
- Grief – hopelessness; from
- Gestures, makes – mouth; movements of – pulling in; lips, of / sticking out; tongue, of
- Haughty – clothes – *best clothes; likes to wear his*
- Hiding – himself
- Instinctive
- Meditating – deeply
- *Meditating – prostration; with extreme*
- Mistakes; making – calculating, in
- Mistakes; making – writing; in – omitting – letters
- *Observer* – being an
- *Order* – desire for
- Nostalgic
- Resolving – conflicts; internal
- Positiveness
- Postponing everything to next day
- Repeating
- Theorizing
- Threatened; feels
- Tidy – appearance; in one's personal
- Unconsciousness – sensation of
- *Wildness*

Dreams

Accidents – car; with a / Animals / Animals – domestic animals – pets / Bathing / Camping / Car / Care-taking / Cliff / Delivering a baby / Disease / Driving – car; a / **Drowning** / **Escaping** / Excrements – smeared with excrements; being / Excrements – soiling himself with excrements / Flying / Food – preparing food – desserts / Haemorrhage / House / House – youth; like the house of her / Obese; being / **Pursued**; being / Reading / Repeating / Running / **Spiders** / **Suicide** / Unremembered

Physicals

- **Skin**
  - Itching
    - § changing place – rapidly
    - § Scratching – must scratch
    - § Wandering
- **Generals**
  - Side – alternating sides
  - Air; open – desire for open air
  - Change – symptoms; change of
    - § Constant
    - § Rapid
  - Complaints – appearing – suddenly – disappearing; and – suddenly
  - **Electricity**; sensation of static
  - Motion – desire for
  - Pain
    - § Appear suddenly – disappear; and – suddenly
    - § Wandering pain – suddenly
  - **Sudden manifestation**
  - **Zigzag** sensation or appearance

Provers speaking as one

⸋ No logic, no creativity. Instead I felt **animal**, **predator**, but no level of threat, except I was hungry. . . . I wanted to sit up high and observe things. . . to recline up high so I could see what was going on around me. **Not feeling threatened**. . . . Strange sort of light **alertness** and quickness . . . in amongst the **slowness** and **heaviness** all around them – like *a separate brain within a brain* . . . came across a martial arts site that talked of the ultimate 'no mind' state essential to the art as one of **descending into the reptilian brain**. . . .

Much of the **conspiracy** theory, reptilian-type stuff has slithered away now . . . the inertia is back. Difficult to get motivated. Want to hibernate and hide from the world. Need a shower more than anything. . . .

$ **Feeling like coming out of hibernation. I'm abandoning my cage, not going back. I'm done with that part of my life for now.** . . . I am not a neat individual, *but I groomed myself.* I wore a brown belt. Haven't worn a belt in decades. Slick hair, smoothed it down . . . Did a *serious cleaning of my office.* Remedy had an organizing influence . . . I felt better outside, more **liberated.** Inside a friend's house, I felt suffocatingly hot in here. **Couldn't get out fast enough . . . Confinement is an issue.** . . .

$ I am usually **gregarious**; this has an element of **frantic** to it. . . . Feeling so much more comfortable in social groupings than I normally do . . . Irritable. **Bitey.** Almost like "I'll never laugh again". Like the character, Scrooge . . . *Discontented, displeased, dissatisfied, disconcerted, disgruntled* – in short, **full of crap.** Which is no surprise after two days without a stool. I don't like this. It feels like total **stasis.** . . .

$ Everything is **threatening** around me. . . . It is like an **Anacardium war – the good side talking to the bad side.** . . . In myself are competing activities – money is good, money is bad, wrong. There's a dialogue; one says **good**, one says **bad**. *Two energies interfere with my life.* The proving resolved this polarity. . . .

$ Dream: Of being in a **forge** where many **swords** were being made, named and dedicated.

$ Dream: Sitting in the bath, notice lots of **spiders** overhead. . . . All of a sudden, one of the huge spiders **dashes** across the room on its web across the ceiling at a **phenomenal speed** and falls in the bath water beside me. It is upside down and I can see a tiny human-like mouth in a tiny human-like face **gasping for breath.** . . . It is obvious it is going to **choke** and **drown.** I just sit there and watch it. . . . Everything has a **clarity**, a sharpness to everything I see has sharply **defined edges** and stands out from everything else. Physically I feel wonderful. No aches and pains. Feel joyful, full of life, content, peaceful. Just great.[12]

PARASITES

Any organism with a blood stream is a target for blood-sucking parasites. These remedies give a feeling of dependency; greed; laziness; taking without giving back; annoying, irritating; constantly bugging you. Another common theme is an offensive odour.

Galla quercina ruber (Knopper oak gall)

The morbid growth produced on the cupules of *Quercus pedunculata* by the larvae of the wasp *Cynips calicis.* In early Summer, the wasps lay eggs in the developing cupules of Quercus robur, stimulating the oak tree into producing a gall rather than a cup and acorn. The gall provides developing knopper gall wasps with a safe refuge during the most vulnerable time of their life cycle. Galls are sticky and green, later becoming woody and brown, and smell oddly sweet and rancid. They have a ridged and horned hood of smooth green wood. Even though knopper gall wasps have little effect on the general health of a tree, galls can reduce reproduction in the oak host thereby making the gall a potential threat to the reproduction of the tree.

Proving by: **Misha Norland and Peter Fraser, Czech Republic and UK (1998).**[16]

It is interesting to note how the tables are turned between plant and insect in this remedy in relation to Drosera, where the insect is duped by the plant.

- Delusions
  - Banished; she is
  - Clouds – black cloud enveloped her; a heavy
  - *Hand – amputated, she has no hands; as if*
  - Hated; by others
  - **Parasite; she is a**
  - **Sucked up; she is being**
  - Suffocating; as if

- Mind
  - Fear – infection; of
  - Hatred – humankind; of
  - Jesting – black humor
  - **Loathing – oneself**
  - Smiling – *force people to smile; wants to*
  - Suspicious – **plotting against his life; people are**

Proving Themes[16]
- **Flying**, **Floating**, Blown upwards.
- **Nakedness**, **Sexuality**, Pregnancy.
- Anger, Violence, Recklessness.
- Insecurity, **Ugliness**, **Criticised**.
- **Homesickness**, Homelessness, Lack of space.
- Emptiness, old and tired.
- **Curtain, Fence, Separation.**
- **Ostracism and Exclusion.**
- Death, Black humour.

Mind
"Felt that I was one of a large string of beads, suspended in space. . . . One member of the group was **ostracised**, being called a **parasite**. She did not dare even to use a pen for fear of being further ostracised. . . . They perceive me as a user of people – do things to get what I need at their expense. **Felt that I hated all people and also myself.** . . . Felt that **I did not have the right to be with others**. I feel that I'm **sucking them out. Throwing my dirt** at others."[16]

Sensations
- Heat radiating out from body / Coldness on the surface of my entire body.
- Pulling sensation in my head.

- As if could not breathe.
- Pulsations in whole body.
- Coldness of finger tips and hands. Coldness of back.
- Pressure on chest.

Curative effects

"Prover X seemed to be the only unreservedly happy person during the week of the seminar, for as the days progressed a growing sense of **homesickness and a feeling of not belonging, of exclusion**, inexplicably pervaded many of us. Prover X, who customarily felt excluded, began to feel increasingly confident, even cherished. She has been a lifelong eczema sufferer, **feeling disfigured by it, ugly and undesirable**. She often **feels she is the most repulsive person**, that no one could possibly find her acceptable. During the seminar these feelings abated, her skin cleared up, and she was approached by a man who revealed his attraction for her! After the proving her condition gradually deteriorated and she naturally enough requested that I send her another dose. This I did and she took it, yet with little therapeutic effect."[16]

Cimex lectularius (Bedbug)

Phylum: Arthropoda.
Class: Insecta.
Order: Hemiptera.
Family: Cimicidae.

Cimex lectularius is found all over the world in almost every area that has been colonised by humans. In the past, bed bugs were particularly an affliction of the poor and occurred in mass shelters. However, in the early part of the modern resurgence it was the tourist areas that were most impacted. If feeding regularly, a female bed bug can lay between two and three eggs per day throughout her adult lifetime, which may last several months, allowing one female to produce hundreds of offspring under optimal conditions. It is one of the world's major "nuisance pests".

Provings by: **Joseph Wilhelm Wahle (possibly Rome c1845).**

Reference

Bradford T Lindsay. *Pioneers of homeopathy. John Wilhelm Wahle (1794–1853).* Available online at: http://www.homeoint.org/seror/biograph/wahle.htm (Accessed 29th September 2020)

Keywords

Fetid / Musty / Violent / Breaking / Destructiveness

Burnt gum, palate, tongue / Coldness, skin / Fatigue, limbs / Gagging, cough / Gum, itching / Gums, burnt / Gums, scalded / Joints, shortened / Shortness, tendons / Sleep, insufficient / Sleepiness, irresistible / Strained, liver / Swollen, tongue / Weariness, lumbar

A common theme of the parasitic insects is an offensive odour.

"Violent, poor, defenceless and unable to relax. . . . [Their] violence is a clear sign of being desperate and of having no place where they can stay. . . . [They] **compete to an extreme because if they don't win it is like being nobody.** It is as if they have no better access to the world than passing through the stool and being a professional stinker!" _{Mangialavori}[24]

Rubrics

- **Mind**
  - *Anger – violent – breaking everything*
  - Delusions – *creep into his own body*; he would crouch together as much as he could and
  - *Destructiveness*
  - *Disgust*
  - Rage
  - Tearing – things in general
- **Stomach**
  - Appetite – increased
  - Eructations; type of – sour
  - Gagging
  - Hiccough – painful
  - Thirstless – fever; during
- Vomiting – cough – during – agg.

- **Fever**
  - Dry heat – night – **gagging**, with spasmodic
  - Heat – absent
- **Larynx and Trachea**
  - Tickling – larynx, in – fever; during
- **Cough**
  - Drinking – after – agg.
  - Violent
- **Respiration**
  - Arrested – drinking agg.
  - Difficult – drinking – agg.
  - Impeded, obstructed – gagging – esophagus; in
- **Perspiration**
  - *Odour – fetid / musty / offensive / sour*

Pulex irritans (Human flea)

Phylum: Arthropoda.
Class: Insecta.
Order: Siphonaptera.
Family: Pulicidae.

Pulex irritans is a holometabolous (metamorphic) insect with a four-part lifecycle consisting of eggs, larvae, pupae, and adults. Flea saliva contains anticoagulants – bites generally cause the skin to raise, swell, and itch. Plague, a disease that affects humans and other mammals, is caused by the bacterium Yersinia pestis. The human flea can be a carrier of the plague bacterium.

Proving by: **W.A. Yingling, USA (1891).**

Themes Mangialavori[24]

Parasitic themes of selfishness, greed, disgust; doing things for their own gain.

A common theme of the parasitic insects is an offensive odour.

- **Female Genitalia / Sex**
  - *Cotton in vagina; as if*
  - **Leukorrhea**
    - § Copious / greenish / greenish yellow / offensive / putrid / purulent.
    - § Staining linen – colours the clothes, difficult to wash off
  - **Menses**
    - § Green / late, too / staining – colours the clothes, difficult to wash off
  - **Pain** – Vagina – burning

- **Bladder**
  - Urination – interrupted – sudden – followed by – pain
  - Involuntary – delayed; if
  - Urging to urinate
    - § Frequent / menses – before – agg.
    - § Sudden – hasten to urinate or urine will escape; must
  - Weakness

Proving extracts[25]

⨎ Feels a **heat** or **glow** all over, like being over **steam**, yet no sweating, but skin is moist. On going to bed had a warm feeling like heat or a glow for a short time. . . . **Electric shocks** all through system, at times start in body, at others in head; generally come from motion. (*cf. Doryphora*)

⨎ Feeling that a bullet, or something similar, fell in bladder to its outlet.

⨎ **Intense burning of vagina**, esp. toward external parts and meatus; burns as if **scalding steam** were pouring into vagina – continuous without intermission.

⨎ Diarrhoea very urgent, copious, dark brown, muddy, very foul penetrating odour.

⨎ **Prickly itching** all over, but more esp. on hands and feet, between fingers and toes.

⨎ Skin emits **foul odour**.

⨎ Very rapid growth of finger – and toenails; very thin, almost like is in glass; easily blackened by a bruise.

Natural behaviour

Jumping / Sucking / Piercing / Escaping / Puncture wounds / Feeding off a host / Parasitic

cf. Yersinia pestis.

Insecta / Insects

Pediculus capitis (Head louse)

Phylum: Arthropoda.
Class: Insecta.
Order: Phthiraptera.
Family: Pediculidae.

Head lice are wingless blood-sucking parasites who spend their entire lives on the human scalp and feed exclusively on human blood. They use their snout armed with minute teeth to grip the host's skin, thrusting needle-like stylets into the skin and injecting saliva into the wound to prevent blood from clotting. To attach an egg, the adult female secretes a glue from her reproductive organ. This glue quickly hardens into a "nit sheath" that covers the hair shaft and large parts of the egg. After hatching, the louse nymph leaves behind its egg shell (usually known as a "nit". The empty egg shell remains in place until physically removed, or until it slowly disintegrates – which may take 6 or more months.

Proving by: **Benoit Jules Mure, Brazil.**

Pathogenetic Ward[23]
Blood, pimples / Brain, compressed / Bristle, hairs / Chewing jaw / Lice, scalp / Lifted, hair / Nettles, popliteal / Pimples, back / Pin, arm / Weeping, eyes / Worms, nose

Mind
- Ailments from – joy – excessive
- Anger – causeless
- Gestures; makes – lively
- Heedless
- Hurry
- **Industrious**
- Laughing – trifles; at
- Malicious
- Mocking
- Moral feeling; want of
- Propensity – to work
- Sadness – causeless
- Suicidal disposition – drowning; by
- Thoughts – rapid

Clinical Ward[23]
Children – diseases of / Colic / Diarrhoea / Ganglion – foot, of / **Hair – falling of** / Irritation / Oedema / Psora – hereditary / Skin – affections of / Stammering
   Disposition for study; quick of apprehension; eager for work; writes with feverish rapidity. (Stammering improved.) Clarke[26]

Themes from cases by Massimo Mangialavori[24]
Industrious in order to reach a goal / Unable to connect with others / Dissatisfaction / Disregard for others; omnipotence / Inner perception that something is wrong with them / Seductive appearance / Focus on fitness and looking good. **A greed to live all the possibilities that life can offer.**

Female
- Very painful **lancinations**; great **heat** and **itching** in uterus.
- Shifting pain in uterus; she cannot lean upon it, evening.
- Painful stitch in uterus.
- Leucorrhoea.
- **Urine** – Odour – strong. Colour – greenish / red / pale
- **Bladder** – urging, to urinate – frequent, urination

Natural behaviour
Parasitic / Blood sucking / Makes you feel lousy

LEPIDOPTERA (BUTTERFLIES AND MOTHS)

Themes of the group expressed in rubrics

Mind
- Absentminded – dreamy
- Activity – desires activity – creative activity
- Affectionate
- *Ailments from – responsibility*
- Amusement – desire for
- Awareness heightened
- Beautiful things – awareness of; heightened
- *Beautiful things – yearning for*
- Benevolence
- Carefree
- Cares; full of – others; about
- *Change – desire for – life; in*
- Cheerful – lightness; with sensation of
- *Childish behaviour*
- *Clothes – luxurious clothing, finery; wants*
- Colours – bright – desire for
- Colours – desire for
- Concentration – difficult
- Confidence – want of self-confidence – support; desires
- *CONFLICT – higher consciousness and worldly existence; between*
- Confusion of mind
  - Identity; as to his – duality; sense of
  - *Identity, as to his – sexual identity*
- Contradictory – actions are contradictory to intentions
- Contradictory – impulses
- Countryside – desire for
- Dancing
- **Delusions**
  - Danger; impression of
  - Divided – two parts; into
  - Double – being
  - Double – existence; having a double
  - *Protection, defense; has no*
  - Small – body is smaller
  - Trapped; he is
- Dream; as if in a
- *Dress – extravagant*
- Dullness
- *Duty – aversion to*
- *Duty – too much sense of duty*
- Elegance
- Emotions – strong; too
- *Extravagance*
- ***FORSAKEN FEELING***

- *Fragile people*
- *Freedom*
- **Frivolous**
- Grounded – not grounded
- **GUIDANCE; NEED FOR**
- Helplessness; feeling of
- *Idealistic*
- **Impressionable**
- Inconstancy
- Insecurity; mental
- Irresolution
- **Mirth**
- Mood – alternating / changeable
- **Naive**
- Nature – loves
- Overwhelmed
- Perfume – loves to use perfume
- **Persisting in nothing**
- Playful
- Prostration of mind
- **Responsibility – aversion to**
- **Responsibility – taking responsibility too seriously**
- *Scattered*

- **Sensitive**
  - External impressions; to all
  - Noise; to
- *Shameful – sexuality; about*
- Spaced-out feeling
- Spirituality
- Squandering
- *Suggestible*
- *Sympathetic*
- Thinking – aversion to
- *Time – fritters away his time*
- *Truth – telling the plain truth*
- *Undertaking – many things, persevering in nothing*
- *Vulnerable*
- Wilderness – desires
- **Dreams**
  - *Metamorphosis; about*
  - **Sexual identity; ambiguous about one's**
  - *Women – he is a woman*
- **Generals**
  - Delicate constitution
  - Food and drinks – liquid food – desire
  - Food and drinks – sweets – desire

Limenitis bredowii californica (California sister butterfly)

Phylum: Arthropoda.
Class: Insecta.
Order: Lepidoptera.
Family: Nymphalidae.

The scaly wings of *Lepidopteran insects* come in 2 pairs and are often colourful. They have large compound eyes, with a simple eye above called an ocellus. Their mouthparts are formed into a sucking tube, or proboscis, which is used to drink nectar. The larvae [caterpillars] have chewing mouthparts and are herbivorous. It is named 'sister' for its black and white markings on the forewing that resemble a nun's habit. The usual host plants for the larvae are several species of oaks – this diet makes them unpalatable to predators, which might explain why so many other species have formed a mimicry complex around it. There are four larval instars. After fourteen days, the final instar will pupate whilst attached to tree trunks by large silken webs. When the adults finally emerge, the development time from egg to adult will have taken 65 days (*Theme – extended juvenile period*).

Proving by: **Nancy Herrick, USA (1996).**[14]

Nucleus in rubrics
- *Conflict – higher consciousness and worldly existence; between*
- Communicative – heart; desire to be from the
- Comprehension – heart; of everything from the
- **Delusions**
  - Alien; she is
  - Work – accomplish her work; she cannot

SRP rubrics
- Acceptance
- Cheerful – lightness; with sensation of
- Children – nurture; desire to
- Discipline – want of
- Emotions – spontaneous and natural
- Joy – spontaneous feelings of pleasure
- **Love – children; for – yet naive about responsibilities**
- Love – coming towards her and from her; feelings of love
- **Love – exalted love – humanity; for**
- Pleasure – spontaneous feelings of
- Responsibility – give up her responsibility; wanting to
- *Spaced-out feeling – desire to have*
- *Theorizing – philosophical matters; mind dwells on*
- *Thinking – mundane; is*
- Thoughts – one thought excludes all other
- Thoughts – speculative

Important themes
- *A child feeling unprotected by adults.*
- Desire to be magnetised.
- Emotions, not the mind. Loving feelings.
- Sexuality / Body awareness / Sensuality.
- Mother / Father / Family.
- Buildings (cocoon).
- Affectionate. Cheerful. Spontaneous. Benevolence.
- *Naive. Aversion to responsibility.*
- Sensation of heat.

Characteristic physicals
- **Head** – Pain
  - Chronic – lasting four days
  - Occiput – extending to – Back & Neck
- **Eye**
  - Awareness of
  - Band around the eyeballs; sensation of a
  - Pain – forenoon – pressing pain
  - Twitching
- **Vision**
  - Accommodation – defective
  - Wavering
- **Ear**
  - Pain – extending to – Gums and Teeth

- **Nose**
  - Coldness – Inside – menthol; as if had smelled
  - Smell – acute – flowers
- **Face**
  - Cracked – Mouth; corners of
  - Eruptions – acne – Chin
- **Mouth**
  - Swelling – Palate and Tongue – sensation of
- **Throat**
  - Prickly
  - Swelling – sensation of
- **Stomach**
  - Appetite – relish; without
  - Jumping; sensation of
- **Abdomen**
  - Conscious of the abdomen
- **Respiration**
  - Asthmatic – night – sitting up in bed – must sit up
  - Wheezing – night
- **Chest**
  - Convex
  - Expansion; sensation of – Heart
  - Feathers or petals; sensation of – overlaying chest
  - Open; sensation as if – chakra; heart

- Palpitation of heart – night – waking; on
- **Back**
  - Pain – Cervical region – extending to – Ear – Behind – left
  - Pain – Sacral region – standing – agg. – long time; for a
- **Extremities**
  - Pain – dislocated; as if
  - Paralysis – sensation of – night
- **Sleep**
  - Sleepiness – driving – air; in open – amel.
- **Fever**
  - Internal heat – evening
- **Perspiration**
  - Clammy – evening
- **Skin**
  - Cicatrices
    - § painful
    - § red; become
- **Generals**
  - Heat – sensation of – fever – sensation as from
  - Shuddering, nervous – emotions – from; as if
  - Weakness – evening – 20.30 h

The naive and childlike qualities brought out in this proving are unique and characteristic features of the Lepidoptera class to which the following remedy summaries will attest.

Acherontia atropos (Death's head hawkmoth)

Phylum: Arthropoda.
Class: Insecta.
Order: Lepidoptera.
Family: Sphingidae.

Unlike most moths, which generate noise by rubbing external body parts together, all three species within the genus Acherontia can produce a "squeak" from the pharynx – sucking in air to cause an internal flap between the mouth and throat to vibrate at high speed. The genus name Acherontia relates to Acheron, a river located in Epirus, Greece. Atropos was one of the three Moirai – goddesses of fate and destiny. According to Greek mythology, the three Moirai decide the fate of humans, making them a lesser symbol of death. It gets its name from the sinister-looking skull shape on its back. In many cultures it is thought to be an omen of death. It was featured in the Hannibal Lecter film 'The Silence of the Lambs', and appears on the poster. In the film, the serial killer Buffalo Bill uses the moths as calling cards, stuffing them into his victims' throats.

Proving by: **Patricia LeRoux, France (2009).**[27]

Extracts:

⨎ "Pleasure boat attacked by pirates – captain jumps overboard and abandons us."[27]

Peter pan, Tinkerbell and, to an extent, captain Hook seem to be important mythological characters in Lepidoptera consciousness – covering the themes of an extended juvenile period, lightness of being and fairy consciousness under the threat of an authority figure.

⨎ Dream of men wearing flowery women's dresses in a formal council hearing.
⨎ "A night fright – wake suddenly, jumping out of bed, in the grip of a feeling of being **violently suffocated**. . . . Dream – A swarm of bees flies into the garden. . . . They start stinging me. I pull off my clothes, scratching, **scratching**, then I am **suffocating**. . . . I'm attacked by a cloud of heavy, ponderous butterflies. They are soft when they touch me. Feeling of profound **disorientation** and **abandonment** – no-one comes to help me . . . my way is **blocked** . . . I am completely **shut in**, in the **dark**, I can't get through any doors. . . ."[27]

Mind
- Anguish
- **Checking** – twice or more; must check / **Conscientious** about trifles (*OCD tendency*)
- Concentration – difficult
- Delusions – light = low weight – is light; he
- **Euphoria**
- Excitement – working; when
- **Forsaken feeling**
- GUIDANCE; NEED FOR
- *Materialistic*
- Orientation; sense of – decreased
- Rest – cannot rest when things are not in the proper place
- **Squandering – money**
- Time – quickly, appears shorter; passes too

Dreams
Bees / Boat – foundering / Closet / Doctors (*cannot be trusted*) / **Forsaken; being** (by the captain of a boat) / **Funerals** / Insects / Pirates, attacking the boat / Sea / Stung by an insect; being / Suffocation / Trap – being trapped

Physicals
- **Head** – Pain – cutting pain / sharp / **vice; as if in a**
- **Face** – Itching – Cheeks
- **Throat** – Inflammation – Esophagus – reflux esophagitis / Lump; sensation of a
- **Rectum** – Diarrhea
- **Respiration** – Difficult / Suffocation; attacks of
- **Chest** – Palpitation of heart
- **Sleep** – Falling asleep – difficult / Waking – sudden

Generals
- Energy – excess of energy
- Food and drinks – honey – desire

Apeira syringaria (Lilac beauty)

Phylum: Arthropoda.
Class: Insecta.
Order: Lepidoptera.
Family: Geometridae.

Geometridae is the second largest family of moths after Noctuidae or owlet moths. All geometer moths undergo complete metamorphosis with 4 life stages: egg, larva, pupa, and adult. The caterpillars feed on members of the Caprifoliaceae and Oleaceae, upon which they are well camouflaged. This species overwinters as a larva.

Dream proving by: **K.J. Müller, Germany (1998).**
Clinical observations by: **J.P Jansen (2001).**

Mind
- Ailments from joy
- **Delusions – guardian angel; is a**
- **Forsaken feeling – guided by parents, feels not**
- Guidance; need for
- Horrible things, sad stories affect her profoundly
- Introverted
- Mistakes; making – speaking, in – words – misplacing words
- Timidity – public; about appearing in; talk, to
- Weeping – music; from; romantic
- Weeping – thoughts; at sad

Physicals

- **Head**
  - Pain
    - § Pulsating – light, bright, agg.
    - § Pulsating – noise agg.
    - § Shocks – electric, like
- **Face**
  - Pain – stitching pain
- **Stomach**
- Nausea – *Chilliness – with*
- **Cough**
  - Tickling
- **Expectoration**
  - Lumpy / viscid / yellow
- **Chill**
  - Warm – desire for warmth which does not relieve

Dreams

Animals / Birds / **Car** / Coloured / Coloured – green / Crime – committing a crime – he had committed a crime / Dogs / Flying / Gardens / Horses / Money / Remorse / Swimming / Water

Dreams from Filip Degroote's repertory[17]

- Bees – attacking a witch
- Clothed in – black – people – with black hats
- Diaper – **dirty** – change a dirty diaper; has to
- Failure – because of not having the proper equipment and skill
- Forsaken, being or feels – **friendless; feels**
- Injection – receiving an – above middle of right eyebrow
- **Transsexuality** – girl seems afterwards to be a boy
- Proving: "I dream that the bottom of my Renault Clio has fallen out, and I must drive by running myself, like Fred Flintstone".

Natural behaviour

Camouflaged / Nocturnal / Anchoring themselves / Fluttering / Swaying

Bombyx chrysorrhoea (Brown tail moth)

Phylum: Arthropoda.
Class: Insecta.
Order: Lepidoptera.
Family: Lymantriidae.

Members of the Lymantriidae family are also termed tussock moths. This common name refers to the larvae which have prominent tufts of hairs, or tussocks, on the back. These stinging hairs are also incorporated into their silken cocoon, protecting the pupa from potential enemies. In autumn, colonies of larvae build webbed nests in trees constructed from a single leaf wrapped tightly with white silk. The larvae feed on many species of trees and shrubs, especially members of the Rosaceae. As moths, they are attracted to light.

Symptoms and themes
- Pricking, burning pains in the eyes
- Dreams – needing to **escape** from a cave full of moths flapping their wings
- Feeling **trapped. Refusing help**
- **Themes** – Camouflage (*life is better when hidden*)
- Freedom, Liberty, Abandonment (forsaken)

"The characteristic urticaria of Bombyx shows hard, large tubercles with a red areola. The tubercles are most marked near the joints. There is a sensation of a foreign body under the skin, with itching of the whole body. The itching gets worse in the evening but is not relieved in any way. There is a burning heat everywhere." Master[28]

- **Mind**
  - Runs about – things; runs against
  - Shrieking – sleep, during
- **Eye**
  - Eruptions – Lids – **vesicles**
  - Inflammation – Conjunctiva
- **Face**
  - Eruptions – pimples – Nose – tip
- **Chest**
  - Discolouration – **redness**
- **Back**
  - **Heat** – Cervical region
  - Pain – extending to – Arms

Dreams
Amorous / Banquet / Car / Danger / Dead bodies – returning to life / Dogs – bitten by dogs; being / Dogs – black / Fights / Flood / Flying / Horses / Journeys / Jumping – water – he is jumping into / Murdered – being / Pursued, being / Spiders / Urinating / Water

Bombyx processionaria (Oak processionary moth)

Phylum: Arthropoda.
Class: Insecta.
Order: Lepidoptera.
Family: Thaumetopoeidae.

The oak processionary is a moth whose caterpillars can be found in oak forests. The larvae construct communal webbed nests of white silk from which they crawl at night in single file, head to tail in large processions to feed on foliage in the crowns of trees, returning in the same manner. The eggs are enclosed in an anally spun web that can cause irritation to the skin and eyes of human beings. They pupate either in the web or underground.

Proving by: **Didier Grandgeorge, France (1991).**[27]

Themes

- Follow the leader / pied piper.
- During a proving by D. Grandgeorge (1991), one prover admitted themselves to hospital suspecting they had a twisted testicle. Upon investigation, it was found that nothing was wrong.
- Strong sense of feeling under imminent attack, as the dream of arrows piercing muscles testifies.

Dreams

Arm – cauterizing of / Arrows – piercing muscles / Children; about / Children; about – newborns / Coffins / Dead bodies / Falling – height; from a / Flying / Skeletons / Water

Physicals

- **Head**
  - Pain – Temples – stitching pain
- **Throat**
  - Pain – stitching pain
- **Stomach**
  - Nausea – morning
- **Chest**
  - Heart – stitching pain
- **Extremities**
  - Itching – Hands
  - Tingling – Feet / Hands

- **Sleep**
  - Sleepiness
  - Waking – frequent
  - Yawning
- **Skin**
  - **Body were under the skin; as if a foreign**
  - **Itching of the whole body**
  - **Urticaria**
- **Generals**
  - Pain – **stitching** pain

Clinical Clarke[26]

Contact with the caterpillars or the emanations from a nest of them causes intense irritation, and hard, large, areola-formed tubercles, with a red areola, so thick as to leave hardly any space between. Sometimes they are linear formed; most marked near joints. Sensation as if a foreign body were under the skin. Itching of whole body – evenings; not relieved by anything.

Toxicological Allen[3]

If a nest of the insects is touched or stirred up, persons within reach of the emanations will be attacked with a papulous eruption, more or less confluent which will last several days and be attended with violent itching.

Euphydryas aurinia (Marsh fritillary)

Phylum: Arthropoda.
Class: Insecta.
Order: Lepidoptera.
Family: Nymphalidae.

This species lives in calcareous grassland, woodland clearings, damp marshy areas and heathland dominated by tussock forming grasses. Their eggs are laid in one large batch on a carefully chosen site; they therefore spend a long time choosing this and are very selective when looking for a host plant. There are six instars. The first three instars, which are gregarious, form a communal web around the food plant *Succisa pratensis* (*Caprifoliaceae*) and feed on the host plant for about three weeks. In the spring, the fourth instar emerges from hibernation. All three of the post-hibernation instars bask in the sun – helping to increase body temperature, promoting faster development. At the end of the sixth instar (spring), pupae start forming. Adult butterflies emerge to undergo the flight period between May and June feeding opportunistically on nectar from varied plants.

Proving by: **Patricia LeRoux, France (2007).**[27]

- **Mind**
  - Business – aversion to
  - **Carefree**
  - Concentration
  - Difficult
  - Impossible
  - Excitement
  - **Playful**
- **Head**
  - Pain
    § Forehead – pressing pain – **band**; as from a
    § Temples – **pulsating** pain
- Temples – **warm** – applications – **amel.**

- **Eye**
  - Discolouration – red
  - Heat in
  - Inflammation – Lids (Blepharitis)
  - Pain
    § Burning
    § Burnt; as if
- **Skin**
  - Eruptions – Discharging / Itching
  - Itching – warm – bathing – amel.
- **Generals**
  - Food and drinks – spices – desire
  - Warm food – desire
  - Light; from – **amel. – sunlight**

Gonepteryx rhamni (Brimstone butterfly)

Phylum: Arthropoda.
Class: Insecta.
Order: Lepidoptera.
Family: Pieridae.

The brimstone relies on two species of buckthorn plants (Rhamnaceae) as host plants for its larvae. Adults show sexual dimorphism in their wing colouration; males have yellow wings and iridescence whereas females have greenish-white wings and are not iridescent. The butterfly inhabits wetlands during the mating and breeding season, as they provide ideal areas for oviposition due to an abundance of host plants. They are one of the longest-living butterflies, with a life expectancy ranging from 10 months to a year. Due to its hibernation and life cycle, it has one generation per year. Development from the laid egg to the emergence of the imago is approximately 50 days.

Proving by: **Patricia LeRoux, France (2007).**[27]

- **Mind**
  - Benevolence
  - Helping others
  - Orientation; sense of – decreased
  - Sadness
  - Sitting – inclination to sit – still
  - Tranquillity
- **Head**
  - Pain – Forehead
- **Eye**
  - Inflammation – Conjunctiva
- **Extremities**
  - Eruptions – itching
  - Hands – Back of hands – itching

Skin
Itching – scratching – unchanged by scratching

Dreams
Airplanes / Beautiful dreams (does not want them to end) / Beauty / Children; about – newborns (wrapped in swaddling clothes) / Flowers / Journeys / Light; of / Peaceful / Women (*beautiful, graceful and delicate*)

Graphium Agamemnon (Tailed jay)

Phylum: Arthropoda.
Class: Insecta.
Order: Lepidoptera.
Family: Papilionidae.

Graphium agamemnon is a predominantly green and black tropical butterfly that belongs to the swallowtail family. They mostly fly among the tree-tops but can descend to ground level in search of flowers or host plants. Because of their relatively fast life cycle (just over one month from egg to adult), tailed jays may produce up to seven or eight broods per year. They are strong and restless fliers, fluttering their wings constantly even when at flowers.

Proving by: **Chetna N. Shukla, Mumbai, India (2001).**[29]

Mind

- Aggression
- **Amusement** – desire for
- Anger – trifles; at
- Anticipation
- Confident
- Confusion of mind – identity; as to his – **sexual identity**
- Dress – **cross dressing**
- Dress – girlish; in boys
- Dress – **womanly**
- **Ennui**
- Exertion – physical – desire
- Fear – Cockroaches; of / Insects; of / Lizards; of
- Indifference – business affairs; to
- Jesting
- Mental exertion – desire for
- Restlessness
- **Unification** – sensation of unification
- Weeping

Dreams

- Identity – girl says she's a boy
- Kissing – somebody passionately
- Genitals – sex change – her vulva becomes a penis
- Penis – coming out of vagina
- *Transsexuality* / *Transvesty*
- Women – penises; with

Skin eruptions

Inachis io (European peacock butterfly)

Phylum: Arthropoda.
Class: Insecta.
Order: Lepidoptera.
Family: Nymphalidae.

The peacock butterfly is a colourful butterfly found in Europe and temperate Asia. The name is thought to be derived from Greek mythology, meaning Io the daughter of Inachus. The adult butterflies drink nectar from a wide variety of flowering plants including buddleia, willows, dandelions and more. Due to their life cycle in which females are receptive only after over-wintering, they employ a monandrous mating system – mating with one partner at a time. Therefore, holding a desirable territory increases the male's likelihood of finding a mate, but this needs to be weighed against the costs of defending such a territory. Their primary anti-predator defence stems from the four large eyespots that they have on their wings – when attacked, they open their wings exposing the eyespots in an intimidatory display of threat. It is thought that by imitating the eyes of the avian predators' natural enemies, they can ward off such attackers. They also use crypsis; blending into their environment by mimicking a leaf whilst immobile with wings closed.

Proving by: **Patricia LeRoux, France (2006).**[27]

Polarities
- *Meditating* vs. *Internal restlessness*
- *Doubtful* vs. *Egotism*

Mind
- Anger – **alternating** with – tranquillity
- Anticipation
- **Awareness heightened – body; of**
- Capriciousness + Mood – alternating
- Confidence – want of self-confidence
- Contradiction – intolerant of contradiction
- Escape; attempts to
- Impatience + Industriousness
- Sensitive – noise; to
- Singing
- Tidy
- Time – quickly, appears shorter; passes too
- Tranquillity – incomprehensible
- Truth – telling the plain truth

Dreams
Accidents / Anger / Animals / Anxious / Birds / Boars, wild / Buildings / Buildings – big; seeing / Business / Car / Cares; full of / Children; about – **newborns** / Confused / Disconnected / Dogs / Driving – car; a / **Enemies / Escaping / Falling** / Falling – height; from a / Falling – water; into / Fantastic / Fights / Flies / Flowers / Flying / Flying – airplane / Friends / Friends – meeting friends / Friends – old / Gardens / Helping – people / Horses / House / **Hurry** / **Jealousy** / Journeys / Landscape – **beautiful** / Many / Parties / People / People – crowds of / Pleasant / **Pursued**, being / Quarrels / **Relocation**; of / Remembered / Riding / River / Shopping / Smoking / Solemnities / Stairs / Swimming / Swinging / Theft / True on waking; dreams seem / Unpleasant / Visits – making visits / Vivid / Water / Wedding / Women / Women – old women / Worms / **Worms – creeping**

Dreams – masks, wearing – venetian[27]

Physicals
- **Head**
  - Heat
  - Noises in head – roaring
  - Pain
    - § Morning – pressing pain
    - § Forehead – pressing pain
    - § Pulsating – morning
  - Tingling
- **Eye**
  - Discolouration – red – canthi
  - Inflammation – lids
  - Fullness; sensation of

- **Ear**
- Noises in – whistling
  - Pain
    - § Drawing / stitching / pressing
    - § Night
  - Wind – sensitive to
- **Skin**
  - Burning
- Coldness
- Discolouration – red – spots – itching
- **Eruptions** – Blotches – itching, oozing / Patches / Pimples / Red / Urticaria
- **Itching** – Crawling / Intolerable / Scratching – agg.

Morpho menelaus occidentalis (Blue morpho)

Phylum: Arthropoda.
Class: Insecta.
Order: Lepidoptera.
Family: Nymphalidae.

Morpho menelaus is unique because of its iridescent blue colour and large wingspan. They are one of the most familiar and recognisable neotropical insects. Both sexes have a slow and floppy flight pattern and feed on rotting fruit that has dropped to the ground. Caterpillars are covered with bristles that release an irritant upon contact. The peak of the caterpillar is in the dry season, a climate that is unsuitable for most animal communities. These caterpillars will enter diapause or suspend development and can delay pupation in order to survive this harsh period. Adult eyespots are usually formed of dark circles surrounded by a brighter outer layer. The 'pupil' of the eye has a sparkle that mimics the natural reflection of the cornea. These eyes are thought to deflect a predator's attack away from more vital organs and toward the spot on the wings.

Provings by: **H. Renoux, Paris (2010).**
Proving under hypnosis by: **E. Chamurliyska, Sofia (2012).**

- **Delusions** (*Renoux*)
  - Legs; belong to her; do not
  - Legs; give away
  - **Light**, incorporeal, immaterial; he is
  - Poisoned; has been, he; drugged
  - **Spirit**; he is a
  - **Ugly**; is
  - Waves; of
  - Wings; has
- **Delusions** (*Chamurliyska*)
  - Arms – belong to her; arms do not
  - Bird – seeing birds – eagles
  - Body – out of the body
  - Buried
  - Butterflies; of
  - Dark
  - Enclosed; she is – cave; in a – womb; as if
  - Existence – begun his existence; he had just that moment
  - Existence – own existence; he doubted his

- Floating – air; in
- lying
- Identity – errors of personal identity
- Legs – belong to her; her legs don't
- Light = brightness
- Paralyzed; he is
- Pulled – he was – upwards
- Swinging; he were
- Waves; of
- Whirling
- Wings – has wings; she
- Wolves; of

Mind

Renoux proving

- Absent-mindedness – driving; while
- Cheerfulness – dancing, laughing, singing, with
- Company – aversion to; solitude, desire for
- Confusion of mind – location, about; loses his way in well known streets
- Death; thoughts of – waking; on
- Detached – observing from the outside; as if
- Distance; inaccurate judge of – cannot judge distance to ground
- Duty – aversion to
- Euphoria
- Harmony – sensation of
- Organised and methodical; desire to be
- Sensitive –
  - Disorder; to / Impressions; to all external / Odours
- Shame
- Thoughts – persistent – past; of the
- Thoughts – wandering
- Warmth – amel.
- Work – impossible

Chamurliyska proving

- Anxiety – causeless
- Blissful feeling
- Communicative
- Confusion of mind – identity; as to
- Content
- Depersonalisation
- Elated
- Joy
- Merging of self with one's environment
- Peace – heavenly peace; sensation of
- Power – sensation of
- Tranquillity – settled, centred and grounded

Dreams

Abortion / Accidents; of – car, with / **Adolescence**; of / Adoption; of / Animals; of – devouring her or him / Apocalypse – end of the world / Blood – bleeding; that she is / Bombs – detonating / Cats / Children – **adopting a child** / Children – **newborns** / Children – danger; in / **Children – protecting** / Crypts / God – deities / Hair – cut / Journey – travelling / **Metamorphosis** – about / People; of – naked / **Pregnant – of being; abort; wants to** / Pursued – of; murderers; by / Rape – children; of / Remorse – of; want of / Restaurant – expensive / Saving others / **Scarf that might suffocate her**; an orange / Scorpions – burn; tries to / Searching – unsuccessfully / Spiders – attacking ants / Storms – ship; while aboard a / **Surgery; of – enlarge a girl's vagina; to** / Turkish delights – eating / Underground / Water – sea, ocean; of / Wolves – licking her neck

Physicals

- **Vertigo**
  - Lying – down; must / Sitting – amel.
- **Head**
  - Shivering
- **Eyes**
  - Convulsions – Lids / Quivering
  - Pain
    - § Applications – cold – amel. /
    - § Burning, smarting, biting – soap; as from
- **Ears**
  - Eruptions – pimples
  - Pain – pinching
- **Hearing**
  - Whistling – obstruction; with
- **Nose**
  - Discharge – purulent – green
  - Epistaxis, haemorrhage – bathing, washing – agg.
- **Smell**
  - Acute – perfumes / strong odours
- **Face**
- Desquamation / Eruptions – herpetic / Itching – nose / Numbness, insensibility / Warmth – amel.
- **Mouth**
  - Discolouration – Tongue – red – Sides
- **Neck**
  - Torticollis – drawn to side
- **Stomach**
  - Nausea – riding in a carriage or on cars – agg. / Motion-sickness
- **Abdomen**
  - Bending – amel. – double

- **Rectum**
  - Constipation – dryness of rectum; from
  - Hemorrhoids – itching
  - Pain – tenesmus, painful urging
- **Female**
  - Dryness – vagina / Stitching – vagina
- **Larynx and trachea**
  - Tickling in air passages – throat-pit
- **Respiration**
  - Difficult – lying – amel.
- **Cough**
  - Itching, tickling; from – throat-pit, in / Whistling, wheezing
- **Chest**
  - Eruptions – **blotches** / Water – sensation / Water – sensation – drops
- **Back**
  - Coccyx / Eruptions – patches – pink / Pain – cervical region – motion – agg. – head, of – backward
  - Stiffness – sitting – while
- **Extremities**
  - Numbness / Pain – pinching / **Paroxysmal** / Wandering, shifting / Redness – hands
- **Skin**
  - Eruptions – blotches / Eruptions – papular – itching / Eruptions – patches
- **Generals**
  - **Fluttering** sensation / Pain – **burnt**, scalded / **Quivering** / Trickling; as from drops of water

Natural behaviour

Iridescence / Shimmering / Blue / Flashing of wings

Pieris brassicae (Cabbage white butterfly)

Phylum: Arthropoda.
Class: Insecta.
Order: Lepidoptera.
Family: Pieridae.

Caterpillars live in groups in their early stages, becoming solitary later on in life. The larvae have four moultings and five instars. In the third instar, they are observed to eat voraciously, and cause significant amounts of damage to their host plant (*Brassicaceae*).

Proving by: **K.J. Müller, Germany (1996).**

Mind
- *Amusement* – desire for
- Anxiety – conscience; anxiety of
- *Change* – desire for
- Delusions
  - Floating – air; in
  - Turn – she – was turning
  - Dream; as if in a
- Fear – fire
- Frightened easily
- Laziness
- Loquacity
- Mood – alternating
- Occupation – amel.
- *Playing* – desire to play
- *Sentimental*
- Singing
- Talking – amel. the complaints
- Talking – desire to talk to someone

Dreams
Balls / Banquet / Beetles – manure beetles / **Carousing** / Country – foreign / Dogs / Forest / **Gypsies** / Journeys / Many / Parties / People / People – crowds of / **Rats** / Skeletons / **Solemnities** / Worms, maggots and flies

Physicals
- **Vertigo**
  - Exertion – agg.
  - Intoxicated; as if
  - Turning; as if – everything were turning in a circle; as if
  - Warm – room
  - agg. – entering a warm room; when
- **Head**
  - Constriction – band or hoop
  - Heaviness – warm – room – agg.
  - Lump; sensation as from a
  - **Pain**
    § Boring / Pressing / Grasping / Pressing / Stitching pains
    § Bending – head – forward – agg.
    § Motion – agg.
    § Thinking of the pain – agg.
    § Temples – extending to – occiput and vertex
    § Vertex – pressing pain – weight; as from a
- **Eye**
  - Agglutinated – morning
  - Discharges
  - Heat in
  - Heaviness – Lids
  - Inflammation – Conjunctiva

- ○ **Pain**
  - § Air; in open – amel.
  - § Burning
  - § Swelling
  - ○ Twitching – Eyebrows and Lids
- • **Female**
  - ○ Menses – scanty / Short; too
  - ○ **Pain**
    - § Ovaries – left – stitching pain
    - § Ovaries – stitching pain
    - § Uterus and region – bearing down
    - § Vagina – coition – during
- • **Generals**
  - ○ Activity – amel.
  - ○ Air; in open – amel.
  - ○ Bending, turning – forward – agg.

- ○ Dry sensation – Internal parts; in
- ○ Efficiency – increased
- ○ Exertion; physical – agg.
- ○ *Formication* – External parts
- ○ Hair – sensation of a
- ○ Heat – lack of vital heat
- ○ Heaviness
- ○ Pulse – frequent
- ○ Sleep – short sleep – amel.
- ○ Stoop shouldered
- ○ Tension
- ○ *Twitching*
- ○ Twitching – sleep – during – agg.
- ○ Warm – agg.
- ○ Wet – applications – cold wet applications – amel.

REPERTORY ADDITIONS FOR INSECTS
(made to existing rubrics in Synthesis[30])

MIND
- ○ ABSORBED – business matters; in
- ○ ACTIVITY – desires activity
- ○ AILMENTS FROM
  - § abused; after being
  - § humiliation
  - § mortification
  - § rejected; from being
  - § reproaches
  - § sexual excesses
  - § shame
  - § violence
- ○ AMBITION – increased
- ○ ANGER – sudden
- ○ ATTACK OTHERS; desire to
- ○ ATTRACTING OTHERS
- ○ BUSY
  - § fruitlessly
- ○ CHANGE – desire for
- ○ CLEANNESS – mania for
- ○ COLOURS
  - § bright – desire for
  - § desire for

- ○ CONFUSION OF MIND – identity, as to his – sexual identity
- ○ DELIRIUM – erotic
- ○ DELUSIONS
  - § abused; being
  - § appreciated; she is not
  - § attacked; being
  - § body – ugly; body looks
  - § consciousness – higher consciousness; unification with
  - § crushed
  - § dirty – he is
  - § insulted; he is
  - § insulted; he is – looked down upon
  - § invaded; one's space is being
  - § metamorphic
  - § parasite; she is a
  - § pursued; he was
  - § repulsive fantastic
  - § separated – group; he is separated from the
  - § small – body is smaller

§ small – he is
§ torture
§ torture – tortured; he is
§ trapped; he is
§ wrong – suffered wrong; he has
- DESIRES – full of desires
- DESTRUCTIVENESS
- DIRTY
- DISGUST
§ body; of the
- DISTURBED; AVERSE TO BEING
- EFFICIENT, ORGANISED
- ESCAPE; ATTEMPTS TO
- ESTRANGED
- EXTRAVAGANCE
- FANCIES – lascivious
- FASTIDIOUS
- FEAR
§ attacked; fear of being
§ death; of
§ death; of – sudden death; of
§ death; of – suffocation; from
§ dirt; of
§ disease; of impending
§ escape; with desire to
§ hurt; of being
§ injury – being injured; of
§ narrow place; in
§ poverty; of
§ suffocation; of
§ violence; of
- FIGHT; WANTS TO
- FLOATING SENSATION
- GREED, CUPIDITY
- HAUGHTY
- HUMILIATED; FEELING
- HURRY
§ aimless
- IMPULSE; MORBID
§ sexual
§ violence; to do
- IMPULSIVE
- INDUSTRIOUS
- KILL; DESIRE TO
- LASCIVIOUS
- LIBERTINISM

- LOVE – perversity; sexual
- LUXURY, DESIRE FOR
- MATERIALISTIC
- MOOD – repulsive
- NYMPHOMANIA
- OBSCENE, LEWD
- OCCUPATION – amel.
- ORDER – desire for
- ORGANISED AND METHODICAL; DESIRE TO BE
- POWER – sensation of
- PROSTRATION OF MIND
- RAGE
- RAGE – kill people; tries to
- RAGE – violent
- RESPECTED – desire to be
- RESTLESSNESS
§ busy
§ internal
- RICH; TO BE – desire
- SATYRIASIS
- SELFISHNESS
- SENSITIVE – colours; to
- SHAMEFUL
§ sexuality; about
- SHAMELESS
- SIMPLE PERSONS
- SPEED – desire for
- SQUANDERING – money
- STRIKING
- TALKING – business; of
- TASK-ORIENTED
- THOUGHTS – rush
- THOUGHTS – wandering
- UNDERTAKING – many things, persevering in nothing
- UNREFINED
- VIOLENCE
- VIOLENT
• **HEAD** – HAIR – falling
• **EYE** – PHOTOPHOBIA
• **STOMACH**
- APPETITE
§ increased
§ insatiable
• **RECTUM** – CONSTIPATION

- **BLADDER**
  - ○ FULLNESS; SENSATION OF
  - ○ INFLAMMATION
- **KIDNEYS** – INFLAMMATION
- **URETHRA** – PAIN – stitching pain
- **MALE GENITALIA / SEX**
  - ○ ERUPTIONS
  - ○ SEXUAL DESIRE
    - § excessive
    - § increased
    - § violent
- **FEMALE GENITALIA / SEX**
  - ○ SEXUAL DESIRE
    - § increased
    - § violent
- **RESPIRATION** – SUFFOCATION; ATTACKS OF
- **CHEST** – PHTHISIS PULMONALIS
- **EXTREMITIES**
  - ○ INFLAMMATION – Joints
  - ○ PAIN – wandering, shifting pain
- **SLEEP** – SLEEPLESSNESS – anxiety; from
- **DREAMS**
  - ○ ANIMALS
  - ○ ANXIOUS
  - ○ BIRDS
  - ○ BUILDINGS
    - § big; seeing
  - ○ CAR
  - ○ CHILDREN; ABOUT – newborns
  - ○ DOGS
  - ○ FIGHTS
  - ○ HOUSE
  - ○ JOURNEYS
  - ○ PEOPLE
  - ○ RIVER
  - ○ SWIMMING
  - ○ WATER
  - ○ WOMEN
- **SKIN**
  - ○ DISCOLOURATION – red – spots
  - ○ FORMICATION
  - ○ ITCHING – burning
  - ○ LUPUS
- **GENERALS**
  - ○ AGILITY
  - ○ ALTERNATING STATES
  - ○ FORMICATION
  - ○ HEAT – flushes of
  - ○ HEAT – sensation of
  - ○ PAIN
    - § biting pain
    - § burning
    - § stinging
    - § stitching pain
    - § wandering pain
  - ○ TUBERCULOSIS

References

1 Gray AC. Homeopathic Proving of Blatta Orientalis (Indian Cockroach). Sydney, 2002. In: *Experience of Medicine* Book 5 (2nd edn). 2017. (Accessed in RadarOpus.)

2 Gray AG. Homeopathic Proving of Cutex pervigilans (Mosquito). Sydney, 2002. In: *Experience of Medicine* Book 12 (3rd edn). 2020. (Accessed in RadarOpus.)

3 Allen T. *Encyclopedia of Pure Materia Medica, Apis.* New York NY. (Originally published in 1874.) (Accessed in RadarOpus.)

4 Begin M. *The Firefly (Lamprohyza spledidula) – A case and the proving.* (Accessed in RadarOpus.)

5 Rowe T. *A Proving of Schistocerca americana – American desert locust.* Phoenix AZ: AMCH Publishing; 2010.

6 Sonz S, Stewart R. *The Proving of Musca domestica.* New York NY. (Accessed in RadarOpus.)

7 Gray AC. Homeopathic Proving of Blatta Orientalis (Indian Cockroach). Sydney, 2002. In: *Experience of Medicine* Book 5 (2nd edn). 2017. (Accessed in RadarOpus.)

8 Lilienthal S. *Homeopathic Therapeutics* (2nd edn). New York NY: B Jain Publishers Pvt Ltd; 2008 (Accessed in RadarOpus.)

9 Grandgeorge D. *The Spirit of Homeopathic Medicines: Essential Insights to 300 Remedies*. Berkely CA: North Atlantic Books: and Homeopathic Educational Services; 1998. (Accessed in RadarOpus.)

10 Wilson P. *Mantis religiosa – Cosmic transformer – Interhomeopathy*. Available online at: *http://www.interhomeopathy.org/mantis-religiosa-cosmic-transformer* (Accessed 1st September 2020.)

11 Chamurliyska E. *Proving of Coccinella septumpunctata*. (Accessed in RadarOpus.)

12 Grimes M. *Enallagma carunculatum – A Proving of Tule Bluet Dragonfly*. (Accessed in RadarOpus.)

13 Fraser P. *Insects – Escaping the Earth*. Bristol: Winter Press; 2008.

14 Herrick N. *Animal Mind Human Voices*. Grass Valley CA: Hahnemann Clinic Publishing; 1998.

15 Fraser P, Norland M. *Schistocerca gregaria – The Homeopathic Proving of The Plague Locust*. Stroud, 2007. Available online at: *https://www.homeopathyschool.com/the-school/provings/locust* (Accessed 15th September 2020.)

16 Norland M. *Collected Provings – Galla quercina ruber*. Devon, 1998. Available online at: *https://www.homeopathyschool.com/the-school/provings/oak-galls* (Accessed 15th September 2020.)

17 Degroote F. *Dream Repertory*. Ishes (B): Archibel; 2009. (Accessed in RadarOpus.)

18 Sankaran R. *Sankaran's Schema* (2nd edn). Mumbai: Homoeopathic Medical Publishers; 2007.

19 Joshi B, Joshi S. *Quick Book of Minerals and Animals*. Mumbai: Serpentina Books; 2013.

20 Shah N. *Proving of Culex musca*. Available online at: *https://hpathy.com/drug-provings/culex-musca-mosquito*

21 Begin M. *Transforming the insanity and poison of Solanaceae: a case of Doryphora*. July 2012. Available online at: *http://www.interhomeopathy.org/transforming-the-insanity-and-poison-of-solanaceae-a-case-of-doryphora* (Accessed May 36th 2021.)

22 Sherr J. *Calopteryx splendens – Banded Damselfly The proving*. Malvern; 2002. Available online at: *http://homeopathyforhealthinafrica.org/product/calopteryx-splendens*

23 Ward J. *Unabridged Dictionary of the Sensations "as If"*. Noida UP: B Jain Publishers; 1995.

24 Mangialavori M, Burley V. *Koiné seminar – Identity and Individualism*. Bologna: Matrix; 2004.

25 Vermeulen F. *Vista Vintage – Proving of Pulex irritans by W.A. Yingling. Homeopathic Physician*. 1892; 12 (5). (Accessed in RadarOpus.)

26 Clarke J.H. *Dictionary of Practical Materia Medica* (Vols 1–3). Mumbai: B Jain; 2005. (Work originally published in 1900.) (Accessed in RadarOpus.)

27 LeRoux P. *Butterflies: An Innovative Guide to the Use of Butterfly Remedies in Homeopathy*. France: Narayana verlag; 2009.

28 Master F. *Diseases of the skin*. Mumbai: (Accessed in RadarOpus.)

29 Shukla C. *The Soul of the Spirit in the Substances*. Delhi: Indian Books and Periodicals Publishers; 2001.

30 Schroyens F. *Synthesis 9.1* (Treasure edn). Ghent: Homeopathic Book Publishers; 2009 (plus author's own additions).

31 Roberts H. *Sensations "as if" – A Repertory of Subjective Symptoms*. Noida UP: B Jain Publishers; 2002.

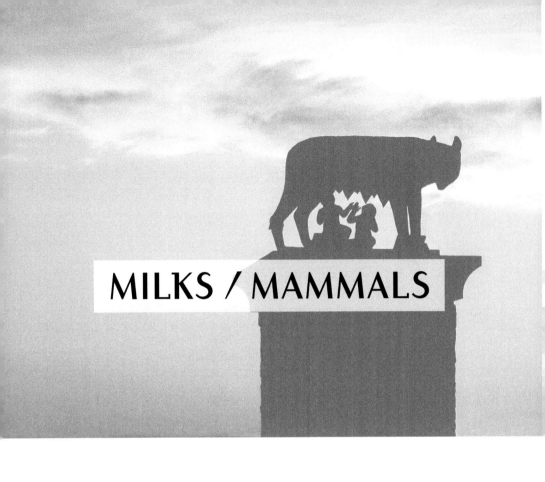

MILKS / MAMMALS

MYTHOLOGY

The Astrological Moon is a clear astrological symbol for Milk remedies, relating directly to your experience of the mother archetype – the kind of relationship to your mother, and how you take on the role of caring for and nurturing others. The moon rules: the mammae (and nutrition from mother's milk); how you bond with others; how you react on an instinctive level; your habits, subconscious, routines and cycles. It is naturally reflective of the light of the sun (consciousness) and is constantly changing shape in response to sunlight. This equates to an innate adaptability and changeability. For a Lunar type, partnerships and relationship revolve around the need to create a safe family environment. A negatively aspected Moon can lead to dependency issues and an inability to stand on one's own two feet, as well as a desire to be mothered or to be the constant care-giver oneself.

The lunar goddess Artemis is an important mythological symbol for the Milks; as soon as she is born she helps her mother give birth to her brother Apollo, highlighting the importance of nurture and childbirth amongst this group of remedies. Problems connecting with the mother at this early stage of development may be an important indication for the Milks, taken together with the totality of characteristic themes and symptoms.

*As soon as **Artemis** was born, she helped her mother give birth to her twin brother, thereby becoming the protector of childbirth and labour. She asked her father to grant her eternal chastity and virginity, and never gave in to any potential lovers; devoted to hunting and nature, she rejected marriage and love.*[1]

Hecate reflects the shadow side of the Lacs, the one for which there are feelings of shame and disgust, or of being an outcast. She was Persephone's escort to and from the underworld, which could be seen as a symbol for the more base or animal nature reflected in the substances.

Moon

Cyclical, Reflective, Soulful, Fertile.
Yin, Emotional, Sense of self, Place at home.
Inward, Mother, Union, Subconscious.
Uncompensated, Feelings, Responsive, Receptive, Reactive.
Flowing, Oversensitivity, Family, Nurture.
Creature comforts, Habitual, Instinctive.
Caring, Sensitive, Touchy, Moody, Waxing and Waning.

Lunar Affinities
Oesophagus, Uterus, Ovaries, Lymphatics, Sympathetic Nervous System, Synovial Fluid, Alimentary Canal, Lymph, Chyle, Nerve Sheaths.

Mars – Moon
Fighting mother. Fierce nurturing. Emotional conflict, sensitive to discord.

Venus

Co-operation, Giving, Compromise.
Beauty, Love, Comparison, Art, Taste, Exchanging.
How we seek to make ourselves and others happy.
Pleasure, Sharing, Values, Socialising.
Expressing affection for others, Seduction, Attraction.
Balance, Harmony, Sexual Lust, Flirtatious.
Conciliation, Friendship, Beauty, Desire.
Reaction, Sensation, Relationship, Partner.

The themes of Venus relate to the attractiveness of the animal kingdom – the desire to be beautiful, alluring, and to attract a mate. There is also an urge to maintain balance and harmony within the group, relating more specifically to the Mammals. The qualities of Venus are receptivity, fairness, cooperation, comparison and compromise. Libra (a sign of the zodiac ruled by Venus) is known to be a very tactful and diplomatic type, adept at seeing the other's point of view and letting other's have their voices heard. In a herd animal, these are vital qualities to ensure survival of the group. In Mammal cases, there is always a focus on the group and one's place within it; how the power-struggles between the group play out, and whether one is dominant (Mars) or submissive (Venus).

In Greek mythology, Aphrodite and Ares have many passionate sexual encounters, although officially she is married to the lame smithy-god Hephaestus. The sexual chemistry between the god of war and the goddess of love is very potent and they have countless illicit liaisons. The two planets Mars and Venus have come to represent the archetypal forms of male and female sexual energy.

If Venus is negatively aspected in a chart, this can lead to tension in how one relates to others, whether they can be seen as attractive or 'good relationship material'. There may be an excess of sexual energy, leading to promiscuity or a propensity towards problems with the female sexual organs. Venus rules the kidneys, and so has a strong bearing on the fluid systems of the body as well as the adrenals (fight or flight in herd mammals). Because the keynote of Venus is balance, it is also important in governing homeostatic processes in the body.

Mars – Venus
Assertiveness *vs.* Compromise. Fighting *vs.* Yielding. Competitive *vs.* Balancing.

Venus / Taurus Affinities
Throat, Kidneys, Thymus Gland, Venous Circulation. Warm, Lymphatic, Relaxing, Sedentary. Goitre, Diphtheria, Laryngitis, Tonsillitis, Croup, Polypi, Quinsy, Glandular Swelling of throat, Apoplexy.

MILK REMEDIES IN HOMEOPATHY

Milk, suckling, connection, warmth, fullness

A universally important feature of the Mammals is expressed in the form of **milk**, breasts and suckling; symbolising a flow of unconditional love and warmth between mother and baby. This means; to feel such a strong connection with your child that you would sacrifice your own survival to save them without a second thought.

The benefits of being breast fed can be seen through a study of the signs and symptoms from the provings of Milk remedies. These provide a picture of what happens when this essential early bonding between mother and child is absent, lacking or replaced by formula milk. At the centre of the Milk remedies lies Lac humanum. One could conjecture that there is a 'lack-of-milk disease' currently afflicting developed countries, for which Lac humanum may be *the* polychrest remedy.

The resulting loss of self-esteem, lack of ability to maintain relationships, and porous boundaries suggest that this early experience of being bonded with the mother goes a very long way to informing our ability to make and sustain contact with our group (*Confusion of mind – identity, as to his – boundaries; and personal*). We are after all mammals ourselves, so all the Milk remedies have this common feature of needing to belong to the group, but in some way having to reconcile this with the desire to be independent (especially in the human milks).

The primary physiological role of milk lies in its **nutritive** function. Lack of nutrition results in the characteristic symptomatic response observed through-out the Milk remedies in our materia medicas – *dizziness, ungroundedness, floati-ness, bewilderment, lack of concentration.*

Suckling also sets up an important hormonal function; the **oxytoxin** effect. When the mother produces milk, this hormone helps create the bond of uncon-ditional love; caring for the other more than you care for yourself. The lack of this bond means feeling profoundly alone, abandoned, unsafe; there is no one around to look after you or support you. This situation can lead to utter desolation. One learns to live with it through compensatory behaviours (such as addictions, compulsive caring for others, falling into victim-rescuer dynamics). Such compensations do not heal the wound, and it remains like a bottomless pit in your belly; an emptiness or void that can never truly be filled.

MAMMALIAN QUALITIES

Extended juvenile period

For Mammals, growing up happens once they've been born rather than in utero – therefore parenting is really important. Mother, child and the tribe form a close-knit unit to support the rearing of the young. The community comes together, forming a vital support network where the young are encouraged to discover and experiment through playing, practicing and learning new skills. This leads to great adaptability and inventiveness. Humans are at the top of this evolutionary tree, with a very long period of childhood; even longer than orang-utans and chimps. Learning means you are not pre-programmed; you become more adaptable and are able to squeeze into more niches than any other species – hence our success. If you're more primitive, you live according to a set of hard-and-fast rules. Humans are *the most* adaptable, and so we are currently endanger-ing the earth through overpopulation.

> *Mammals were the latest class of vertebrate to evolve and, following the demise of the dinosaurs, became the biggest animals on the planet. Physiologically they differ from other animals in that they feed their young with milk excreted by the mammary glands, giving perhaps the closest bond between mother and offspring of any creature. The vast majority are fertilised internally and give birth to live young usually covered in fur. One of the factors that have made mammals so successful is their ability to regulate their internal heat at a constant temperature despite changes in external conditions. This means that they have been able to colonise every habitat on the planet, adapting to every extreme of climate. Some groups also make seasonal adjustments, either migrating to a warmer area for part of the year or lowering their metabolism sufficiently to allow hibernation during the coldest months.*[13]

With the animal milks such as Lac-leo, Lac-c, Lac-f etc. there is more of an issue of who is the dominant one – the **aggressor** and who will **submit**. Victim consciousness is very often a central component in the pathology of types who respond to homeopathically prepared Milk remedies. There is a sense of martyring themselves, of caring for the needs of others; running themselves into the ground by not considering their own emotional needs. There is a parallel here with Sea animal remedies, especially Sepia which continues to be such a useful remedy for burnt-out caregivers.

These qualities of becoming the carer for others, or the advocates for people who have been under cared for, or under nourished, are a type of compensation for the fact that **they themselves did not receive that care when they really needed it**.

*As a group, these remedies focus on issues of **self-worth**, **dependence**, **competition**, **attractiveness**, **nurturing**, **hierarchy**, **territory**, **group acceptance**, jealousy, perform- ing and suffering wrongful acts, and, in our patients, the split between the animal and human side of one's nature . . . [there is] a feeling of having suffered wrong [with] the suppression of natural instincts in order to harmonise with the group to which one belongs.*
Kalathia[2]

MAPPA MUNDI

Choleric / Phlegmatic

Dominant *vs.* Submissive.
Individualistic *vs.* Conforming to the group.

Fire / Air

Connected, fulfilled *vs.* Isolation, neglect.
Warm Fullness *vs.* Cold Emptiness.
Unconditional love *vs.* Forsaken and unloved.

Earth / Water

Hierarchy and Supremacy *vs.* Softness and Nurturing.
Nutrition, digestion and elimination.

THEMES

Family, society, the group *vs.* The individual

Family and community are important themes in Mammal remedies; the herd, group or tribe are absolutely intrinsic to survival. The group stands for *protection, nurture, nourishment and care* but also implies *hierarchy* in which one has to find one's place. 'Do I lead, or am I happy being led? Am I being treated fairly by the others? Do I back down or stand up for myself?' The issue of **Self *vs.* Group** becomes apparent in the core experience of the patient. There arises a tension between suiting one's own needs *vs.* conforming to peer pressure in order to be

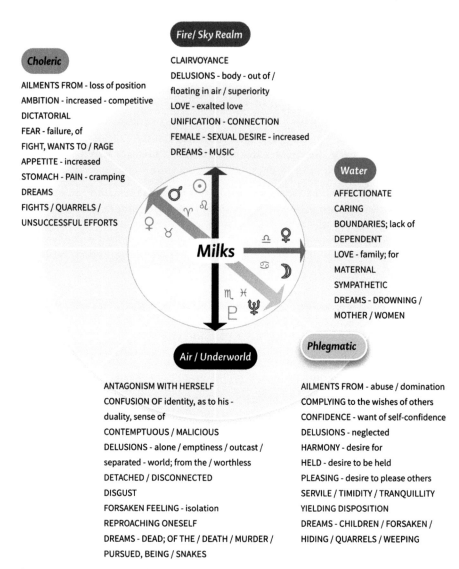

Fire/ Sky Realm

CLAIRVOYANCE
DELUSIONS - body - out of /
floating in air / superiority
LOVE - exalted love
UNIFICATION - CONNECTION
FEMALE - SEXUAL DESIRE - increased
DREAMS - MUSIC

Choleric

AILMENTS FROM - loss of position
AMBITION - increased - competitive
DICTATORIAL
FEAR - failure, of
FIGHT, WANTS TO / RAGE
APPETITE - increased
STOMACH - PAIN - cramping
DREAMS
FIGHTS / QUARRELS /
UNSUCCESSFUL EFFORTS

Milks

Water

AFFECTIONATE
CARING
BOUNDARIES; lack of
DEPENDENT
LOVE - family; for
MATERNAL
SYMPATHETIC
DREAMS - DROWNING /
MOTHER / WOMEN

Air / Underworld

ANTAGONISM WITH HERSELF
CONFUSION OF identity, as to his -
duality, sense of
CONTEMPTUOUS / MALICIOUS
DELUSIONS - alone / emptiness / outcast /
separated - world; from the / worthless
DETACHED / DISCONNECTED
DISGUST
FORSAKEN FEELING - isolation
REPROACHING ONESELF
DREAMS - DEAD; OF THE / DEATH / MURDER /
PURSUED, BEING / SNAKES

Phlegmatic

AILMENTS FROM - abuse / domination
COMPLYING to the wishes of others
CONFIDENCE - want of self-confidence
DELUSIONS - neglected
HARMONY - desire for
HELD - desire to be held
PLEASING - desire to please others
SERVILE / TIMIDITY / TRANQUILLITY
YIELDING DISPOSITION
DREAMS - CHILDREN / FORSAKEN /
HIDING / QUARRELS / WEEPING

Figure 5.1 Mappa Mundi dynamics for the Mammals

accepted. This could also be expressed as a conflict between living as a self-determined individual, i.e. *following one's own path vs.* subjugating oneself to the group/ family i.e. *fitting in.*

> *Feels good to be part of the group yet still have my own space; yet I felt I had* **surrendered** *to the group . . . feeling the need to look around the group; to* **connect** *with others.* lac-h.[3] *Obsessed about* **individuality** *vs. group* **conformity.** *In a dilemma whether I should give more importance to my individuality and speak and question freely, or keep quiet like the rest of the group.* lac-h.[4]

This tension between autonomy / individuality and conforming to the group is one of the essential features of the mammal group. *cf. Lanthanides – where the issue of autonomy is also central.*

The patient whose central state revolves around how *other people perceive them* may find a healing response from a Mammal remedy.

> *It felt like I was having to **chase after them**, in a '**please like me**' kind of way. . . . I feel as though people don't like me, turn their back on me; are critical, making nasty jokes, shutting me out. It is a very dark place – if I am not liked it is a big deal. . . . I wasn't their type of person. My response is, 'don't reject me, what can I do to change?' Feels desperate, isolating, horrible.* lac-leo.

Rubrics
Company – desire for – group together; desire to keep | Comply to the wishes of others; feeling obliged to | Harmony – desire for | Desires – suppressing his desires | Yielding disposition | Undertaking – things opposed to his intentions | Sociability | Pleasing – desire to please others | Friendship – maintain; need to | Dependent of others

Rejection means becoming the outcast; isolated and alone

A close-knit group has community spirit; the group defends its members against outside attack. Inside it you are **safe**, but you must conform to the rules and submit to peer pressure. If you're forced out for being too non-conformist, or for an undesirable character trait, or simply for not fitting-in, then you are forced to survive outside this protective circle. This is often a lonely and isolating experience and may lead to attempts to gain favour again by being over-friendly or not being true to yourself.

> *I felt **separated** from the **group** . . . Like outside a window, looking in . . . Feeling like an **outsider**, or outcast . . . Wanted to be with people, but felt **shunned**.* lac-del.[6] *I felt like an **outsider** to my **family**, that I didn't **belong**. Also that they did not even care to hear my viewpoint. It made me feel unimportant and incidental.* lac-lup.[7] *I felt I didn't belong and that they were just inviting me to be nice. I felt an **outcast** . . . **It is not ok to be just me, I don't fit in** . . . Felt like crying all day; felt sad and **isolated**. With friends, I didn't get the jokes, felt different, isolated, **stuck in self**."* phasco-ci.[8] ***Invader;** he is an – he feels unwelcome wherever he goes; an outcast or **scapegoat.*** lac-lup.[7]

Especially for teenagers, there is nothing worse than 'losing face', being the weird odd one out, or the butt of jokes because of a 'mistake' one has made. The extreme peer pressure of modern social media is likely to bring out Mammal themes in the young people of today; there is currently a crisis in adolescents developing mental health disorders such as self-harming, anorexia and body dysmorphia. These behavioural patterns act as an escape or release valve from the *incessant **comparing of oneself to others*** through digital platforms that appears to be leading to such extreme measures being taken up by so many young people.

Does this remedy resolve old shock conditions or remind us of those situations in which we must survive without the protection of a group?. . . **Those who are not normal are expelled by the group because only normal people belong to the group.** *You are alone and you must die. You are* **hunted.** *The group can kill you, they won't let you live because you are different – or you live in isolation and die by yourself.* lac-h.[9] *Sensitive to criticism, Was shopping and sales lady asked my size and said, you're much broader than that. Normally, I brush it off but kept thinking about it.* lac-lup.[7]

Rubrics
Delusions – outcast; she were an | Delusions – family, does not belong to her own | Delusions – separated – group; he is separated from the | Forsaken feeling – friends or group; by | Delusions – looked down upon; she is | Delusions – neglected – he or she is neglected

Within the hierarchy – who is dominant and who is submissive?

This polarity is expressed in the rubrics;
Ailments from – domination and abuse *vs.* Complying to the wishes of others, feeling obliged to.

The delusion of a patient needing a Milk remedy is that there is someone in a dominant position; they might picture themselves in this position (Lac-leo), or that others dominate them unfairly and 'lord it over them' (Lac-c). There may be quarrels, arguments and fights to establish dominance and these experiences permeate their life. There is a need to find and maintain one's position within the hierarchy.

The alphas engage in ritualistic altercations with their lower-ranked pack mates to demonstrate their **dominance.** *. . . The beta submits and rolls onto its back with tail between legs, all the while whining, smiling, and urinating on itself . . . afterward[s], the pack will mob the alpha to show its* **support** *and* **submission.** lac-lup.[7]

The one who becomes dominant is the leader, the chief who gets all the privileges and maintains the status quo in the group. In the mating season there will be disputes with other males who feel they have a claim to the position of alpha male. There is always a chance of an opportunist power-grab from one of the subordinates. This **posturing for supremacy** can lead to a test of one's strength in combat, and even a fight to the death if each competitor is too evenly matched to settle the conflict without violence. This contrasts Insect super-societies which are essentially a Monarchy, where the workers carry out their duties under strict pheromonal control.

Over-reacted when I thought my servant was being haughty, too **dominating** *and trying to point out my mistake. Was boiling with anger and had the* **malicious** *plan of removing her from my service. Started to talk behind her back, but did not* **confront** *her.* lac-leo.[10] *Seeing others of his group being* **beaten** *and* **abused** *by other people /* **authority**, *but being helpless against it.* lac-d.[22]

In mammals, there is a fight between males to claim dominance and to have breeding rights. This alpha is the only male who will reproduce with the hareem. This is in contrast to birds who tend to form lasting partnerships when caring for their young and sea animals for whom the parental role is rather non-existent. In mammals, the main caring role is taken by the mother and this could account for the single-parent-family phenomena observed by Philip Bailey[12] in 'Lac Remedies in Practice'.

In human terms, this may be expressed in compulsive competitiveness; feeling as though one constantly has to prove oneself, fending off perceived competitors, and maintaining high standards of appearance to remain attractive.

Rubrics
Anger – authority; against | Ailments from – abused; after being | Ailments from – domination | Ailments from – suppression | Delusions – looked down upon; she is | Delusions – wrong – suffered wrong; he has | Ambition – increased – competitive | Anger – authority; against | Malicious | Submissive | Servile

Belonging, inclusion and connection vs. Isolation, estrangement and separation

One of the fundamental dynamics expressed in mammal cases is the polarity between feeling *included and connected with others*, *vs.* the opposite feeling of *estrangement and disconnection*. The vital sensation may be expressed as warmth and contentment, alongside expressions such as *cuddly, playful, furry, nurturing, fulfilling*. The opposite is *cold, isolated, uncared for, unappreciated, distant, ignored*. "Mammal remedies are indicated in people who are particularly influenced by the group or family and are sensitive to the idea of whether they are being looked after or look after others." Fraser[13]

> *Feeling **love** and **openness** towards my friends. I am **accepting** myself more. I am enjoying life and what it brings, good and bad.* lac-lup.[7] *Love, security, **humanity**, caring, being **connected**, oneness are all attributes I symbolically equate with mother's milk. But the sickness of Lac humanum shows a cruel picture. We find the shadow in inhumanity, lack of feeling, hardness, cruelty, hunger, violence, **neglect** and **addiction**.* lac-h.[9] *Felt **disassociated**, not connected to my body. **Disconnected** from emotions, from things going on around me. Things were happening but I was apathetic.* lac-lup.[7] *Feeling, on being scolded, as if **people don't care**, or as if I am **alone**. I feel they can't understand me and that I should commit suicide because it does not make a difference whether I live or die.* lac-h.[4]

Rubrics
Connection; sense of | Content | Unification – sensation of unification | Tranquillity *vs.* Detached | Disconnected feeling | Estranged | Delusions – neglected – he or she is neglected | Delusions – separated – world; from the – he is separated

Nurture *vs.* Neglect

In remedies made from milk, the central problem can be traced back to the experience of nurture; whether this was taken away too early, missing entirely, or given in too much abundance so as to be over-bearing. A common compensation is to respond to this situation by **giving too much to others,** or finding a partner who needs rescuing so one can vicariously make up for the care that was missed out on in one's own upbringing. Unfortunately, this situation perpetuates the imbalance in the Lac patient's life; whilst lavishing care on the needy partner, they don't receive anything in return. A strong theme in the proving of Elephant's milk was a desire to care for others by feeding them, brought out in the following dream.

> *Dream: I want to take care of this boy and his companions. I feed them with food from my mother's kitchen, but they are greedy and grab it . . . broken, desperate, hungry, poor.* lac-loxod-a.[14] *Dream: My next-door neighbour asked me to take care of the little baby she is being a foster parent for. I was mildly annoyed at the imposition, but agreed. Once she brought him over, I was very solicitous of him and found him very cute. I really felt fond of the little boy.* lac-del.[6]

Rubrics
Nursing others | Responsibility – taking responsibility too seriously | Maternal instinct; exaggerated | Cares, full of – others, about | Caring | Duty – too much sense of duty

Warmth *vs.* Coldness

Mother's milk represents unconditional love; a sensation of warmth and fullness, nurture and nourishment. The opposite sensation is of a cold and empty space; a void that can never be filled.

> *The desire for suckling – the physical closeness, **warmth and contact,** both to have it and to give it – is extremely powerful in mammals . . . [it is a] warm, comforting feeling. . . . Nourishment helps to make the young child (and the adult into which it will grow) feel **content, happy and secure.** If this process is in some way disturbed then the opposite is the case – the individual can feel **profoundly unfulfilled, empty and insecure.*** Hardy[15]

Rubrics
Content | Cuddle – desire to be cuddled | Contact; desire for | Affection – yearning for affection | Affectionate | Benevolence | Held – desire to be held | Love – exalted love *vs.* Delusions – emptiness; of | Stomach – emptiness | Insecurity; mental | Delusions – forsaken; is | Forsaken feeling – isolation; sensation of

Floaty, light-headed, ungrounded, bewildered

Lack of nutrition results in the following 'floaty, spaced-out' symptoms seen in the Milk remedies.

- **Delusions**
  - Floating – air, in
  - Float; he was so light he could
  - Is light; he
  - Grounded – not grounded
  - Bewildered
  - Concentration – difficult
  - Confusion of mind – identity, as to his – boundaries; and personal
  - Spaced-out feeling
  - Vertigo

Such floating sensations may also refer to the gestational period that mammals spend in utero. Beginning their life in the amniotic fluid of the womb makes sense of the floaty, weightless feelings expressed in the provings.

Compensations and addictive behaviour

A difficult relationship to the mother / nurturing archetype may lead to compensatory behaviours to fill the void; pets can become the recipient for the kind of unconditional love that the patient craves for themselves. Eating disorders may also be an important component of remedies prepared from milk; compulsive eating also fills the void where they feel they have missed out on nourishment. *(Earth-Water axis of nutrition, digestion and elimination.)* This may go back to the primary bond with mother, where there should be feelings of *safety, connectedness, fulfilment and unification*. The opposite is a feeling of being *disconnected, forsaken, unloved, alone, hungry, distanced, in a void or incubator.*

The mother needs mothering

The patient's family history and particularly the relationship with their mother may be seen in Homeopathic terms as the 'never been well since' symptom. "The child is very attuned to their mother and will be very supportive and caring from a young age, forcing them to grow up too soon. A pattern commonly observed in single parent families . . . [these patients may end up] **wanting to nurture the whole world because they themselves missed out on it.**" Bailey[12] "Patients needing milk remedies are somewhat immature emotionally – they often **regress into a child-like state** under stress. They are self-conscious and shy. It is common to see a history of poor bonding with a parent, especially the mother. . . . There [can be] a feeling that siblings were preferred to them." Hardy[15]

> *My relationship with my mum is the same; betrayal. Enormous sense of disappointment, and not being valued, being rejected. Not being supported. My dad filled up the gaps and he is not there anymore. Huge sense of loss . . . I was the replacement daughter. A lot of feelings of not being valued. Parents rejected me . . . Mum was totally useless to me. Her grief took precedence over my needs.* lac-lup. *Furious and violent with my mum. How dare you! I get this feeling when anyone cuts me down in any way. It is a red rag to a bull. You'll be the one who's cut off not me.* lac-leo.

Rubrics
Affectionate | Ailments from – neglected; being – mother; by one's | Attached | Cares, full of – relatives, about | Delusions – family, does not belong to her own

| Dependent of others | Estranged – family; from his | Forsaken feeling – beloved by his parents, wife, friends; feeling of not being | Maternal instinct; exaggerated | Mother complex | Nursing others

Shame / split between human and animal, low self esteem

Conflict with oneself regarding control of sexuality, sexual guilt. Self-critical, self-contempt, looking down upon himself. Delusions – dirty – he is. As with Ana-cardium, Snakes and Aurum salts, there can be a feeling of *antagonism within themselves*, as if they are somehow at odds with the different aspects of their psyche.

> *Haven't got confidence to go out – people are going to judge me . . . it does not take much for me to feel mortified, shamed. Great sense of shame. I can't go into a group of people and stand up and be a person. Deep sense of shame and guilt.* lac-d.

Rubrics

Ailments from – shame | Antagonism with herself | Confidence – want of self-confidence – self-depreciation | Conflict – within oneself | Contemptuous – self, of | Delusions – body – ugly; body looks | Delusions – despised; is | Delusions – dirty; he is | Delusions – worthless; he is | Dirty | Disgust – oneself | Loathing – oneself | Reproaching oneself – sexual thoughts; about | Shameful

Headaches

This is one of the most common physicals amongst the milk remedies. Below is a selection of rubrics where 3 or more Lacs can be found in the Head and Vertigo chapters of Synthesis repertory.

VERTIGO
- ACCOMPANIED BY – Head – pain in head

HEAD
- CONSTRICTION – Forehead
- HEAVINESS – Forehead
- PAIN
  - accompanied by
    - § nausea
    - § vomiting
  - jar agg.
  - pressure – amel.
  - Forehead – Eyes – above
  - Occiput
  - Temples – pressing pain
  - Vertex – pressing pain
- PULSATING
  - Forehead
  - Temples

lac-c.	lac-h.	lac-d.	lac-leo.	lac-cp.	lac-lup.	lac-del.	lac-e.	lac-f.	lac-loxod-a.
1	1								1
1	1				1				
1		2	1					1	
2	1	2							
2	1	2							
1	1	1							
1	1	2							
3	1	2							
3	1	1	1	1		1			
1	1				1		1		
1	1			1					
2	1	3	1						
2	1	1							
1	1	1	1	1	1	1	1	1	1

Figure 5.2 Rubrics containing at least 3 Lac remedies from Vertigo & Head chapters

Female hormones

Rubrics where 3 or more Lacs can be found in the Chest and Female chapters of Synthesis.

- **CHEST**
  - SWELLING – Mammae – menses – before – agg.
- **FEMALE**
  - LEUKORRHEA – yellow
  - MENSES
    § clotted
    § copious
    § early; too
    § frequent; too – day – two days too early
    § frequent; too – week – one week
    § painful
    § scanty
  - PAIN – Ovaries
  - SEXUAL DESIRE
    § diminished / increased

lac-c.	lac-leo.	lac-lup.	lac-d.	lac-h.	lac-loxod-a.	lac-e.	lac-f.	lac-v-f.	lac-cp.
2				1			1		
1			2				1		
2				1	2				
2		1		1	2			1	
1					2	1			
1	1		1						
1	1							1	
2	1	1					1		
1		1	1						1
2		1	1						
	1	1			1	1			
2	1			1		1			
1	1	1	1	1	1	1	1	1	1

Figure 5.3 Rubrics containing at least 3 Lac remedies from Chest & Female chapters

Digestive problems, food intolerances, metabolic disturbances

Rubrics where 3 or more Lacs can be found in the Stomach and Abdomen chapters of Synthesis.

- **STOMACH**
  - APPETITE
    - § increased
    - § wanting
  - DISORDERED / DISTENSION / EMPTINESS / ERUCTATIONS / NAUSEA – morning
  - PAIN
    - § burning
    - § cramping
    - § eating – after – agg.
  - THIRST – large quantities; for – often; and
  - VOMITING; TYPE OF – food
- **ABDOMEN**
  - DISTENSION / FLATULENCE / HEAVINESS
  - PAIN
    - § cramping
    - § dragging, bearing down
    - § Hypogastrium
    - § Inguinal region

lac-c.	lac-d.	lac-h.	lac-del.	lac-e.	lac-leo.	lac-f.	lac-loxod-a.	lac-lup.	lac-cp.
2	1	2	1				2	1	
1	1				1	1			
1	1		2						
	2	1		1		1			
3		1					1		
1	2	1	1	1	1	1	1		
2	2		1		1				
2		1	1	1			1		
	2	1						1	
2			1					1	1
1	2	1							
1	2	1							
2	2	1		1	1		1		
2	2	1	1	1		1			
	1	1							1
2		1				1		1	
2	1							1	
1	1			1					
2	1	1		1					
1	1	1	1	1	1	1	1	1	1

Figure 5.4 *Rubrics containing at least 3 Lac remedies from Stomach & Abdomen chapters*

Differentiating mammals

Mahesh Gandhi has done some ground-breaking work in helping Homeopaths differentiate between the vast Animal kingdom. Regarding the mammals, he first places them into the *terrestrial* realm, before dividing the Orders based on an Elemental understanding, using Water (Cetacea – sea mammals), Earth (prey mammals) and Fire (predatory mammals). Further divisions are made using the Eriksonian model of psychosocial development (as pioneered in Homeopathy by Michal Yakir). The only drawback is that, in order to use this model, one does need to have a good grounding in Erikson's theory. *Peter Fraser*[36] also had some very interesting thoughts on this subject;

Rudolf Steiner saw the body as divided into three cavities, each containing one of the main systems. The Cranium contains the Brain and the Nervous system; it is the best armoured of the cavities. The Thoracic cavity is protected by the ribs and contains the Rhythmic systems; the Lungs and Heart. The Abdominal cavity is much less protected and contains the Digestive system [these mammals are preyed upon by the carnivores].

In humans, these three systems are in balance whereas in most mammals one of the systems strongly predominates. This allows for a threefold division: the Rodents – in which the Nervous system and the Senses predominate; the Carnivores – in which the Rhythmic systems predominate; and the Ungulates – in which the Digestive system predominates.

Schad (continuing in Steiner's footsteps) looks at the mammals in a Goethean manner and identifies several notable features of each group. The teeth are an example: in the Nervous mammals, the incisors dominate; in the Rhythmic mammals, the canines dominate; and in the Digestive mammals, the molars dominate. There are many other such examples; the food they eat, their size, limbs, colouration, antlers and tusks, etc. These all provide a way of dividing and classifying the mammals.

Within each of the three groups, there can be a further threefold division according to the importance of the systems in their makeup. For example, the most Nervous of the Carnivores are the Bear-like animals, the most Carnivorous are the Cats and Dogs, whilst the most Digestive are the Sea mammals. Within the Bear-like animals, the Bears are the most Digestive and the Mustelids the most Nervous. Within the Mustelids, the Weasels are the most Nervous, the Martens and Otters the most Carnivorous and the Badgers the most Digestive.

This process of sub-division can be carried on right down to the level of species. It is therefore possible to place the mammals on a complete spectrum; from the Rodents, in which the nerves and senses predominate, down to the most Digestive of the Herbivores. Schad outlines not only the way the individual species can be divided but also the features that are found within them. Thus, at one extreme the most Nerve-dominant Mouse can easily die of simple fright whilst at the other extreme, the Digestive-dominant Sloth can be shot in the heart and will still take several days to die.

There are a few mammals in which two systems predominate. For example, the Pachyderms, as herbivores, are Digestive-dominant but their excessive noses and ears show that the Senses are also important. The Insectivores, such as Moles and Anteaters, are also Sense-dominant (Anteater's nose) but they are Carnivorous in their diet and in other aspects. Applying the same understanding to our patients can help us to see much more clearly which parts are out of balance in the human three-foldness and therefore to see the indicated remedy. [This of course relies on good provings bringing out the physical symptoms so one can differentiate based on the physical affinities.]

Summarising and adapting these innovative ideas into an Elemental model lead to the following:

Mutable / Air = Nervous (Rodentia)

Focus
- Nervous, scurrying, busy.
- Escaping from danger, hiding, senses acute.

- Fear, fright.
- Gnawing.
- Pests – trapped, poisoned, eliminated from our homes.
- Rats thrive in the shadows – in the dark sewers.
- Mutable energy operates chiefly through the mental channels – it is a strongly mercurial dynamic, requiring movement, adaptation and changeability. Gemini (Mutable Air) rules the central nervous system.

Contains
Rats, Mice, Beavers, Squirrels, Chipmunks, Guinea pigs, Porcupines.
Possibly include – Rabbits, Hares, Talpidae?

Fixed / Fire = Rhythmic (Carnivora)

Focus
- Roaming to find their prey. Difficult to find food – scarcity.
- Special, talented.
- Fast and fierce attack.
- Pack or solitary.
- Domesticated / Abused. Independence traded for security and an easy life.
- Fixed types are intensely focused on their task – as is certainly necessary to be a successful predator. Leo (Fixed Fire) rules the Heart area.
- *Cats* – Territorial, grooming, preening, fast, agile, prowling, lounging.
- *Dogs* – Hunting as a pack, teamwork, roaming as a unit.
- Both – Hierarchy, cuddling, playful, sudden pouncing, torn-apart, cut-down, the chase.

Contains
Cat-like (including cats, hyenas, mongooses, viverrids)
Dog-like (including dogs, bears, wolves, foxes, raccoons, badgers, seals and mustelids)

Cardinal / Water and Earth = Digestive (Ungulata)

Focus
- Grazing, big bodied, terrestrial mammals – preyed upon.
- They do the hard graft – converting grains and grasses into big units of muscle which the predator takes advantage of (theme of letting themselves be taken advantage of).
- Food is in abundance, but they are always in danger of being attacked and predated upon.
- Need the group for safety.
- Agriculture, intensively farmed, caged, liberties taken.
- Sea mammals returned to the ocean with an evolutionary advantage – becoming carnivorous.
- Cardinal types provide initiatory energy – converting food into energy in the digestive tract.

Contains

Equidae, Camelidae, Suidae, Cetacea, Ruminantia (for example, Bovidae, Cervidae etc.)

Source words

Warm, Furry, Burrowing. Pouncing, Scratching, Claws, Cut down, Ripped apart.
Playful, Posturing. Fighting, High speed chase.
Milk, Suckling, Closeness. Caring, Cuddling.
Herds, Packs, Prides. Migration, Territorial. Fluffy, Friendship. Adaptable.

Differential Diagnosis

Sycotic, Malarial and Ringworm
  Miasms
Matridonals
Malvales (attached)
Scrophulariaceae (bonded)

Leguminosae (unified)
Conifers (cut-off)
Molluscs (home and house)
Prey Mammals – Stages 2–4
Predators – Stage 10 and 11

REMEDIES

MAMMALIA (MAMMALS)

Kingdom: Animalia.
Phylum: Chordata.
Class: Mammalia.

ac-alc, lac-as, lac-buf-xyz, *LAC-C*, lac-ca-b, lac-ca-dr, lac-cav-p, lac-cn-l, lac-cp, lac-cp-m, **lac-d**, lac-d-i, **lac-del**, LAC-E, lac-eleph-m, **LAC-F**, **LAC-H**, lac-h-f, lac-h-m, lac-hyae, lac-lam, lac-lem-s, **lac-leo**, lac-lep-eu, lac-loxod-a, **lac-lup**, lac-mac-m, **lac-mat**, lac-mc-gg, lac-mr-l, lac-o, lac-od-z, lac-odo-v-v, lac-oryc, lac-p-d, lac-pan-p, lac-pan-tr, lac-ph-v, lac-phas-c, lac-pr, lac-pum-cc, lac-sui, lac-sui-sc, lac-urs, lac-v-b, lac-v-c, lac-v-f, lac-v-fe, lac-vul-v.

Human Milks

It is useful to look at the human milks (maternum and humanum) when gathering general themes for the lac remedies as they do not have the animal themes as well.

Lac humanum (Human milk)

Breast milk is the primary source of nutrition for newborns before they are able to eat and digest other foods. Human milk contains 0.8% to 0.9% protein, 4.5%

fat, 7.1% carbohydrates, and 0.2% ash (minerals). It also contains as many as 600 different species of various bacteria and a unique category of sugars – human milk oligosaccharides (HMOs) – which are not present in formula. HMOs are not digested by the infant but help to make up the intestinal flora. The level of Immunoglobulin A in breast milk remains high from day 10 until at least 7.5 months post-partum. All mammalian species produce milk, but the composition of milk for each species varies widely. Human milk is less rich and more watery than the milk of mammals whose young nurse less frequently than our own.

Provings by: **Rajan Sankaran, India (1998),**[4] **Elizabeth Schulz, USA (1996).**[9] **Patricia Hatherly, Australia (2005)**[3] **and Jackie Houghton, UK (1991).**[5]

Keywords
Alone / Betrayed / Body – ugly / Neglected / Domination / Rats / Unreal / Violence / Worthless / Neglected / Friendless / Antagonism / Will – contradiction of / Benevolence / Disgusted at oneself / Reprimanded – mother; by / Nakedness – alone / Not feeling guilt / **Individuality** *vs.* **Conformity** / Sacrificed / Cut off

Mind
- **Delusions**
  - Alone, being – *always alone*
  - *Betrayed*; that she is
  - Body – ugly; body looks – fat; too
  - *Born into the world; he was newly*
  - Crime – committed a crime; he had
  - Faces, sees – distorted
  - Fire
  - *Friend – unwanted by friends*
  - *Friendless; he is*
  - Injury – about to receive injury; is
  - Invaded; one's space is being
  - Mice – sees
  - *Neglected* – he or she is neglected
  - *Nesting*; as if she is
  - Poisoned – he – has been
  - Rats; sees
  - Trapped; he is
  - Unreal – everything seems unreal
  - Violence, about
  - *Worthless*; he is
  - *Wrong – done wrong; he has*

- **Ailments from**
  - Abused; after being – children
  - Abused; after being – sexually
  - Domination – long time; for a
  - Embarrassment
  - Neglected; being
  - Neglected; being – mother; by one's

- **Fear**
  - Attacked; fear of being
  - Authority; of
  - Cancer; of
  - Crowd, in a
  - Dark; of
  - Death; of – alone, when
  - Disturbing someone; of
  - Dogs; of
  - Failure; of
  - **Life; of embracing**
  - Mistakes; of making
  - Murdered; of being
  - Noise, from – sudden, of
  - Sudden

- **Italic-type mentals**
  - Alert
  - *Antagonism with herself*
  - Benevolence
  - Detached
  - Indifference
    - § Everything; to
    - § Suffering; to – others; of
  - *Will – contradiction of*

- **Italic-type dreams**
  - Cousin
  - *Forsaken; being – friends; by*
  - *Helping – friends; his*
  - Journeys – train
  - Relatives
  - Snakes
  - Vivid

Unusual dreams

Buildings – collapsing / **Childbirth** – distressing / Children; about – captive; held / Cliff – edge of a; he is at the / Cousin – **handicapped** – helping; she was / **Disgusted – herself**; with / Fun – hurting others; by / Guilt – **not feeling guilt** / Leg – eruptions; covered with / Men – obnoxious – held back by / **Men – obnoxious** – macho; big – suitcase; in a small / Milk – lake of white milk / **Mother – milk**; asking for / **Nakedness – alone**; being naked when / **Reprimanded – mother; by** – rude behaviour; for / Rescued; being – brother; by / **Revered person is sexually abusive** / **Snakes** – converted into liquid / Snakes – killing / Snakes – surrounded by / **Tyrant** – power of a; being under the / Unsuccessful efforts – swim; to

Characteristic physicals

- **Head**
  - Pain
    - § Shooting pain – pulsating pain
    - § Occiput – extending to – Eye – left eye
    - § Pulsating – pressure – agg.
    - § Pulsating – Occiput – afternoon
- **Eye**
  - Lachrymation – wind agg.
- **Nose**
  - Odours; Imaginary and real – nauseating – milk, of – mother's milk
- **Face**
  - Eruptions – Rash – Menses amel.
  - Pain – Jaws – Dislocated; as if
- **Throat**
  - Catarrh – Adherent
  - Tingling
  - External Throat – Eruptions – red
- **Gastro-intestinal**
  - Heaviness – Eructations – amel.
  - Vomiting – Frequent
  - Stool – Tarry-looking
- **Female**
  - Leukorrhea – cream-like
  - Metrorrhagia – ovulation; during
  - Pain – Ovaries – ovulation – menses; from ovulation until – sharp
- **Chest**
  - Discharge from nipple – milky – male; in
  - Pain – Mammae – Stitching pain – milk would appear; as if
- **Generals**
  - Food and drinks
    - § Alcoholic drinks – agg. – intoxicated; easily
    - § Milk – desire – warm
  - Periodicity – hour – 12 hourly
  - Varicose Veins – congested

Obsessed about individuality *vs.* group conformity [Sankaran][4]

In a dilemma whether I should give more importance to my individuality and speak and question freely, or keep quiet like the rest of the group.[4]

   Delusions – friend – unwanted by friends. Detached – ego; from.

Provers speaking as one

§ Isolated feeling as if **no one cares for me**, or as if there is no one to look after me. I feel all are busy in their own lives. . . .

§ Felt very angry at parents for doing something against my wish. Felt I had many times **sacrificed my desires** for them and had done things against my wishes for them. Wept a lot, feeling as if I was all alone in the world. . . .

§ Angry at husband for returning late; shouted at him, **clenched teeth, pounced on him**, asked him to kill me because I could no longer bear to live alone waiting for him. . . .

§ **Feeling "cut off" from my friend circle; I don't want to be with them, or I am unable to maintain a relationship with them.** . . .

§ "Wild" with anger with friends when they neglected me and sat amongst themselves. Felt ignored, like I had no value. Felt that people don't understand or consider me although I try to help them in many ways. Felt the need of someone who understands me. . . .

§ I felt it's preferable to stay alone and concentrate on your aim, **because then you have a position and people appreciate you.**[4]

Lac maternum

(Milk of 9 different women from day 3 (colostrum) to 10 months following parturition)

During the first few days after delivery, the mother produces colostrum – a thin yellowish fluid that sometimes leaks from the breasts during pregnancy. It is rich in protein and antibodies that confer passive immunity to the baby. Colostrum also delivers nutrients to the newborn's small and immature digestive system in a very concentrated low-volume form whilst having a mild laxative effect to encourage the passing of meconium. A number of cytokines (small messenger peptides that control the functioning of the immune system) are found in colostrum, including interleukins, tumour necrosis factor, chemokines, and more. It also contains many growth factors.

Proving by: **Patricia Hatherly, Queensland, Australia (2001).**

Mind

- Alienation – feelings of
- Antagonism with himself
- Individuality *vs.* Group
- Estranged – friends; from

- Forsaken feeling – isolation, sensation of
- Misunderstood; feelings of being.

Dreams
- Friends – estranged from;

Synthesis of Lac maternum from Inspiring Homeopathy Smits[19]
- **Want of self-esteem**; *Has been put down from a young age – told it is not OK to be the way that they are, so the delusion that something is implicitly wrong with them becomes manifest.*
- **Neglects oneself.**
- **Martyr** – *'I would prefer to look after the wishes and needs of another rather than myself.'*
- **Poor boundaries.**
- Feeling of not fulfilling the expectations of life, of others, her husband / his wife;
  Delusions – despised; is / Repudiated; he is – relatives; by his
- Feeling of not being considered, of no longer being physically attractive; *Unacknowledged.*
- Trying to fulfil the expectations of others; *cf. Carcinosin – also derived from breast tissue.*
- Never angry; avoiding conflicts. *cf. Natrums, Magnesiums, Staphisagria, Muriatic Acid.*
- *cf.* Lac Humanum – There is a Hydrogen quality to Lac Maternum – *They're not grounded, don't know how to be here, or cope with the world, like they haven't fully incarnated.*

ANIMAL MILKS

Lac caninum (Bitch's milk)

Phylum: Chordata.
Class: Mammalia.
Order: Carnivora.
Family: Canidae.

The dog (*Canis lupus familiaris* when considered a subspecies of the wolf) is a domesticated carnivore. Their long association with humans has led them to be uniquely attuned to our behaviour and needs. They perform various roles, such as companionship, hunting, herding, pulling loads, guarding, assisting police, as well as aiding disabled people and providing therapy. They have proven themselves to be incredibly versatile, highly adaptable (to which the plethora of different breeds attests) and sociable – forming very close bonds within their human 'packs'. They have sophisticated forms of social cognition and communication within the hierarchy, which may account for their trainability, playfulness, and ability to fit into the human world as 'man's best friend'.

Man's best friend, but at what cost?

Fundamental delusions of Lac caninum

Looked down upon; she is.
- A feeling of being diminished, of low self-worth; that one has allowed one's very nature to be dominated by another.

Lie; all she said is a.
- They have lost so much faith in themselves that they cannot even trust what they say. They must suppress their own nature to please the other.

Prostitute, is a.
- This expresses a similar theme of subjugation in order to survive; selling oneself to gain favour.

Nose – someone else's nose; has.
- The nose gives a dog its most powerful sense; the means by which it can sniff out prey and therefore succeed as a predator. With someone else's nose, their innate abilities have been stripped.

Themes

Instinctual urges suppressed – the wild beast has to be controlled in order to retain favour with his master so that he may continue to live the easy life of being fed and looked after, to be accepted as part of the human pack. **The dog's place by man's side makes him the most controlled of any mammal, subjugating his wild instincts in order to please.**

This desire to please, to be loyal, faithful and controlling of one's animal instincts (suppressing anger, aggression, a need for dominance) must be at the heart of the remedy made from bitch's milk. Allied to this comes a feeling of shame at having allowed oneself to undergo such cruel treatment as a trade-off for security; think of the countless breeds of dogs who have been experimented on to accentuate desirable behavioural qualities or aesthetic attributes. No wonder the remedy is listed under – Delusions – Nose – someone else's nose; has.

Philip Bailey[12] talks about Lac-c types as being very well suited to family life, as they can get the kind of unconditional love that they crave from their children upon whom they are very doting. They may have endured relationships in which they have given a great deal, and suffered through mistreatment out of their **submissiveness and dependable nature**.

They are so controlled that they will not voice their misgivings over the way they are treated, and are therefore **susceptible to being used as a doormat**; the innate fear is that they will lose their place of security if they let their anger or displeasure be known to the partner. One situation he describes is that of the male Lac-c type being very nerdy, the type of person who may find their partner through internet dating after a succession of relationships that didn't work out, or where their reliable nature might have been taken advantage of by a stronger partner.

Dogs will submit to the alpha male, the pack leader, the one with the loudest bark and the sharpest teeth. They can have strong feelings of shame, much like Thuja, regarding their suppressed sexuality, or have feelings of self-loathing about the way they look – no matter how hard they try, **they will find themselves in situations where they are belittled by an alpha type who senses their susceptibility to being brought down a peg or two to the level of a lowly dog.**

SRP Rubrics
- **Delusions**
  - Body – out of the body – crazy if she could not get out of her body; she would become
  - Diminished – short, he is
  - Disease – loathsome, horrible mass of disease; he were a
- Hysteria / Insanity – orgasm; at the height of
- **Writing – meanness to her friends**

Important Mind rubrics
- **Delusions**
  - Clouds – black cloud enveloped her; a heavy
  - *Dirty* – he is
  - *Floating* – air, in
  - Mind – out of his mind; he would go
  - Snakes – in and around her
- Ailments from – abused; after being
- Company – desire for
- Death – desires
- *Disgust*
- **Fear**
  - Duty – unable to perform her duties; she will become
  - falling, of – descending stairs; when
  - Insanity
  - snakes, of
- Grief – waking, on
- Hatred
- Idiocy
- Loathing – life
- Malicious
- Offended, easily
- Perseverance
- Rage – contradiction, from
- Washing – desire to wash – hands; always washing her
- Yielding disposition

Dreams
Devils / Disease / Dogs / Snakes – bed, in / Spiders / Unsuccessful efforts – finding; in – toilet; the / Urinating / Vermin / Vivid

Bold type physicals
- **Vertigo**
  - Lying – agg. – touch the bed; as he did not
  - Walking – *gliding in the air;* with sensation of – feet did not touch the ground; as if
- **Head**
  - Pain
    - § Occiput – morning – waking; on
    - § Sides – alternating sides

- **Mouth**
  - Taste – salty – only salty food tastes natural
- **Throat**
  - Liquids taken are forced into nose
  - Membrane – pearly
- Paralysis – post *diphtheritic*
- **Female**
  - Menses – membranous
  - *Ovulation – during*
  - Pain
    - § Ovaries – extending to – Other ovary; from one to the
- § Uterus – stitching pain – upward
- **Chest**
  - Mammae; complaints of – menses; before
- **Skin**
  - Shining
- **Generals**
  - Side – *alternating sides*
  - Whiteness – Parts usually red; of

Lac caprinum (Goat's milk)

Phylum: Chordata.
Class: Mammalia.
Order: Artiodactyla.
Family: Bovidae.
Subfamily: Caprinae.

Goats are among the earliest animals domesticated by humans. Neolithic farmers began to herd wild goats for easy access to milk and meat, as well as to their dung which was used as fuel. Their bones, hair and sinew were put to use in the making of clothing and tools. They naturally have two horns and as ruminants, four-chambered stomachs. A buck in rut will display lip curling and urinates on his forelegs and face. Sebaceous scent glands at the base of the horns add to the buck's odour, making him more attractive to the does. Unlike grazing cattle and sheep, they prefer to browse on vines, shrubbery and weeds. They are curious escape artists – nimble and agile – able to climb to steep and precarious places. They tend not to herd as closely together as sheep.

Provings by: **Rajan Sankaran, Mumbai, India (1994)[28] and Kees Dam, Holland (1994).**[29]

Mind

- Addicted; tendency to become
- *Adulterous*
- *Adventurous*
- Ailments from
  - *Position; loss of*
  - Responsibility
- Ambition – increased
- Amorous
- Anarchist
- <u>*Anger – easily*</u> (*Nux-v.*)
- Anger – interruption; from
- Anger – trifles; at
- Anger – uncontrollable
- Answering – snappishly
- Antagonism with herself
- *Audacity*
- Censorious
- *Chaotic*
- Clinging – grasps at others – angry; when
- Company – aversion to
  - bear anybody, cannot
  - *desire for solitude*
- Complaining
- *Contemptuous*
- Delusions
  - Body – out of the body
  - Talking – people talk about her
  - Unreal – everything seems unreal
- Fear
  - Approaching; of
  - Blood; fear when looking at
  - Heart – disease of the heart
- Pins; of
- Sudden (panic attacks)
- Touched; of being (*Arnica*)
- *Fearless – danger; in spite of* (*Tungsten*)
- Fight, wants to
- Forebodings
- *Hurry – everybody – moves too slowly* (*Iridium., Med., Tarent.*)
- Indifference – others, toward
- Indignation
- Malicious
- *Rebellious*
- *Responsibility – inability to take*
- Restlessness
  - Drives him from place to place
  - *Move – must constantly*
- *Satyriasis*
- Serious
- *Shameless*
- *Spirituality*
- Starting – waking, on
- Striking – desire – strike; to
- Sulky
- Suspicious
- *Threatening*
- Truth – telling the plain truth
- Unconsciousness – *frequent spells of unconsciousness – injuries to head; after* (cf. *Nat-s.*)
- Undertaking – many things, persevering in nothing
- Witty

Dreams

Advice – not heeding / Amorous – pollutions, with / Animals **Antisocial** elements / Arguments – friends; with / *Attacked, of being – knife; with a* / Bed – narrow; too / *Bed – place to sleep; she had to hunt all night for a* / Brakes – find while driving; cannot / Caught; of being / **Cockroaches** – trousers; in her / Court; judicial / *Dead; of the – relatives* / **Deceit** / **Deceived**; being / Devils / **Drowning** / Flowers / Friends – old / Fruits / **Games – sex**; of – aunt; with / Girl – attention of a; trying to attract the / Girl – beautiful girls; of / **Girl – running after** / Goats / Guests – bed by guests; deprived of their / Guests – unable to ask a guest to stop what he is doing / Horrible / Insects – trousers; in her / Kissed – he was kissed – black figure; by a – pink lips; with / Lascivious / Locked up – half-open gate; with

/ **Pursued**, being / **Pursuing**; of / Quarrels / Rabbits / Resolving / Sexual – rain; having sex in the / *Sexual – sexual activity – broadcast on television; being* / **Shameless** / Shameless – behaviour of guest / Struggling; of / **Urgency**; of / Vegetables / Wolves / Women

Characteristic physicals

- **Vertigo**
  - Objects – turn in a circle; seem to – room whirls
- **Head**
  - Fullness – Forehead – Eyes – Above – pulling hair amel.
  - Pain – Closing the eyes – must close the eyes
- **Stomach**
  - Pain – eating – after – agg. – burning
- **Urine**
  - Burning

- **Male**
  - Pollutions – dreams – with
- **Female**
  - Menses – scanty – profuse flow; with sensation of
- **Skin**
  - Itching – burning
- **Generals**
  - Cold – bathing – desire for cold bathing
  - Covers – aversion to
  - Pain – wandering pain
  - Strength, sensation of

Lac vaccinum defloratum (Skimmed cow's milk)

Phylum: Chordata.
Class: Mammalia.
Order: Artiodactyla.
Family: Bovidae.

Cattle are large quadrupedal ungulate mammals with cloven hooves and are commonly raised as livestock for their meat, milk, and hides. They are also put to service as draft animals – oxen or bullocks pull carts, ploughs and other implements. They can therefore be classified as *beasts of burden*. They are also ruminants; their digestive system is highly specialised to accommodate the ingestion of poorly digestible plants. Vision is the dominant sense in cattle, and they obtain almost 50% of their information visually.

Proving by: **Dr Swan, USA (1871–72) and Rajan Sankaran, Mumbai, India (date unknown).**[22]

Fundamental delusion
- *Dead – friends are dead and she must go to a convent; all her*
- She is separated from her group, and is forced into a community to which she feels she does not belong. This leads to the following symptoms:
  - *Delusion – Separated – group; he is separated from the.*
  - Company – desire for – group together; desire to keep.

Keynote
Anger – authority; against

Delusions
- Die – about to die; one was
- Flesh was off bone and edges sticking out
- Objects; about – tossed up from below in every direction; objects were
- Pursued; he was

Suicidal disposition – thoughts – *meditates on easiest way of committing suicide*

Mind
- Abusive
- **Ailments from – abuse**
- **Company – aversion to – sight of people; avoids the**
- *Coquettish* – too much
- *Estranged – family; from his –* strangers, but not with his entourage and his family; being kind with
- **Fear**
  - *Narrow place, in*
  - *Suffocation, of*
  - *Toilet; in*
- Fight, wants to
- Hysteria – fainting, hysterical
- *Loathing – life*
- Maternal instinct; exaggerated
- Prophesying – predicts the time of death
- Suicidal disposition – thoughts – meditates on easiest way of committing suicide
- Vivacious
- Weary of life

Dreams
Adoption – dogs; injured / **Anger – authority; against** / Animals – beaten / Animals – tied / Animals – wild / Attacked, of being / **Beaten**, being / **Cheated**; being / Children; about – dirty / Coloured – green / Crippled man – carried on his back / Danger / Death – relatives; of – brother; of his / **Dirt** / **Disgusting** / Dressing up / **Embarrassment** / Face – emotionless face / Forsaken; being – helpless; and / Friends – meeting friends / Friends – old / *Friends – save her friends; attempting to* / Friends – separated from her friend / Frightful / Hiding – danger; from / Homesickness / Journeys / Lascivious / Missing – train; the / Mother / **Neglected** being / **Pursued**, being / Robbers / **Separated**; being / Snakes / Statue – life; coming to / Tigers – surrounded by / Wedding

Characteristic physicals
- **Vertigo**
  - Closing the eyes – amel.
  - Turning in bed agg.
- **Head**
  - Lifting up; sensation of – Skull
  - Pain – periodical – week – every
  - **Pulsating** – Vertex
- **Eye**
  - Band around the eyeballs; sensation of
  - Photophobia – light; from – artificial light – agg.
- **Vision**
  - Complaints of vision – head; pain in – during
- **Mouth**
  - Froth, foam from mouth – talking agg.
- **Throat**
  - *Lump; sensation of* a – rising sensation
- **Stomach**
  - Nausea – riding – carriage; in a – agg.
  - Nausea – *seasickness*
- **Stomach**
  - Thirst – large quantities; for – often
  - Vomiting; type of – bile – headache; during
- **Kidneys**
  - Pain – Region of – *burning*
- **Urine**
  - Copious – headache – during
- **Female**
  - *Heaviness – Ovaries*
  - Menses
    - § Late, too – seven days
    - § Suppressed menses – shock, from mental – suddenly
- **Chest**
  - *Milk – disappearing*
- **Chill**
  - Chilliness – headache – during
- **Skin**
  - Sensitiveness – cold; to
- **Generals**
  - *Fatty degeneration – Organs*
  - *Sleep – loss of sleep; from*
  - Wind – sensation of – cold

Themes[22]
- Being **abandoned**, forsaken or neglected by friends and community.
- Compensate by doing things for one's friends in order to feel included.
- Strong sense of **community spirit**.
- Need to be **helpful** and kind to by accepted by the group.
- Witnessing members of his group being **beaten / abused** by authority figures; feeling **helpless** against it.
- Feeling **suppressed, of no importance: having no voice**.
- Being **forced** to do things. Reacting with anger against authority.
- Mothering. Adoption. Not being cared for by the person who should be caring.
- Embarrassment.
- Feeling **fat, ugly, dark, dirty**. Suicidal disposition.
- Attractiveness.
- Violence. Sense of fear and danger. Being beaten with sticks.
- Green colour.

CASE 5.1 Gout, night-watching and ailments from grief

Patient: Female, age 70
Prescription: Lac-d 1M

Primary themes
∫ Feeling as though she can't be herself in a group.
∫ Fear she will be judged, they won't like her, that she will be exposed, trapped; a sitting target.
∫ Dreams of beating up her friends.
∫ Sent to a convent despite belonging to the Church of England.

Secondary themes
∫ Two / Dichotomy.
∫ Wants to be loyal in relationships.
∫ Rape / Abuse.
∫ Judging herself, ashamed.
∫ Caring / rescuer / adopting.
∫ Estranged from her own family.

Physicals
∫ Gout, rheumatic pains.
∫ Vertigo – Agg. in open spaces.
∫ Endometriosis.
∫ Constipated as a child.

Generals
∫ Loves sweets, spices. Warm agg., Sun agg., Cheese agg.

		caust.	ign.	lac-d	cocc.	cupr.	nux-v.	sep.	
		1	2	3	4	5	6	7	
		15	14	14	14	14	13	13	1
		18	26	23	21	19	24	20	1
1. MENTAL QUALITIES - Divided / Doubled / Duality*	(221) 1		2		1			1	
2. MENTAL QUALITIES - Low self esteem etc.*	(402) 1	2	2	1	2	2	2	4	
3. MENTAL QUALITIES - Trapped etc.*	(282) 1	2	3	2	2	3	2	2	
4. THEMES - DOMINATED – ABUSED	(105) 1	1	2	1		1	1	1	
5. THEMES - DUTY – RESPONSIBILITY	(231) 1	1	1		2	1	1	2	
6. MIND - FEAR - crowd, in a	(134) 1	1		1	1		2	1	
7. VERTIGO - TURNING; WHEN - head; or moving the	(74) 2	1	2	2	1	1		1	
8. HEAD - PAIN - Sides - one side	(218) 2	1	2	2	1	1	2	2	
9. KIDNEYS - PAIN - Region of	(137) 1	1		2		1	1	1	
10. EXTREMITIES - PAIN - Feet	(326) 1	2	1	1	1	2	2	1	
11. GENERALS - REST - amel.	(191) 1	1	1	1	2	2	3	1	
12. GENERALITIES - Night watching, mental strain, ill effects	(14) 3	1	2	2	2	1	2		

Figure 5.5 Analysis

	lac-d.
	1
	1
	3

1. MIND - AILMENTS FROM - abused; after being	(79) 1	1
2. MIND - CONFIDENCE - want of self-confidence	(224) 1	1
3. MIND - DEATH - desires	(108) 1	1
4. MIND - DELUSIONS - convent, she will have to go to a	(2) 1	1
5. MIND - FEAR - crowd, in a	(134) 1	1
6. MIND - FEAR - narrow place, in	(123) 1	2
7. MIND - MATERNAL INSTINCT; EXAGGERATED	(11) 1	1
8. MIND - SUICIDAL DISPOSITION	(215) 1	2
9. MIND - YIELDING DISPOSITION	(84) 1	2
10. VERTIGO - VERTIGO	(630) 1	1
11. VERTIGO - MOTION - head; of - agg.	(72) 1	2
12. VERTIGO - TURNING; WHEN - head; or moving the	(74) 1	2
13. RECTUM - CONSTIPATION - difficult stool	(232) 1	3
14. EXTREMITIES - PAIN - rheumatic	(304) 1	1
15. EXTREMITIES - PAIN - Feet	(326) 1	1
16. EXTREMITIES - PAIN - Feet - broken; as if	(7) 1	1
17. EXTREMITIES - TOES - first	(3) 1	3
18. GENERALS - EXERTION; PHYSICAL - agg.	(230) 1	2
19. GENERALS - PERIODICITY	(197) 1	1
20. GENERALS - SLEEP - loss of sleep; from	(62) 1	2

Figure 5.6 *Symptoms covering the case using reverse repertorisation*

Lac delphinum (Dolphin's milk)

Class: Mammalia.
Order: Artiodactyla.
Infraorder: Cetacea.
Family: Delphinidae.

Dolphins are descendants of land-dwelling mammals of the artiodactyl order (even-toed ungulates). They are aquatic mammals within the infraorder Cetacea and are sleek, fast moving, efficient hunters; often skilled in aerial display. Mother-calf bonds are very strong and long-lasting. A calf typically stays with its mother for 3 to 6 years. Milk is composed of 33% fat, 6.8% protein, 58% water, and low in lactose. This rich milk helps the baby rapidly develop a thick blubber layer which in turn aids their buoyancy. Breathing involves expelling stale air in an upward blast through their blowhole followed by inhaling fresh air into the lungs. The dolphin ear has specific adaptations to the marine environment; it is acoustically isolated from the skull by air-filled sinus pockets, allowing for greater directional hearing underwater. Dolphins send out high frequency clicks from an organ known as a melon, allowing them to produce biosonar for orientation.

Proving by: **Nancy Herrick, USA (1994–5).**[6]

Themes
Alert / Playful / Thrill-seekers / Enjoying danger and seeking it out / Milk + Sea animal themes.

SRP delusions
- *Danger – impression of; yet remains calm*
- Surrounded – enemies, by (*cf. Merc., Anac., Crot-h., Stage-12*)
- Safe; she is not (*cf. Sea animals, Latex.*)
- Alone – in the world (*cf. Androc., Plat., Kola., Stage-10*)
- Outcast; she were an (*cf. Leprosy miasm, Hura., Crotalidae, Liliales, Germanium*)
- Separated – group; he is separated from the (*cf. Milks, Musca-d.*)
- Big – everything seems
- Vehicle coming at me in the wrong lane

Mind
- Affectionate
- *Amusement – desire for*
- Antics; playing (*Solanaceae, Veratrum, Saccharum album*)
- Confidence – want of self-confidence – ***inferior; feels***
- *Fearless – waves; plunged through big*
- Mother fixation
- Sensitive – noise, to – sleep, on going to
- Sentimental – music; with
- Spaced-out feeling – *fog between self and other; sensation as if*
- Swimming – desires

Characteristic dreams
Circle – centre of – he is in / Circle – going clockwise toward a / Circle – standing outside a circle – looking in / Circle – walking in a / Encircled tightly, being / Flood – *calm* in a / Flood – house is in a / Horses – racing / House – community centre – rundown

Characteristic physicals

- **Vertigo**
  - Accompanied by – vision – dim vision
  - Spaciness; with
  - Turning; as if – he turns in a circle
- **Head**
  - Pain
    - § Occiput – dull pain
    - § Temples
- **Eye and Vision**
  - Photophobia
  - Vision
    - § Acute – objects; for small
    - § Blurred – large objects seem
- **Ear**
  - Stopped Sensation
- **Nose**
  - Catarrh – Postnasal – watery
- **Mouth**
  - Aphthae
- **Throat**
  - Pain – lump

- **Stomach**
  - Appetite – relish, without
  - Nausea – morning
  - Pain – gnawing pain
- **Rectum**
  - Constipation – bowels – action lost – sensation as if
  - Haemorrhoids – painful – burning, smarting
- **Urine**
  - Odour – offensive
- **Male**
  - Sexual desire – increased
- **Larynx and trachea**
  - Tickling – Air passages – talking agg.
  - Voice – lost – excitement agg.
- **Sleep**
  - Semi-conscious – hears everything
- **Skin**
  - Itching – burning
- **Generals**
  - Exertion; physical – desire for
  - Weakness – heat – sun; of the – agg.

Provers speaking as one

⨎ Dream: House flooded and had to use rowboat to get to friend's house. I was using a rowboat to get to and from classes and visit friends and go back and forth. Water was everywhere, and this was my mode of transportation. **Calmness, no sense of** danger. . . .

⨎ Desire to **touch** people, be near them, **feel** their presence, feel **connection**, to have **fun** with them, to laugh with them. . . . Feeling of **separation**; I felt separated from the group during the proving. Feeling like an outsider, or outcast. Pervasive feelings lasted over three months. Wanted to be with people but felt **shunned**. Like outside a window, looking in. Like standing outside a circle. Very profound. Every time I talk about it, the feelings are very intense. . . .

⨎ Psychic ability and **intuition** heightened. . . . While in the midst of a conversation, I couldn't remember whether I had spoken some of my ideas or merely thought them. This never happens to me, and it felt very unusual and unnerving. . . .

⨎ Obsession about alarm systems and protection; **she felt a constant, unnamed threat all around her**.[6]

Lac Equinum (Mare's milk)

Class: Mammalia.
Phylum: Chordata.
Order: Perissodactyla.
Family: Equidae.

The horse is an odd-toed ungulate mammal and has evolved over the past 45 to 55 million years from a small multi-toed creature into the large single-toed animal of today. Humans began domesticating horses around 4000 BC, eventually leading to their varied use in warfare, sporting and non-competitive recreation, police work, agriculture, entertainment, and therapy. Horses are adapted to run, allowing them to quickly flee from predators. They possess an excellent sense of balance and a strong fight-or-flight response. Related to this need to flee from predators in the wild is the unusual ability to sleep both standing up and lying down. Mares carry their young for approximately 11 months, and a young horse – called a foal – can stand and run shortly following birth.

Proving by: **Nancy Herrick, USA (1994).**[20]

- The nucleus of the remedy revolves around these fundamental delusions:
  - **Hindered; he is**
  - Fail; everything will
  - Hardship; life is
- The feeling of Lac equinum is that they are burdened or hindered, that life is a series of hardships that she must endure; she is trapped by them and feels like all her efforts will fail. The delusions below reveal her response to this central idea:
  - *House – surrounded; house is (cf. Arsenicum)*
  - *Stalked; he is being*
- The house is a symbol for one's self; so she is not only trapped but surrounded, with a feeling as of being stalked (where someone is following you or approaching with stealth behind you). This gives a feeling of being chased, pursued or hunted. The remedy state is given further expression in the following delusions:
  - *Delusions – Control; out of – organisation; losing control over one's*
- This sense of loss of control could give a hint of the cancer miasm; where one is faced with a state of chaotic disorganisation and responds by trying to control everything (*Arsenicum*).
  - *Delusions – Sinking; to be – quicksand; in*
- The sense of sinking in quicksand is reminiscent of the feeling of 'time running out' in the tubercular miasm, where drastic, revolutionary efforts are needed to recover one's position of safety.

Other important symptoms

- **Delusions**
  - Control; out of – *organisation; losing control over one's*
  - **Insulted**; he is
  - **Neglected – duty; he has neglected his**
  - Trapped; he is

- **Anxiety**
  - Breathing – suffocative
  - **Conscience; anxiety of**
  - Expected of him; when anything is
  - Family; about his – safety of family; for
  - Secrets revealed
  - Time is set; if a

Mind

- Ailments from – embarrassment – poor job performance; of
- Ambition – increased
- *Anger – touched; when* (Bold type)
- Anger – traffic; in
- Censorious
- Children – loves profoundly her beautiful daughter
- Contradiction – intolerant of contradiction – **rules; intolerant of inflexible**
- Cursing – desire to curse
- Dictatorial
- Duty – too much sense of duty
- Efficient, organised – clutter; bothered by
- Escape, attempts to – family and children; attempts to escape from her
- **Estranged – family; from his**
- **Fear – control; losing**

- Impatience – boredom; with
- Intolerance – ambiguity
- Irritability – business – proceed fast; when does not
- *Love – children; for – daughter; for – limited in expression of it; but*
- Rest – cannot rest when things are not in the proper place
- Restlessness – anxious – fresh air amel.
- *Revealing secrets – impulsively – own; her*
- Riding – horseback; on – amel.
- Sadness – menopause, during
- Sensitive – noise, to
- Struggle – everything is
- Touched – aversion to be
- Travelling – desire for
- Truth – telling the plain truth
- Unconsciousness – unable to mediate between loved ones; when

The mental picture draws comparisons to *Arsenicum, Carcinosin, Natrum mur and Sepia.*

Dreams

Accidents – car; with a – hit-and-run / Adolescents – time of / Adventurous / Alien from outer space – psychic / Bathrooms – cannot find the bathroom / **Betrayed, having been** / Bored – people are / Cats / *Children; about – mutilated* / Children; about – precocious and arrogant / Confidence; breach of / **Escaping – danger; from** / Frustration / Groups – screwed over by attorney / **Groups – working well together** / Guilt / Helping – rejected by those he tries to help / Hiding – danger; from / Horses / Indignation / Killing – idea of; but did not like the / Mammae / Moral feeling – lack of – others; in / People / People – native –

Americans / *Precision* / Pursued, being / Rabbits / *Rejected; being – helped; by those he had* / Seduction – unwanted / Shameful / Singing / Sports / Teaching / Teamwork / Traffic / **Unsuccessful efforts** – do various things; to

Characteristic physicals

- **Female Genitalia/sex**
  - Orgasm – delayed
  - Pain – Ovaries – alternating sides – menses; after
  - Sexual desire – increased – menses – after – agg.
  - Tingling, voluptuous – Ovaries – left – menses; after
- **Generals**
  - Evening – amel.
  - Clothing – intolerance of
  - Convulsions – heat; during
  - Pulse – frequent – motion agg.
  - Tension – Muscles; of
  - Weakness – warm – bathing; after
- **Head**
  - Pain – Gnawing pain
- **Eye**
  - Pain – Stinging
- **Mouth**
  - Aphthae – Palate
  - Bleeding – Gums – easily
- **Stomach**
  - Disordered – excitement agg.
  - Hiccough – eating – after – agg.
- **Abdomen**
  - Distension – night
- **Stool**
  - Flatulent
- **Chest**
  - Pain – Mammae – menses – before – agg.
- **Back**
  - Pain – Lumbar region – rising – sitting; from – agg.
- **Extremities**
  - Eruptions
  - Forearms – desquamation, bran-like
  - Forearms – urticaria
  - Pain – Knees – ascending – stairs – agg.
  - Restlessness – Feet
  - Shaking

Lac felinum (Cat's milk)

Phylum: Chordata.
Class: Mammalia.
Order: Carnivora.
Family: Felidae.

The cat is a domestic species of small carnivorous mammal in the Felidae family. They have a strong flexible body, quick reflexes, sharp teeth and retractable claws suited to killing small prey. They have excellent night vision, a keen sense of smell and are very communicative with a variety of vocalisations and body-language. They are a social species apart from when hunting, at which time they are solitary. They are most active at dawn and dusk, sleeping or grooming themselves for large parts of the day. The cat's tongue has backwards-facing spines called papillae which act like a hairbrush. When cats become aggressive, they try to make themselves appear larger and more threatening by raising their fur, arching their backs, turning sideways and hissing or spitting.

Proving by: **Divya Chabra, India (1994).**[26]

SRP Rubrics
- Cleanness – mania for
- Curious
- Fear – falling, of – descending stairs; when (*cf.* Lac-c)
- *Haughty – clothes – best clothes; likes to wear his*
- Jewellery – desire to wear
- Libertinism
- Magnetised – easily magnetised
- *Order – desire for*
- *Touched – aversion to be*

Themes Chabra[26]
- **Desires freedom, aversion to any restrictive relationships.**
- **Conflict between dependency and independence.**
- Low self-esteem, feeling ugly.
- Feels neglected / abused but wants to be independent and free from norms.
- Feeling of **having to prostitute oneself to have her needs met.**
- Morbid conscientiousness; every little fault appeared a crime. (Clinically verified by Swan.)
- "Proud behaviour of the cat; sensuality; intolerance of hunger"
- Dreams of sexual intercourse; many dreams of being pursued for rape, even by relatives.
- Desire to be **pampered** *vs.* **desire to be independent.**
- Sensual behaviour; passionate, expressive.
- Fear of falling downstairs, but without vertigo.
- Fear of pointed things.
- Region – Nerves. Female organs. Head. Eyes. Left side.
- Piercing pain over the left eyebrow – like a needle (or claw).
- **Severe darting, cutting pain through centre of eyeball or in back of orbit to some point in head.**

Characteristic physicals
- **Head**
  - Formication – Vertex
  - Heat
    - § Flushes of – headache; before
    - § Vertex – extending to – left side of head and face
  - Looseness of brain; sensation of
  - Pain
    - § Forehead – Eyes – Above – left – stitching pain
    - § Vertex – extending to – Ear
- **Eye**
  - Asthenopia
  - Inflammation – Iris – chronic
  - Lachrymation – pain; from – eye, in

- Pain
  - § Cutting pain
  - § Jerking pain
- **Rectum**
  - Constipation – difficult stool – recedes; stool (*Silica*)
- **Female**
  - Itching – voluptuous
  - Pain – Uterus and region – standing – agg. – bearing down
- **Chest**
  - Inflammation – Bronchial tubes – alternating with – colds / cough
  - Swelling – Mammae – menses – before – agg.
- **Skin**
  - Eruptions – rash
- **Generals**
  - Allergic constitution – cats; to
  - History; personal – abuse; of

Dreams

Animals, of – rats / Animals, of – snake/s – bed, in / *Appearance; concern about* / **Clothes, clothing – fur** / Inadequate, feels / Penis – penis; huge / Pregnant – **pregnant rat** / **Prostitute**; *prostitution* / **Rape** – that he has committed / Sexual – **brothel**; home of a friend, is a / Sexual – eunuchs, assaulted by; feeling of revulsion / Sexual – naked; observed undressing; man, by / Sexual – rape – *pursued for the purpose of rape; relatives, by* / **Woman – prostitute**

Provers speaking as one

ϕ Dream: I was changing in the bathroom when I realised that there was no window and instead there was a gap in the wall from where I could see the adjoining room. *The hostess' grown-up son was looking at me changing.* I hid myself and shouted to him to go away. But he tried to put his hand through the opening in the wall. I shouted and said that If he did not leave I would call out to his mother. He only smiled and said. "Go ahead, call out". I had a **conflict**. *Should I call out and spoil the relations with the family?* **I felt I almost submitted myself.** I felt terrible that I could do such a thing. *For the sake of the relations with the family, how could I submit myself.* The same prover developed a complete aversion to touch by any male, even by her boyfriend who accidentally touched her elbow as they were sitting for a lecture together. **The feeling was hate and a dirty feeling; "Don't touch me".** . . .[26]

ϕ This was an animal remedy with a **dirty feeling** about oneself, a feeling of **not being respected**, of being **treated contemptuously**. The feeling arising from a conflict and a choice. The conflict of **submitting oneself, of degrading oneself** to save relationship or for money. The theme of the prostitute who submits her body, her respect for money. The theme of the eunuch who behaves in an obscene manner, creating disgust and revulsion to get money. How bad they must feel about themselves to behave in this manner.[26]

Lac Leoninum (Milk of the lioness)

Phylum: Chordata.
Class: Mammalia.
Order: Carnivora.
Family: Felidae.

The lion is a muscular, deep-chested cat and the only member of the cat family to display obvious sexual dimorphism; males have broader heads and a prominent mane. The presence, absence, colour and size of the mane are associated with genetic precondition, sexual maturity, climate and testosterone production. Lions spend much of their time resting; they are inactive for about 20 hours per day. The lion is the most social of all wild felid species, living in a 'pride' of related individuals and their offspring. Males spend years in a nomadic phase before gaining residence in a pride. The lion is a generalist hypercarnivore and is considered both an apex and keystone predator due to its wide prey spectrum. Young lions first display stalking behaviour at around three months of age, although they do not participate in hunting until they are almost a year old. Their attack is short and powerful; attempting to catch prey with a fast rush and leap. They usually pull it down by the rump and kill by a strangling bite to the throat.

Provings by: **R. Sankaran, India (1994)**[10] **and N. Herrick, USA (1998).**[21]

Fundamental delusions
- **Great person; is a** (*cf. Series-6, Coca., Plat., Gadolinium., Lach., Lycopersicon*)
- **Hindered; he is** – everyone; by (*cf. China., Malarial miasm, Mosch.*)
- Attacked; being (*cf. Animals, Arizon-l., Dysprosium., Granitum*)
- Criticised; she is (*cf. Lac-lup., Dysentery co., Carneg-g.*)
- Laughed at and mocked at; being (*cf. Barytas, Adamas*)
- Neglected – he or she is neglected
- **Persecuted** – he is persecuted
- **Strong**; he is
- Thieves – seeing

SRP rubrics
- Anxiety – future, about – waking; on
- **Benevolence – children; towards**
- Desires – group together; to keep (*Milks*)
- Forsaken feeling – friends or group; by
- Helplessness; feeling of – sensitivity to
- *Sensitive – people's inner nature's; to*
- Unification – sensation of unification – animals; with

Syphilitic expression
- Abusive
- Anger – violent
- Company – aversion to – desire for solitude
- Contemptuous
- Deceitful
- Fight, wants to
- Hard-hearted
- Hatred – husband; of
- Jealousy
- Malicious
- Strange – things; impulse to do strange
- Suspicious
- Threatening

Sycotic expression
- Ailments from
  - Contradiction
  - Egotism
  - Honour; wounded
- Change – desire for
- Clairvoyance
- Coquettish – too much
- Dictatorial – talking with air of command (*Lyc.*)
- Egotism
- Escape, attempts to
- Offended, easily
- Playful
- Sensitive
  - Cruelties, when hearing of
  - Emotions; to
  - Reprimands, to
  - Strange – things; impulse to do strange

Proving by Rajan Sankaran[10]
- Feels **put down; Inferior and foolish**, as if being laughed at. *cf. Bar-c and Lac-c.*
- Feels wrongly **blamed, criticised, neglected, forsaken.** *cf. Palladium.*
- Delusion, being **taken advantage of**; that others interfere in her life.
- People try to **cheat and trap** her deceitfully. *cf. Snakes, Droseraceae.*
- Punching those she imagined were attacking and admonishing her. *cf. Med, Tub, Snakes, Insects.*
- Being treated below her standard. *cf. Platina.*
- Reproaches others; they are selfish and hinder her. *cf. China, Moschus, Malarial miasm.*
- Resents the fact that they feel weak, fragile, timid, and dependent of others.

- Feeling of danger, being attacked, beaten up, as if there were robbers around, and she was alone against them. *cf. Lac-del, Stramonium, Fungi.*
- Feels **caged**; *Independence threatened.*
- Anger with violent impulses. Quarrelsome. Malicious. Loud. Rude, uncivil behaviour. *cf. Androctonus, Anacardium, Nux vomica, Nitric acid, Veratrum album, Solanaceae.*
- Egotism; Ego hurt. Love of power. *cf. Series 6, Stage 11–12, Sulphur, Lycopodium.*
- Sympathy, caring; Wants to help relatives and protect children. *cf. Aves, Milks, Carcinosin, Causticum.*

Proving by Nancy Herrick[21]
- Problems with authority figures
- *The feeling of being unjustly accused or blamed for a bullshit crime evokes a feeling of rage and indignant feeling: "F – You! Don't control me! You have no right!"*

Dreams
Adolescents / **Anger – indignant** – event she is unable to stop; over / Animals – wild / Boyfriend – old boyfriend – amazed at how hairy he'd become / Bridge – building bridges; of / Cares, full of – children; about one's / Cats – gone crazy; from being alone all night / Cats – kitten / Danger / Eating – night; at / Friends – old **Hair – body hair – grooming** / Hair – body hair – licking / House – country; in the / Kidnappers / Nakedness / *Responsibility – adults; towards disabled young / Speech; making a – inspirational / Stealing – impulse to* / **Teaching – adolescents** / Theft – accused of; being – wife accused of theft / Tigers

Characteristic Physicals
- **Head**
  - Heaviness – Forehead – morning
  - Pain – Occiput – extending to – Neck – down back of neck
- **Throat**
  - Foreign body; sensation of a
  - Lump; sensation of a
  - Pain – Morning – waking; on
  - External Throat – clothing agg.
- **Gastro-intestinal**
  - Stomach – Thirst – large quantities; for
  - Rectum – Pain – morning – 7 h
  - Stool – Odour – Sulphur; of
- **Female**
  - Menses
    - § Dark – pitch; like
    - § Frequent; too
- **Larynx and trachea**
  - Voice – loud
- **Cough**
  - Spasmodic
  - Violent
- **Extremities**
  - Eruptions – Thighs
    - § Burning
    - § Urticaria
  - Itching – Forearms
  - Numbness – sleep agg.; during
- **Generals**
  - Fanned; being – amel.
  - Heat – sensation of
  - Hunger – agg.
  - Sluggishness of the body
  - Warm – clothing – agg.

CASE 5.2 Bereavement

Patient: Female, age 39

Prescription: Lac leoninum 1M

∫ Losing a parent is massive.

∫ I am pretty **fiery, easy temper, big ideas, charismatic**.

∫ Less akin to but closer to my mum. Family is fragmented. I keep it together because *my mum can't step up. She's pathetic*, physically weak but emotionally strong; resilient in her own world.

∫ Dizzy, tired – *it* takes all my energy. Feeling depressed and like it is never going to end. Feel disassociated and over-sensitive. Don't want son to touch me – **can't take being jumped on**. Feels like my heart would give way. Just being here is all I can do. . . . I have pushed myself too hard, now my body has just given in. . . . Feels gripping – **it takes over my** whole body. In a bad phase of work where I had to negotiate for a contract – *it almost finished me off* . . . (*syphilitic miasm*)

∫ It felt like I was having to **chase after them**, in a **'please like me'** kind of way. Had to chase money every time. My son has started school. It was better before because **I was in charge**, things were more in my control. The **regimented structure** (of school) is really inconvenient for work.

∫ Felt amazing during the pregnancy; I had **long nails, full hair and felt energetic**.

∫ Feel **shackled** by rules, worried that people can't cope with me. Talking to my counsellor a lot about *being rejected*. Even my first counsellor found me too challenging. I feel as though **people don't like me, turn their back on me; are critical, making nasty jokes, shutting me out** (*being shut out by others is a mammal sensitivity*). It is a very dark place – if I am not liked it is a big deal . . . I wasn't their type of person; 'you're not my type'. My response is, '**don't reject me, what can I do to change?**' Feels **desperate, isolating, horrible.** (*Syphilitic miasm is strong.*)

∫ I am a big character – it is OK if people don't like me (contradiction). People can't cope with me. I find it hard to cope with myself. I go from feeling really buzzing to *'life is awful, nobody likes me, can't bear restrictions'*. Feel buzzed, surging energy – I can feel my blood vessels when excited. As if they are opening wide . . . feels really *addictive*.

∫ **Furious and violent** with my mum. How dare you! I get this feeling when anyone **cuts me down** in any way (*Cat sensation*). It is a red rag to a bull. You'll be the one who's cutoff not me. If somebody cuts me down, I must get them back (*Syphilitic animal*). Not happy with 'No'!

∫ I like problem solving and getting the job done. **I am not afraid of confrontation in a professional environment.** Military provides you with safety especially in a crisis. If it does not require authority, I don't appreciate it. (*Sensitive to and dislikes others authority, but wants it for herself.*)

	lyc.	stram.	anac.	staph.	merc.	sep.	thuj.	calc.	ign.	nat-m.	tub.	lac-leo.	med.	ruta	bell.
	1	2	3	4	5	6	7	8	9	10	11	12	13	14	15
	7	7	7	7	7	7	7	7	7	7	7	7	7	7	6
	20	18	15	15	14	14	14	13	13	13	12	11	11	9	17
2. Clipboard 2 ×															
1. MENTAL QUALITIES - Big ego (241) 1	4	4	2	4	4	2	3	3	2	2	1	3	3	1	3
2. MENTAL QUALITIES - Low self esteem (276) 1	4	2	4	2	3	4	4	2	2	2	1	1	2	2	2
3. MENTAL QUALITIES - Trapped (244) 1	2	3	2	2	2	2	2	2	3	2	2	1	1	2	4
4. MIND - AILMENTS FROM - domination (66) 1	2	1	2	2	1	1	1	1	2	1	1	2	1	1	
5. THEMES - Fighting – Violence – Brutality (186) 1	2	3	2	1	1	2	1	1	1	2	2	2	1	1	3
6. THEMES - Offended Easily – Criticized (224) 1	3	2	1	3	1	2	1	3	2	2	4	1	2	1	2
7. MIND - RAGE (192) 1	3	3	2	1	2	1	2	1	1	2	1	1	1	1	3

Figure 5.7 *Repertorisation*

Lac loxodontum africanum (Elephant's milk)

Phylum: Chordata.
Class: Mammalia.
Order: Proboscidae.
Family: Elephantidae.

Elephants live in a complex matriarchal society normally composed of 8 to 15 related members led by a dominant cow. Males leave the matriarchal herd when reaching adolescence to form bachelor herds – later disbanding to lead a solitary life, approaching the female herds only during the mating season. They become extremely aggressive during musth (a state of increased testosterone), at which time they may: spray urine on their hind legs; walk with head held high and swinging; pick at the ground with his tusks. The trunk, also called a proboscis, is used for breathing, bringing food and water to the mouth, and grasping objects. Tusks, which are derived from the incisor teeth, serve both as weapons and tools. The large ear flaps help communicate and maintain a constant body temperature. The pillar-like legs carry their great weight. Calves are the centre of attention in their family groups and rely on their mothers for as long as three years.

Elephants can live up to 70 years in the wild. They communicate by touch, sight, smell, and sound; using infrasound and seismic communication over long distances. Elephant intelligence has been compared with that of primates and cetaceans – showing self-awareness and empathy for dying / deceased family members. The observed phenomena of the excellent elephantine memory could be based on their having cognitive maps which allow them to remember large-scale spaces over long periods of time.

Proving by: **Nancy Herrick, USA (1998).**[24]

Mind

- *SRP – Tranquillity – conflict; during*
- Cursing – desire to curse
- **Delusions**
  - Emptiness; of
  - Faces, sees – ugly – coming out at him
  - Sea – immersed in the sea; being
  - Despair
- **Destructiveness**
- Ease; feeling of
- Elated
- Expansive
- Fight; wants to
- Euphoria – alternating with – weariness
- Hurt feelings – sarcastic remarks, at
- Impulsive
- Industrious
- Intuitive
- Itching – voluptuous
- Loquacity – alternating with – detachment
- Quiet disposition
- Reflecting
- Spaced-out feeling (*Milks*)
- *Squandering – money*
- *Theorizing*
- *Time – timelessness; sensation of*
- Violent

Fundamental delusion	
• Old – timeless, ancient feeling; having a	*Lycopodium also has this theme, coming as it does from the carboniferous era, where it was once mighty and tall. Actinides and Ancient plants may also express a similar quality.*

SRP Delusions	
• Body – lighter than air; body is • Tall; taller, he is	*"Felt very tall and high off the ground. Looking far down as though looking far down to the ground. Felt very airy, high in the air. In motion, but stillness."*
• Sea – immersed in the sea; being • Air; hovering in, like a spirit	*These give a sense of the life-cycle of mammals; beginning in the amniotic fluid of the womb makes sense of the floaty, weightless feelings expressed in the provings. Lac caninum also produces an array of such symptoms.*

Important dreams • **Mother – old; being.**	
• Children; about – abused; being • Feeding – people • Homeless – people are • Suffering – others; of	*These dreams reveal a strongly-held sense of duty and a desire to help others who are suffering. There was a strong theme of homelessness in the dreams of the provers, suggesting a connection with the actual loss of habitat of elephants in the wild.*

"It may be that in the near future, the only elephants to be found will be in zoos and formal "wild" parks, where people pay to ride through and observe animal behaviour. As this possibility comes closer to reality, *more and more humans will take on elephant energy* (thus the theme, ***people as animals***)."[24]

Starvation, hunger and lack of food to go around

Dreams	
• Poverty • Hunger – people; of hungry • Starved; his cells are being	*The hunger is so severe that it is felt even at the cellular level. Many dreams of hunger, or not enough food to go around.*

Forced into violence

Dream

⨎ Someone I do not know but am friendly with and I am helping him with some task. I feel **he is dangerous and should not be trusted and then he turns on me and we fight using our fists.** He has so much hate. **I am forced to protect myself and I hit him with a broomstick ruthlessly,** and he breaks his wrist and falls down. He is defeated. The feeling is: **'I do not want to fight but I must or I will die.'** A friend who becomes a foe. . . . I am scared but at the same time ruthless.[24]

Dreams

Amorous / Animals – fetuses / Boat / Cattle / *Children; about – abused; being* / ***Children; about – starving*** / Computers – broken / Cooking / Crime – conceal-ment of / Dead; of the – relatives / Disease / **Disgusting** / Elephants – riding on an elephant's back / Elk / Emotions – without / Evil; of – impending / *Evil – helpless in presence of* / **Feeding – people** / Fighting; one is / Fish / Groups / Hair – cut; having hair / Helpless feeling / *Homeless – people are* / Hopeless / Horses / Hunger – people; of hungry / Lions / **Mother – old; being** / Motorcycles / Murder – violent / Patients – suicidal / Penis – detachable / Poverty / Pursued, being – police; by / Sea / Sick people – relatives / Skunks / **Suffering – others; of** / Trees / Turtles / Unremembered / Walking – nature; in / Water / Weaving / Wonderful

Physicals

- **Vertigo**
  - Accompanied by – Head – pain in head
  - Descending; as if
  - Looking – downward
- **Head**
  - Pain – extending to – Cervical region
- **Eye**
  - Agglutinated – morning
  - Discharges – sticky
  - Tired sensation
- **Vision**
  - Colours before the eyes
- **Face**
  - Expression – sullen
  - Pain – Malar bones

- **Stomach**
  - Emptiness – afternoon
  - Eructations; type of – foul
- **Rectum**
  - Diarrhea / Flatus
- **Female**
  - *Bubbling sensation – Vagina – air or water in vagina; as from*
  - Menses – clotted / copious / early; too
  - Sexual desire – diminished
- **Chest**
  - Conscious of heart's action – accompanied by – body had changed into a big soft bag; sensation as if
  - Perspiration – Axillae – right
- **Back – Pain**
  - Straightening up the back
  - Sacrum – cramping
- **Extremities**
  - Cramps – Thighs
  - Trembling – Legs
  - Weakness – Legs
- **Skin**
  - *Itching – voluptuous*
- **Generals**
  - Exertion; physical – aversion for
  - Lassitude – lying – must lie down
  - Sick feeling; vague – hunger; from
  - *Soft – Body had changed into a big, soft bag; sensation as if*

Provers speaking as one

§ A man was pushing his way through the line. I said, "You can get by me," and he answered rudely and smugly, "Are you confident about that?" *I felt a very violent aggressiveness inside*, like I wanted to *hurt him, kick his ass*. It surprised me. In the restaurant I got up to go to the bathroom and *the light was strange and faces seemed to come out at me*. The people in the restaurant seemed stranger than normal. **Plates of meat and dead carcasses-strange, anguished, unconscious people-so ugly, broken, old, diseased. Like a low realm of life. . . .**

§ Quiet-Deep state of timelessness, present ancient state, staring out the window at the mountains. Feel free and a lot of space around me. No history, no self but self, only peace. It feels like my cured state but does not last. . . . **Dream:** of two teenage girls naked with a poodle. They seemed *homeless, broken and yet surviving*. One girl is *emaciated and had large anus hole*. The feeling is she had been *abused, broken, tormented, no hope*, doing what she had to do to live. She had an *animal look in her eyes, no trust. Weary, hungry, frightened, jumping* around like a primate. . . .

§ Dream – Everyone in the house was suicidal. I woke and viewed the whole family a different way. Lots of *suicidal feeling. Dark, sick unrecoverable*. White broken Jehovah's witness suffering. Broken, white low-class **impoverished: no way out, damaged feeling. . . .**

§ *More emotional and sentimental, grateful for my marriage. Taking things more personally, more vulnerable. Loving feeling.* . . . After taking the remedy I argued with wife, highly unusual. The theme from her end is that **I am too serious** and I do not know how to play. My theme is that *the pace is too fast and I want to slow down* and not do it so fast . . . feel **excruciating restlessness, hyper** as though had three cups of coffee, **wiggling** hands and **jiggling** feet, **impatient**, thinking very clearly. Need to get to destination with sense of **urgency**, to get to the movie in time. Some people called me and while I was talking to them,

I was typing and working crossword puzzles and reading textbooks so only half of me was paying attention. . . .

₰ Dream: *Me and my family are living on an island kingdom with a castle.* **I am the mother** (male prover). My beloved son goes off to the *crusades* and he comes back half nuts, crazy on this *wild stallion that is vital and beautiful and untamed.* It comes running at me in this field and I have this stake and I plant it in the ground and the horse impales itself and dies. My son is very upset. *He embraces me, his mother, and he kisses me and then it becomes sexual and I am willing and aroused.* He says this is not moral and *rejects me* and I go to the beach to hide and find a place to sleep but all the huts are full. I sit on the shore and wait for whatever will come. . . .

₰ Overall feeling: **calm and heavy**. Don't want to do too much and then forced to do too much and become hurried. Effort and heaviness and the conflict between these two. Feeling tired and earthbound.[24]

Clinical

"This is then, perhaps, a remedy for ensuring the well-being of the fœtus and for anxiety associated with an inability to conceive; IVF; threatened miscarriage or proposed abortion (lac-ory)." [Hatherly][25]

Lac Lupinum (Wolf's milk / Tundra wolf)

Phylum: Chordata.
Class: Mammalia.
Order: Carnivora.
Family: Canidae.

The wolf is a very social animal – the nuclear family usually consists of a mated pair accompanied by their offspring. Most lone wolves are only temporarily alone while they disperse to form their own pack or join another one. Wolves define their territories by howling and scent marking using urine, faeces, and anal gland scents. In the right conditions, their howls can be heard over areas of up to 130 km². Other vocalisations include growls, barks and whines. When hunting large gregarious prey, they try to isolate an individual from its group. Once prey is brought down, they feed excitedly; ripping and tugging at the carcass in all directions and bolting down large chunks of it. A large catch can feed the pack for days. Wolves carry ectoparasites and endoparasites, usually without adverse effects, though they may manifest in the sick or malnourished. There is a strong hierarchy within each pack. The alpha male is dominant over all other individuals. The next dominant individual is the alpha female. Rank within the pack determines which animals mate and in who gets to eat first; this is demonstrated by postural cues and facial expressions, such as crouching, chin touching, and rolling over to show the stomach. In human culture, the wolf embodies the shadow side; ferocity, cunning, greed, cruelty, evil, but also courage, victory, and nourishing care. The big bad wolf in Red riding hood is a devouring and sexually predatory symbol.

Proving by: **Nancy Herrick, USA (1998).**[7]

Fundamental delusion:
• ***Belong to her own family; she does not*** (outcast, outsider, scapegoat)

This is reinforced by delusions that
• Invader; he is an – he feels unwelcome wherever he goes; an outcast or scapegoat.
• Looked down upon; she is (*Lac-c*)
• Betrayed; that she is (*Snakes; Boa constrictor, Crot-c, Python regia; Lac-c, Falco-pe*)
• Victim; she is a (*Salmon*)

This situation may lead to positive compensatory delusions such as
• *Depending on him; everything is (Aurum)*
• *Benevolence – fortunate; to others less (Aurum)*
• Enjoying the exposure to danger and when at risk he feels relieved (*Lac-del, Agar*)
• Fortunate; he is
• Love – appreciation for fatherly love – younger and older men; between

Negative compensations
• Burn; desire to
• Censorious, critical – wants to blame others and make them responsible
• Delusions
  ○ Dying – he is
  ○ Living – lack of strength to continue
• Roaming (Chaotic – planning, roaming around; unsure, poor)
• Danger – desire for
• Desires – pain
• Heedless – think; of what others

Secondary delusions
• Murdered – women are by men
• **Suffering – women through the ages; conscious of**

The Milk remedies as a group uncover the hardships suffered by women at the hands of men. The rearing of young is left to the women who are dominated by one alpha-male rather than forming a lasting and cohesive partnership (as with birds who share the responsibilities much more evenly). However, there is a contrasting feeling that came up in the proving, of desiring the warmth of paternal love, free from embarrassment or sexual feeling.

Milks / Mammals

Other important Mind symptoms

- Ailments from – discords – chief and subordinates; between
- Alert
- *Benevolence – fortunate; to others less*
- Censorious – blames others – family; *blames others in her family*
- Delusions – danger – *enjoying the exposure to, and when at risk he feels relieved*
- Mood – stuck and tight
- Self-control – loss of self-control
- Sociability
- "Since there is a lot of domination in the hierarchy pattern observed in the pack. Some members of the pack may have a feeling of being dominated or feeling of being despised or looked down upon. Such type of feeling lead to poor self-confidence and self-image." _{Master}[23]

Provers speaking as one

⨍ **I felt like an outsider to my family, that I didn't belong.** Also that they did not even care to hear my viewpoint. It made me feel unimportant and incidental. . . .

⨍ I need to be **unprotected. Wanting to be raw, not hidden behind anything.** I do not want to be sheltered, kept from anything harmful; wanted to be open to all experience with no boundaries. . . .

⨍ When I am out there at risk, I feel relieved-an exposed state, enjoying the exposure . . . Pursued through old building. . . .

⨍ Dream: **Despair of being trapped** with no way out. . . .

⨍ Realised **I didn't want to pass through emotions. Didn't want to feel them.** . . .

⨍ Ahead of myself, a little **panicky, short-tempered, out of body.** External concerns. Felt off, felt not responding to what was happening in the moment. . . .

⨍ Mind **scattered, thoughts all over the place,** difficult time focusing. I felt anxious, like I need to get something done but not sure what. . . .

⨍ Feel like I must help others less fortunate. I am so lucky, I have so much. I just want to help my friends and try and save their lives-help them have better, easier, healthier lives. . . .

⨍ Dream: Down a water tunnel. I am afraid to go down. I pull the rope back up . . . but it is all tangled. My **breathing is short.** I'm too hot, I can't breathe, I try to unbutton my shirt while I untangle the rope. I know I can do this if I can just. . . . Shallow breath, not claustrophobic. Sensations in the body woke me. . . .

⨍ I saw a man hugging a younger man, a genuine, loving fatherly hug. I felt a sense of appreciation and love for them and that **I was missing some kind of male love and companionship. I wanted a fatherly hug,** as if I saw male love for the first time, without it being tinged with embarrassment or sexuality or fear.[7]

Important Dreams
- **Children**; about – Advent spiral; doing an / Baby-sitting / Birthday party / Danger; in / **Gassed**; being | Hair pulled by violent man; having / Murdered, being / Playing – dangerous liquid; with / Teenager – jumping of building, screaming, dies / **Tortured**; being / **Violated**; being / Weeping.
- **Outsider** – Being an outsider – bystander; he was a | Spirit watching; felt more like a.
- **Fire** – Danger, of – burn down the house; someone wants to / Chasing a group of people; fire / **Fire** – Building on fire / Evil little creature in oven; trying to burn / Fireball / Firetruck – riding on the back of a / Kept fires going.
- **Danger** – Death, of / Impending danger.
- **Fear – falling; of** – Cliff; from a | ravine; into a / Trouble; of getting into.
- **Helping** – trying to help / Helpless feeling / Hiding / **Hiding – danger; from.**
- **Home** / **House** / House – youth; like the house of her /
- **Identity** – lost / Indians, being among
- Poison; of / *Poisoned, being – woman and her children being gassed and poisoned; a /*
- **Precarious position – feeling safe is a.**
- *Revelation – die; we never really / Revelation – intruder in his own world; he was an.*
- Social inferiority; of.
- **Trap – being trapped – water; under.**
- Victim – at the mercy of an amusement park ride operator.
- Water – bottom of / Danger – in water; from danger.
- Water – Swimming in – dove to get friend who went under rough water.

Characteristic physicals
- **Head**
  - Pain
    - § Forehead – extending to – Vertex
    - § Sides – left – then right
- **Eye**
  - Open lids – sensation as if open – wide open
- **Vision**
  - Acute
- **Face**
  - Eruptions – pimples – Jaws – Lower
- **Mouth**
  - Dryness – night
- **Stomach**
  - Nausea – odours – fish agg.; of
  - Thirst – small quantities, for
- **Kidneys**
  - Pain – Region of – aching
- **Female**
  - Pain – Ovaries – *sharp*
- **Chest**
  - Pain – Sternum – cutting pain – *knife* down sternum; like someone took a
- **Fever**
  - Relapsing
- **Generals**
  - Endurance – increased
  - Heated, becoming
  - Stiffness – Muscles

CASE 5.3 Trauma reawakened

Patient: Female, age 39

Prescription: Lac lupinum 200c

Themes
- BETRAYED. REJECTION. LOW SELF ESTEEM. GRIEF. ALONE. UNSUP-PORTED.
- UNDIGNIFIED – not to be humiliated and embarrassed.
- *The wrong daughter, not accepted by mother. . . .*

Animal expressions
∫ If it wasn't for my mammal Brain I would have torn you to pieces. Being polite to the man that ripped me up. I would have ripped him up straight back and would have won that fight.

∫ The body can tell it is being attacked.

∫ So angry I had to grit my teeth and just suppress it – I was beside myself. Just gritted my teeth and waited until I got out . . . more angry than have felt before so far.

∫ Allowing somebody else to make me feel weak lowers my self-esteem. Makes me feel weak.

∫ Feeling under threat.

∫ Just want my normal Self back.

Betrayal, rejection, grief, breaking of trust
∫ Extra support – he was helping me through this but has betrayed me and run off.

∫ I have been betrayed by him. My relationship with parents, especially mum is the same. Betrayal from her. Enormous sense of disappointment, and **not being valued, being rejected**. Not being supported. My dad filled up the gaps and he is not there anymore. Huge sense of loss. . . .

∫ Upset, sad and betrayed. But usually I **cover all those feeling up with anger**. I couldn't speak.

∫ Sense of trust being disappointed by someone who you **trust to look after** / take care of you. Strong sense of betrayal coming in. Over 5 years that trust got stronger and stronger. . . . But **he abused my trust** on that day. Knew I was prepared to open up then he was really insensitive.

Estranged from family
∫ Along with the stuff that exploded (during the treatment with therapist) – it opened up dark memories – my parents lost their first child. Memories of when I was young. The way I behaved, or my mum's expectations of me. . . .

∫ I was the replacement daughter for the one that didn't survive. A lot of feelings of not being valued. Parents rejected me when A was sick. . . . Mum was totally useless to me. My daughter is critically ill in hospital. He (the therapist) was first person to support me.

Safety / Threat

∫ Dreams – keeping the family safe. We found a lovely house next to the sea. I found my dream home – let's buy it. Suddenly the family felt safe. About being home, safe, comfortable, happy.

∫ Dreams – Cat turned into a fox or wolf and then turned into a man who tried to force me up against a wall. Trying to keep it safe then it turned into a threat. Keeping family safe.

∫ We walked into a huge crowd. S wasn't homing in on the dangers. Really unpleasant crowd, S was walking into it blind. I took A from him and asked him to walk in front but he just walked off (abandoned). Didn't stay with us. Just walked through crowd. I started pushing my way through – then lady was trying to start a fight with me. Put blinkers down and started marching through.

∫ When I got through, I lost it and was absolutely furious. Straight away after losing it I couldn't breathe anymore. Shaking, go into a fight or flight. Very angry, can get aggressive. Response to that – breathing will go. Cannot breathe properly. I realise what is happening. Not until the breathing goes, that this is a panic attack now.

Mother / Father

∫ Mum couldn't cope with the emotions (of losing her first daughter). *'What's wrong with you. I could have had somebody else.'* Her grief took precedence over my needs. Feeling – so deep in my stomach; most horrible thing she ever said to me. *'You deserve it.'*

∫ Dad is bullied. She is a bully. V unpleasant for dad.

∫ Dreams – *The opposite male role* – he gave me a really nice paternal hug that was comforting and felt like it had something to do with the chiro giving a hug to say sorry. He smelled nice, and was well kempt. Nothing sexual. Warming cuddle.

∫ Care that mum giving dad is borderline abusive, aggressive, undignified. *Not care.*

Escaping

∫ All of a sudden – I need to run away from this. A need . . . or wish to be back in early 20s.

∫ Obsessively looking at my past from that time – when I just wanted to run away to Brazil and to Carnival – escapism. Longing, itching to go to big party – dance it away and forget it all.

Physicals
- ∫ Head pain. Internal stabbing coming from inside at the top between forehead and crown. Like brain rotting from inside. Outward. Sharp or heavy in the head.
- ∫ Like when you're just about to vomit. Real nervous feeling. Like when had tummy bug, without realising coming on and thought having panic attack.
- ∫ **Breathing speeds up – can't get breaths in quick enough. Sickness, nausea goes across back.**

	adam.	ars.	granit-m.	heroin.	hydrog.	lac-h.	lac-lup.	lach.	lyc.
	1	2	3	4	5	6	7	8	9
	7	7	7	7	7	7	7	7	7
MENTAL QUALITIES - Low self esteem * (402) 1	4	2	2	3	3	3	2	2	4
MENTAL QUALITIES - Victim (374) 1	2	4	2	3	3	2	2	4	4
THEMES - Betrayed – Deceived – Corrupted (84) 1	1	1	1	1	1	1	1	1	3
THEMES - Danger (184) 1	1	2	1	1	1	1	1	2	1
THEMES - Forsaken – Alone – Dependent (343) 1	1	3	1	1	1	2	1	2	3
THEMES - Mother (115) 1	1	1	1	1	1	1	1	1	2
THEMES - Neglected – Rejected – Unappreciated (160) 1	1	1	1	1	1	2	1	1	3

Figure 5.8 *Repertorisation (using Sherr's Q Rep and the author's own Thematic Repertory)*

	lac-lup.
	1
	1
1. MIND - ANXIETY - control over senses is lost; with feeling that (1) 1	1
2. MIND - ANXIETY - sudden (19) 1	1
3. MIND - DELUSIONS - belong to her own family; she does not (4) 3	1
4. MIND - DELUSIONS - betrayed; that she is (53) 1	1
5. MIND - DELUSIONS - looked down upon; she is (7) 1	1
6. MIND - DELUSIONS - victim; she is a (9) 1	1
7. MIND - FORSAKEN FEELING (232) 1	1
8. MIND - LOVE - appreciation for fatherly love - younger and older men; between (1) 1	1
9. MIND - QUARRELSOME - family, with her - husband; to (4) 1	1
10. MIND - SUSPICIOUS (179) 1	2

Figure 5.9 *Rubrics covering the case found by reverse repertorisation in Synthesis*

Lac ovinum (Sheep's milk)

Phylum: Chordata.
Class: Mammalia.
Order: Artiodactyla.
Family: Bovidae.
Subfamily: Caprinae.

Like most ruminants, sheep are members of the even-toed ungulates. A sheep's wool is the most widely used animal fibre and is harvested by shearing. They are strongly gregarious mammals, living within the protection of their flock. This, and their natural inclination to follow a leader to new pastures, are pivotal factors in sheep being one of the first domesticated livestock species. As such an important animal in the history of farming, sheep have a deeply entrenched place in human culture, finding representation in much modern language and symbology. They have good hearing, excellent peripheral vision – with visual fields of about 270° to 320° – but poor depth perception – shadows and dips in the ground may cause sheep to baulk. In general, sheep have a tendency to move out of the dark and into well-lit areas. They also have an excellent sense of smell with scent glands just in front of the eyes, and inter-digitally on the feet. They are herbivorous, grazing on grass and avoiding the taller woody parts of plants that goats readily consume. The bleats of individual sheep are distinctive, enabling the ewe and her lambs to recognise each other's vocalisations. A group of ewes is generally mated by a single ram, who has either been chosen by a breeder or has established dominance through physical contest with other rams.

Proving by: **Eric Sommerman and the Northwestern Academy of Homeopathy, USA (2002).**[27]

Delusions
- **Looking – everyone is looking at her**
- *Martyr*; of being a (*Good samaritan theme, desire to help others*)
- *Suffering* – women through the ages; conscious of (*lac-lup., aster.*)
- *Victim*; she is a

Mind
- Activity – desires activity
- Ailments from – *rejected*; from being
- *Antagonism* with herself
- Cares, full of – others, about
- Company – aversion to – desire for solitude
- Company – desire for – *group together; desire to keep*
- Complaining – never (*stoical*)
- Confidence – want of self-confidence – *failure, feels himself a*
- Confusion of mind – identity, as to his – duality, sense of
- Content
- Despair
- *Disgust* – oneself
- *Duty* – too much sense of duty
- Fear – observed; of her condition being

- Forsaken feeling
- *Grumbling*
- *Harmony* – desire for
- Helplessness; feeling of
- *Hiding* – himself
- Hurried; being
- Hurry
- Injustice; cannot support
- Irritability – overwork; from
- *Looked at; to be – **cannot bear to be looked at***
- Maternal instinct; exaggerated
- Mildness
- ***Nursing (nurturing) others***
- *Overwhelmed*
- *Overworked*
- Peace – heavenly peace; sensation of
- Pessimist
- ***Pleasing – <u>desire to please others</u>***
- Powerless
- Resentment
- ***Responsibility – taking responsibility too seriously***
- ***Selflessness***
- Sensitive
- Sympathetic
- Task-oriented
- Time – quickly, appears shorter; passes too
- **Timidity**
- ***Tranquillity***
- *Will – two wills; sensation as if he had*
- ***Yielding disposition***

Physicals

"It would be surprising to see a Lac Ovinum case without some sort of **headaches**. Characteristically, the headaches are *behind the eyes*, in the *temples*, and sometimes around the *back* of the head (occiput). The second would be **chills**, with cold hands and feet and occasional **flushes of heat**. Cold aggravates. They will tend to think about food a lot, be **hungry often**, and have *difficulty getting full*. They also have many **digestion** symptoms, *rumbling* in abdomen, *gas, eructations*, and *nausea*. They may have **alternating constipation and diarrhea**. They will also be very **thirsty**. **Dryness** in general is a problem, in mouth on skin etc. This may cause **itching**. . . . Strange tingly sensation (almost a chill, or numbness), on the vertex or in extremities. They can also get very **exhausted**. They can experience **weakness** in general, low energy, and *desire naps*. They seem to be ameliorated when they get outside in fresh air or just start moving."[27]

MAMMAL REMEDIES (not prepared from milk)

Castoreum canadense
(European Beaver – secretion from preputial gland)

Phylum: Chordata.
Class: Mammalia.
Order: Rodentia.
Family: Castoridae.

The Eurasian / European beaver was once widespread in Eurasia, but was hunted to near-extinction for both its fur and castoreum. As a keystone species, beavers support the ecosystem which they inhabit; their wetlands create habitat for water voles, otters and water shrews. Coppicing waterside trees and shrubs facilitates their regrowth with greater density, providing cover for birds and other animals. Their dams trap sediment, improve water quality, recharge groundwater tables and increase cover and forage for trout and salmon. They have one litter per year, coming into oestrus for only 12 to 24 hours. Unlike most other rodents, beaver pairs are monogamous, staying together for multiple breeding seasons. Castoreum is a yellowish exudate from the castor sacs of the mature *Castor canadensis* and *Castor fibre*. Beavers use castoreum in combination with urine to scent-mark their territory. Both sexes have a pair of castor sacs and a pair of anal glands, located in two cavities under the skin between the pelvis and the base of the tail. It is used as a tincture in some perfumes and was sometimes used as a food additive in the early 1900s.

Proving by: **Caspari, Russia and Nenning, Austria.**

Mind

- Ailments from – excitement – emotional
- Anger – morning – *waking; on*
- Biting – nails
- **Desires – full of desires – anxious desires; full of**
- Extravagance
- Fear – evil; fear of
- Impressionable
- Industrious / Busy
- Nature – loves
- **Sensitive – sensual impressions, to**
- Sentimental
- Starting – sleep – from
- Talking – sleep, in
  - angry exclamations, with
  - excited
- Weeping – sleep, in

Dreams

- Blisters
  - Arms covered with
  - Burning
- Death – relatives; of – parents; of
- Eruptions
- *Murdering – father, her*
- Water – lake
- *Unsuccessful efforts – shriek; to*

Qualities

Changeable / Capriciousness / Elated / Joyful / Ecstasy / Jesting / Vivacity / Mirth / Quarrelsome / Argumentative / Sentimental / Nostalgic / Thieves / Robbers / Yielding / Timid / Delicate / Mild

Clinical Clarke[17]

Chorea / **Convulsions** / Digestion – disordered / **Dysmenorrhea** / **Eclampsia** / Enteralgia / Flatulence / Gravel / Hernia / Hysteria / Ileus / Paralysis / **Pregnancy – vomiting of** / Reaction, defective / Sexual – organs – inflammation of / Sexual – organs – spasm of / Sycosis / Tetanus / Typhoid fever – lack of recuperation after / Typhus fever / Warts / Yawning

Temperaments _{Clarke}[17]

Abdomen – nervous attacks when the aura starts from / Abdominal soreness / Constitutions: leuco-phlegmatic / Cramps or colic – nervous women with, after severe illness / Hysterical / Illness – severe, women with weakness after / Nervous – attacks when the aura starts from abdomen / Nervous – women – with pains, cramps after severe illness

Characteristic physicals

- **Head**
- Pain
  - Vexation; after
  - Forehead – Sides – sitting agg. – *tearing* pain
  - Temples – *jerking* pain
  - Vertex – eating – after – agg.
- Pulsating
  - Evening – sleep; until going to
  - Bathing – after
- **Eye**
  - Complaints of eyes – alternating sides
- **Vision**
  - Stars
- **Nose**
  - Pain – root – tearing pain
  - Sneezing – concussive
- **Face**
  - Quivering – Lips
- **Mouth**
  - Nodosities
  - Odor – putrid – morning
  - Pain – Tongue – *jerking*
  - Tumors – Tongue – centre, size of pea, sensitive to touch
- **Teeth**
  - Acidity – agg.
  - *Crawling*
  - *Jerks*
- **Throat**
  - *Choking*
- **Stomach**
  - *Contraction* – sitting agg.
  - Emptiness – morning – menses; during
  - Eructations; type of
    - § Fluid – dinner; after

- § Food; tasting like
- Nausea and Vomiting – pregnancy; during
- Vomiting; type of
  - § *bile*
  - § *mucus*
  - § *sour – bitterish*
- **Abdomen**
  - Bending double – amel.
  - Flatulence – painful
  - Ileus
  - Movements in – walking agg.
  - Pain
    - § Menses – during – *cramping*
    - § *Twinging*
    - § *Violent*
    - § Umbilicus – *cutting* pain
- **Rectum**
  - Pain – extending to – Pudendum – stool agg.; after – stitching pain
- **Stool**
  - Watery – night
- **Bladder**
  - Urination
    - § Involuntary – night
    - § Seldom
    - § Urging to urinate
- **Male**
  - Pain – cramping
  - Pollutions – excitability of parts, from
- **Female**
  - ***Uterus; complaints of***
  - Inflammation – Uterus
  - Leukorrhea – burning
  - Menses – painful – warmth – amel.
  - Pain – burning

- **Respiration**
  - Difficult
    - § Evening – 18 h – 18–21h
    - § Lying – back; on – agg.
    - § Lying – side; on – left – amel.
- **Cough**
  - Rawness of larynx excites cough
- **Back**
  - Coldness – dorsal region – Scapulae – between – cold water, as from
- **Extremities**
  - Pain – Hands – Ulnar side – tearing pain
  - Pain – Thighs – Knees; above – tearing pain
  - Twitching – wandering
- **Sleep**
  - Disturbed
    - § Nightmare; by a
    - § Twitching, by
- Interrupted – toothache; by
- Sleeplessness – women; especially in – exhausted
- **Chill**
  - Evening – bed – in bed – agg.
  - Shaking – heat – without subsequent heat – perspiration; or
- **Perspiration**
  - Debilitating – fever; after
- **Generals**
  - Constitution – neuropathic
  - Food – sour food, acids – agg.
  - Jerking – muscles, of – sleep – during
  - Mucous secretions – transparent
  - Reaction – lack of – convalescence, in
  - Shuddering, nervous – stool – during – agg.

Choloepus didactylus (Two-toed Sloth)

Phylum: Chordata.
Class: Mammalia.
Order: Pilosa.
Family: Choloepodidae.

Whilst the name "sloth" means lazy or idle, the slow movements of this mammal are a useful adaptation for surviving on a low-energy diet of leaves. They are so solitary in their nature that it is even uncommon for two to be found together in the same tree. The sloth spends almost its entire life, including eating, sleeping, mating, and giving birth, hanging upside down from tree branches. However, when the time comes for urination and defecation they slowly make their way to the ground. This seems to be rather a behavioural quirk, as whilst earthbound they are almost defenceless. Their shaggy coat has grooved hair which plays host to a symbiotic green algae, providing both camouflage and nutrients. The algae also nourishes moths, some species of which exist solely on sloths. Two-toed sloths have half the metabolic rate of a typical mammal of the same size. This fact, combined with their reduced musculature means that they cannot shiver to keep warm as other mammals do, so their body temperature depends on the surrounding ambience. They are reported to have very poor eyesight and hearing, relying almost entirely on their sense of touch and smell to locate food. When threatened, sloths can defend themselves by slashing with claws and biting with sharp teeth. However, a sloth's main defence is to avoid being attacked in the first place. It's slow, deliberate movements and algae-covered fur make them difficult for predators to spot from a distance whilst their treetop homes are out of reach for many larger predators. They can also survive wounds that would be fatal to another mammal of its size.

Proving by: **Luke and Mani Norland, UK (2018).**

Fundamental delusions
- Outsider; being an
- Possessed; being – evil forces; by
- Victim; she is a
- World – she has her own little
- Invisible; she is
- Above it all; she is
- Clear; everything is too
- Fog – wet mist hanging over everything
- Glass – behind a glass; as if

Characteristic Mind rubrics
- Inactivity – unmotivated; and
- Indifference
  - Desire, nor action of the will; has no
  - Feel almost nothing, seems to
- Animal consciousness
- Confidence – want of self-confidence – support; desires – family and friends; from
- Confusion of mind – unfocused, fuzzy
- Helplessness; feeling of – emotional level; on
- Humiliated; feeling
- Insecurity; mental – hiding it; but is
- Spaced-out feeling – fog between self and other; sensation as if
- Estranged – cut-off; feels
- Fight, wants to – helpless people; for
- Insightful
- Mildness – masking violence
- Alert – waking; on
- Drinking – more than she should
- Ennui – laziness; with
- Looked at; to be – evading the look of other persons
- Love – exalted love – family; for her
- Observer – being an – oneself; of
- Sadness – overwhelming
- Self-indulgent
- Sensitive – pain, to – emotional – others; of
- Stupefaction – debauchery; as after
- Tranquillity – settled, centred and grounded
- Unification – desire for
- Weeping – humiliation; after

Italic Mind rubrics
- Bed – remain in bed; desire to
- Confidence – want of self-confidence – **self-depreciation**
- **Ennui**
- Horrible things, sad stories affect her profoundly
- Impatience – slowly; everything goes too
- Inactivity – unmotivated; and
- Indifference – everything, to
- **Injustice**, cannot support
- **Laziness**
- Postponing everything to next day
- Prostration of mind
- Sensitive
- Slowness
- Tranquillity
- Weeping

Important Dreams

Abused sexually; being / Aids – child having aids; her / Animals – attacked by a wild beast; of being / Animals – killing / Animals – protecting; he is / Armageddon / Attacked, of being / Cannonading / Groups – fit in a group; unable to / Guilt / Isolated; of being – feeling isolated while amongst others / Killing – idea of; but did not like the / Outsider – being an outsider / Rash; body covered with / Sexual / Shameful / Slower; companion is / Swimming – sea; in the / Time – short of time; he is running

Physical Affinities

Skin / Gastro-intestinal / Head / Eye and Vision / Nose and Smell / Ears / Face / Mouth and Teeth / Hands and Feet

Important Physicals

- **Head**
  - Constriction – hat – tight hat; as from a
  - Hair – falling – handfuls, in
  - Turning and twisting sensation
- **Eye**
  - Dryness – sensation of
  - Ecchymosis
  - Pain – foreign body; as from a
    - § grains; as from little
    - § penetrating the eye
- **Ear**
  - Equalizing of pressure is difficult
- **Nose**
  - Odours; imaginary and real
    - § cabbage, of
    - § offensive
- **Face**
  - Eruptions –
    - § acne – painful
    - § acne – Chin
    - § boils – Nose
    - § pimples – Nose – Septum
  - Pain – blow; pain as from a
- **Mouth**
  - Odour – offensive
  - Pain – Gums – ulcerative
  - Saliva – oily
  - Taste
    - § cabbage; like boiled
    - § metallic
    - § offensive
  - § smoky – food tastes
  - Ulcers – Gums – lower
  - Teeth – Pain – pulsating pain
- **Stomach**
  - Appetite – diminished
  - Eructations; type of – water brash
  - Thirst – unquenchable
  - Vomiting – sensation of – eructation; during
- **Rectum**
  - Constipation
  - Inactivity of rectum
  - Stool – balls, like – small
- **Female**
  - Itching – leukorrhea; from
  - Menses – exertion brings on the flow
  - Menses – return – ceased; after the regular menstrual cycle has
- **Cough**
  - Mucus – Throat; in
  - Tickling – Throat-pit; in
  - Expectoration – swallow what has been loosened; must
- **Chest**
  - Conscious of heart's action
  - Ecchymoses – spots
  - Eruptions
    - § acne
    - § desquamating
    - § rash – red
    - § Mammae – under

○ Pain – Sternum – blow; pain as from a
○ Perspiration – Axillae – offensive
- **Extremities**
  ○ Eruptions
    § Knees – rash
    § Thighs – circinate
  ○ Formication – Legs – night
  ○ Itching – Legs – insect bites; as of
  ○ Numbness – Fingers – fourth finger – left
- **Skin**
  ○ Eruptions – red – insect stings; like
  ○ Itching – scratching – must scratch
- **Generals**
  ○ Influenza – sensation as if
  ○ Odour of the body – offensive
  ○ Sluggishness of the body
  ○ Wounds – reopening of old

Ailments
- Respiratory – Dry, unproductive cough / Blocked passage of mucus
- Eruptions – Acne / Ulcers / Abscesses / Pimples / Rash / Itching
- Fatigue / Exhaustion
- Constipation – stool consists of hard balls

Sensations
- As of a blow / Intolerable itching / Eye – foreign body; grit, sand
- Numbness / Acute senses ++ offensive odours.

Dream Themes
- Wedding / Engagement Rings (also irritation of wedding ring-finger)
- Ex-partners
- Fast-paced dreams (Slow paced reality)
- Taking the more difficult path
- Isolated / Excluded

Related remedies
Phascolarctos cinereus (Koala) / Cerium metallicum / Pulsatilla / Salix fragilis / Chocolate / Ambra grisea / Stage 2 / Series 3 / Milks / Sycotic miasm

Proving overview
The Sloth individual conserves energy; moving slowly whilst calmly taking life in. They hang-around, staying safe, alone with their own thoughts – seeing the world clearly. Yet within their bubble they become lonely and isolated, leading to procrastination and boredom (Sloth is of course one of the seven deadly sins, referring to idleness). They may develop a deep sense of shame, self-loathing and fear of criticism; disgusted by their own odour, suspicious that others treat them as an outsider. They hide in the canopy; feeling vulnerable and alert to danger – tending to internalise everything. They witness the violence of the jungle; the bullying, abuse and death. The injustice becomes overbearing and they are compelled to speak up. They have flashes of aggression, anger and violence – they can attack when threatened and even move quickly when excited. For love, warmth and hugs they need a mate; Sloths share the same communal toilet and

return each time. Here, by the 'poo-pile', they may find a sexual partner and feel part of the group for a while. In the absence of the mammal need for warmth and affection, they may develop addictive compensations; seeking comfort in bingeing.

Slowness

"Time feels like it is going on forever . . . the only thing I want to do is slow down and take my time . . . Dream: I am a body guard for the Queen, I must protect her . . . I am surprised by how slowly we must move. It takes ages to get anywhere."

Calmness / Tranquillity

"So relaxed. So peaceful . . . this was the most a meditation has ever worked . . . I am speaking slowly, calmly, taking my time, meaning every word . . . Feeling very grounded; like I am able to cope with anything."

Focus / Clarity / Precision / Insight

"The world looked more precise . . . I have a desire to look deep inside me . . . work[ing] with immense clarity and ability to see objectively . . . everything looks really clear – trees, grass, clouds – even though I haven't got my glasses on. I am seeing people for who they are, good and bad."

Isolation / Exclusion / Bubble / Barrier / Invisible / Alone

"Inside the bubble it is safe, but you can't reach anyone. . . . I broke down in tears. So lonely and unloved . . . Feeling I am very much the odd one out . . . Isolated, as if in a box . . . I feel distant and indifferent . . . I feel unloved, unlovable and unable to love . . . Feeling weirdly isolated, but surrounded by people."

Apathy / Boredom / Procrastination

"Tired and out of it. Bored and intolerant of idiots . . . feeling quite dead inside; no sense of urgency. . . I'm just not bothered or motivated . . . emotional numbness and indifference . . . I feel quite blasé . . . I don't care, I just want to stay in bed, look after myself and do nothing."

Exhaustion / Lassitude

"As if my fuel tank was empty . . . Exhausted, feeling heavy . . . Look old. Aged overnight. I don't want to get up. I wish I could lie here all day and sleep and read, alone."

Disgust / Smelly / Self Loathing / Revulsion

"Belching with slight vomit into mouth. Gross returning symptom . . . Self-loathing. Very uncomfortable. . . . Someone is biting their nails next to me. I feel disgusted and almost sick. . . . Strong body odour under armpits. . . . My breath smells. I keep smelling odd smells."

Weeping / Deep emotions

"Sobbing, feel completely overwhelmed, I cannot take anymore criticism . . . cried so hard; sad that I must hide feelings from mum and dad. . . . I am so near to tears and don't want to cry. Just a huge well of tears."

Confusion / Muddled / Blurred / Foggy / Distant

"Struggled to wake up, feeling very drowsy and confused, in a half-sleep . . . when I awoke I had absolutely no idea where I was. . . . I feel as if boundaries are unclear, blurred, changed . . . Discombobulated, Unable to navigate correctly, keep going the opposite way. . . . My head feels blurred and foggy."

Vulnerability

"Woke up with the word "Submissive" in the air. . . . Must deal with people despite feeling like I want to curl up in bed. Quite a challenge to stay present. Feel vulnerable . . . I find it nearly impossible to watch films that show people being victimised or in a position of vulnerability."

Suspicious

"Slight paranoia about people suddenly not needing a lift with me. . . . Have noticed I've been holding back a lot about how I had been feeling . . . worried about people looking over my shoulder . . . I am still suspicious and on my guard."

Death / Despair

"Dream: my son has aids. I cannot bear to think he will die. . . . I feel like there is a shape in front of me, like a rock or if I am in a tunnel. There is darkness and an emotion I do not understand. . . . Dreamt I was digging up animal corpses and moving them, hiding them elsewhere."

Injustice / Outspoken / Whistleblower

"The issues of stigma, shame and complicity are close to my heart. . . . Generally feel that I am less tolerant of injustice . . . it is not fair on me to do all the jobs by myself . . . being trapped in this fear of what might happen when [one] speak[s] up."

Conflict / Violence / Bullying / Abuse

"Conflict seems everywhere. . . . Must play-act so I don't explode . . . humiliated and bullied and victimised . . . I felt I had lost face. Impossible to watch films that show people being victimised or in a position of vulnerability. . . . I have had some almost vindictive thoughts for no real reason."

Anger / Aggression / Agitation

"I was very agitated and impatient. I rarely feel these emotions . . . Outburst of anger . . . Extremely irritated. Snappy, spiky. I must apologise to a number of people because I have been very short with them."

Active / Industrious / Efficient / Fast

"It is a very fast train! I wonder how to cope with it? It is like understanding everything all at the same time, or a bit like losing the plot. It would be easier to just eat, sleep and have sex and not think so much!"

Superhuman control / Possession

"I don't feel like myself and I want to go back to who I really am. . . . I feel that this remedy has an extremely dark side to it, sometimes it seems as if it is taking over me . . . I cannot shake it. I am taken over by it . . . I feel the 'possession' of the proving substance."

Excess / Addiction / Smoking / Drinking

"I want to drink alcohol a lot at the moment. . . . Had quite a lot of white and red wine to drink; felt as if it wasn't really affecting me. . . . I felt the need to smoke tobacco so I did. It felt like a crutch but didn't really satisfy. I just continued to do it. Almost binge like . . . I am still drinking every day . . . No stop button."

Guilt / Shame / Blame / Fear of criticism

"Dreams – Wanting to have sex with younger man. Feeling guilty about it and stopping half way through. . . . I feel so sick not helping my best friend. Who would leave a friend in need? . . . Inside I am terrified of the criticism . . . So much fear. What have I done? I am still scared of leaving the house. . . . Someone could come and tell me off. . . why is that so scary?"

Groups

"More aware of political manoeuvrings of others. I can see how people jostle for position in organisations and how they subtly push others aside and themselves forward . . . I am reaching out for reassurance to friends via text messages and talking."

Family / Warmth / Love / Hugs

"Amazing loving hug fills me up with love and gratitude for this new family I am a part of. I feel a warm glow inside rising up through me. . . . I realise that making myself really vulnerable [means] those who love you will understand and support you. . . . Dream – He took my hand and he seemed really lovely and full of energy and enthusiasm. He curled up and I sat in his lap also curled up. I felt so safe and comforted. We looked over a balcony and he started sucking on my right nipple. It wasn't sexual at all (more like a child suckling)."

Supplementary themes
- *Animals*
- *Transitions / Change*
- *Drunk / Drugged*
- *Overthinking / Overwhelmed*
- *Senses acute / amplified*
- *Accidents / Carelessness*
- *Amorous / Sexual / Ex-partners*

Meles meles (European Badger)

Phylum: Chordata.
Class: Mammalia.
Order: Carnivora.
Family: Mustelidae.

The badger is part of the same family that includes weasels, stoats and otters. Various subspecies are found in a band that stretches from almost the whole west coast of Europe across Europe, Russia and Asia to the east coast of China. Badgers live in setts – networks of tunnels and chambers that they dig in the earth. These setts can be very extensive and deep. They are extremely territorial especially since these territories may have been established many hundreds or even thousands of years ago, and been walked and marked every night by generations of badgers stretching back to long before the Romans or the Saxons came to Britain. One senior boar rules the sett and, in the same way that he marks the territory, he marks the other badgers with his musk – only those smelling of him are tolerated. Badger cubs are extremely playful and invent complicated ways of playing and enjoying themselves. The adults are extremely stubborn and tenacious. This is one of the reasons that they are so desirable as "sporting" animals; they will fight until the end and never give up.

Proving by: **Misha Norland and Peter Fraser, UK (2009).**[33]

"Badger in The Wind in The Willows [is] **grumpy** and averse to company, a **curmudgeon**, but also **loyal** and kindly and **fiercely defensive** of his friends and of tradition and historical values. Thus the badger has qualities that go beyond its actual nature. These metaphorical qualities are often indicative that the substance will make an important remedy"[33]

Keywords relating to the experience of badger culling:
Blamed / Exterminated / Tuberculosis / Infected / Persecuted / Baiting / Systematically wiped out

Mind

- Ailments from – ***position; loss of***
- *Alert*
- Ambition – increased – competitive
- Anger – alternating with – repentance; quick
- Audacity
- Benevolence
- *Breaking* things – desire to break things
- Cautious
- Company – aversion to – bear anybody; cannot
- Contradiction – disposition to contradict
- Confident
- Courageous
- *Cuddle – desire to be cuddled*
- **Delusions**
  - Accused, she is
  - Carousal / debauch; as if after a
  - Great person; is a / Superiority, of

- Insects; skin crawls with
- Persecuted – he is persecuted – backward; and looks
- Persecuted – he is persecuted – everyone; by
- Trapped; and killed, he is
- Dependent of others (*vs.* Capability increased)
- Desires – *group together; to keep*
- *Disgust*
- Fear – narrow place; in
- *Fight, wants to – space; for one's*
- *Growling*
- *Indignation – territory, intrusion of*
- Impulsive
- Intolerance
- Irritability – disturbed; when
- Jesting – licentious
- *Libertinism*
- Love – perversity; sexual
- Mirth
- Pertinacity
- Playful
- Responsibility – family for
- *Shameless – buttocks, desirable*
- Superstitious
- Suspicious
- *Territorial*
- *Tranquility – confined space, within*
- Truth – telling the plain truth

Dreams

Abdomen – constricted; as if the abdomen was / Amorous / **Anger – seething, with masculine pride** / **Animals – marking territory** / **Betrayed**, having been / **Breast fed** / Bullying / Busy, being / Children; about – looking after / Children; about – lost / Coition / Crime – committing a crime / Cruelty / **Danger** – escaping from a danger / **Darkness** / Death – relatives; of / **Deceived**; being / *Dogs – sexual desire for* / Elephants / *Escaping – to start simple life* / Fighting; one is / **Fights – pummelling, with fists** / Guilt / **Hair – body hair, rubbing chests, competition of** / Helpless feeling / **Hero**; of being the / House – big / *House – community centre* / Lascivious / Lewd / Losing – family; his / Lost; being / Machines – *machine, collaborating as a finely tuned* / **Masturbating** / Mutilation / Narrow place / *Outsider – being an outsider* / People – crowds of – needs space / **Powerful – male feeling – woman; in a** / *Predatory – male, that she is* / Prisoner – being taken a / **Prostitutes** / *Protecting* / Stairs / Stealing / Theft – committed a theft, having / **Tortured**; of being / **Tunnel – dark and glistening** / Watched; being / Water – muddy; of / Wilderness – survival in winter

Physicals

- **Head**
  - Formication
  - Itching of scalp
  - Pain
    - § Clamped together; as if
    - § Pressing pain – vise; as if in a
  - Prickling
  - Tingling
- **Ear**
  - Itching – Meatus – boring with finger – amel.
- **Hearing**
  - Acute
    - § Distant sounds
    - § Noise; to / Echoing
- **Nose**
  - Sneezing – violent
- **Abdomen**
  - Itching – Umbilicus
- **Chest**
  - Enlarged Sensation – Mammae
  - **Pain**

- § Cutting pain
- § Needles; as from
- § Stitching pain
- § Violent
- ○ Palpitation of heart – sleep – going to sleep; on – agg.

- • **Generals**
  - ○ Morning – 8 h – 8–12 h
  - ○ Clothing – intolerance of
  - ○ Electroshock; ailments from
  - ○ Food and drinks
    - § meat – desire
    - § salt – aversion
  - ○ Stretching – amel.
  - ○ Warm – air – amel.

Provers speaking as one

ᛞ Felt as if *I **ruled the world***. A feeling of expansiveness. . . . My colleague looks like a lion, regal, we're *cocky* and *jerky* with each other. . . . Very fair, **magnanimous**, **benevolent** overseer. . . . *I'm unperturbed by people's judgements*, just feel utterly benevolent to them. . . . Don't react when colleagues try to *control me;* feel superior, fatherly. . . .

ᛞ Feel very *creative with science*, physics, electric currents, able to draw diagrams, design a sex-powered electric blanket. . . .

ᛞ Feel ***sexy*** and ***effective*** *and warm towards others.* . . .

ᛞ Alternating feelings of being **dependent** and being very **capable**. . . . I feel different, more **confident**, free to **laugh**, less inhibited, held back. . . . Sudden urge to lie down on floor and sprawl and roll around. . . .

ᛞ **Cuddling** my children feels just great. . . . Want to **snuggle** up to them and smell them . . . **joking** and **wrestling** and playing with the kids. . . . Feature about meerkats. Talks about how they are family orientated and cooperative with different roles.

ᛞ [Feeling] a sense of competition. Who is going to be top dog, a slight challenge of ***social positioning***. . . . I am shocked and disillusioned due to **territorial** behaviour. . . . I am sat next to a man who leans into my personal space with seemingly no regard or knowledge that he is doing so. . . .

ᛞ Feel less inhibited and reticent [during sex]. . . . More **playful**, **impulsive** and spontaneous. . . . Friend holds up a massive bright pink Bratwurst which causes a lot of **bawdy hilarity**. . . . I'm aware of a rather ***maternal acceptance*** of [the] child-like qualities of selfishness and precocity which normally rankle me and now vaguely amuse me. It is a relief, letting g*o of the **cynicism** and **dryness** of old age*. . . . *My boobs feel massive* and people have commented on it. Feel **uninhibited**. Want everyone together, no need for clothes. I feel **I'm lacking human touch**. Want to go home and have a shag. I feel quite lush . . . want to be **bawdy**, have a really good fun **orgy** in the style of Hogarth, lots of *tankards of beer swilling* about with **buttocks** and **breasts** and big, frothy petticoats. . . . The idea of an orgy suddenly seems *good fun and earthy, not sordid and desperate like I usually think* . . . more interested generally in modern world, excited by multiplex cinema, interested in adverts, drawn to city, noise, stimulation.[33]

Mephitis putorius (Skunk – secretion from anal glands)

Phylum: Chordata.
Class: Mammalia.
Order: Carnivora.
Superfamily: Mustelidae.

Skunks are notorious for their anal scent glands which serve as a powerful defensive weapon. There are two glands, one on each side of the anus, which produce the powerful mixture of sulphur-containing chemicals. A skunk's spray is powerful enough to ward off bears and other potential attackers, and the muscles located next to the scent glands allow them to spray with a high degree of accuracy – as far as 3 m. They are crepuscular (becoming active at twilight) and inclined to solitude – during the day they shelter in burrows which are excavated with their powerful front claws. It is advantageous to warn potential predators off without wasting precious scent supplies, and the skunk's distinctive black and white colouration gives a visual warning. Threatened skunks will go through an elaborate routine of hisses, foot-stamping, and tail-high threat postures before resorting to spraying. They are not true hibernators in the winter, but do hunker down for extended periods of time.

Provings by: **C. Hering, USA (1837) and H. Schindler, Germany (1976).**

Mind

- *Cheerful – followed by – melancholy*
- *Communicative*
- Delusions
  - Drunk – is drunk; he
  - Enlarged – head is
  - Unfit – work; for
  - Water – of
- Dreams – Hemoptysis (spitting blood).
- Euphoria – alternating with – sadness
- Fancies – exaltation of
- *Frightened easily – waking, on – dream; from a*
- Gestures, makes – angry – somnambulism; in
- *Indifference – pleasure; to*
- Loquacity – changing quickly from one subject to an other – important matters about; on (*aran., lach.*)
- *Loquacity – nonsense*
- Moonlight agg.

Pathogenetic Ward[18]

Diarrhoea colic / Distended head / **Electric shocks** / **Enlarged** head / Exerting eyes / **Eyes** body / **Flatulence** side / Injected conjunctiva / **Insensible** legs / **Needles** eyes / Pressed occiput / **Stupefied** mornings / Styes lids / Talkative intoxication / **Vibrations** bones

Clinical Ward[18]

<u>Asthma</u> sulphur / Body eyes / Burning lids / Coppery taste / **Cough spasmodic** / Cough sulphur fumes / Diarrhoea set in / **Die coughing** / Distended head / Emptiness stomach / Enlarged head / Eyes foreign body / **Eyes needles** / Eyes

over exertion / Fingers pressing / Fullness head / Head pressing / Heaviness occiput / Insensible limbs / Lameness internal / Legs insensible / **Loquacity intoxication** / Needles eyes / Onions nose / Pinched toe / Pressing eyelids / Pressing head / Pressing lids / Pressure occiput / **Pulsation** head / Stitches eyes / Strained eyes / Stye burning / Stye eyelids / Sulphur fumes / **Talkative drunk** / Taste coppery / Threads head / Trunk threads / **Undulation** head / Vapor asthma

Whooping cough, croup Lilienthal[36]

"Cough purely spasmodic, catarrhal element imperfectly developed, inclined to hoarseness, oftentimes croupy, without being dry; mucous râles through upper portion of lungs; in attempting to swallow, food goes the wrong way; spasms of larynx ending in a long-drawn whoop, with little or no expectoration; child is aroused by sudden contraction of throat followed by rapid spasm; coughing produces a smothering sensation, child cannot exhale (Samb., cannot inhale); vomiting of all food hours after eating; bloated face; convulsions; cough and vomiting agg. at night and after lying down."

Related remedies
aven., castn-v., chlor., cor-r., cupr., dros., ictod., lach., mosch., pert., phos., rumx., samb.

Moschus (Deer musk)

Phylum: Chordata.
Class: Mammalia.
Order: Artiodactyla.
Family: Moschidae.

Musk deer are ruminants, along with cattle, goats, sheep, deer, and antelope. They digest food in 2 steps, chewing and swallowing in the normal way to begin with, and then regurgitating the semi-digested cud to re-chew it to extract the maximum possible food value. They are more primitive than the cervids, or true deer, in not having antlers or facial glands, but they do possess a musk gland – found only in adult males in a sac between the genitals and the umbilicus. They resemble small deer, with a stocky build and hind legs longer than their front legs. They are very shy and therefore difficult to catch – using rocky areas with dense vegetation to escape from predators. Lichens are the main part of Siberian musk deer diet, accounting for up to 99% of the food intake in winter.

Provings by: **C S F Hahnemann, Germany (???), Jörg, Germany (1824), Hromada, Germany (1833) and by E W Berridge, UK (1874).**

Indications
- "Violent spasmodic cough, with rattling of mucus when breathing; great dyspnoea, agg. by being in open cold air, amel. after vomiting large quantities

of thick mucus; cramplike, suffocating constriction of chest. . . . Suitable to **hysterical persons and children**; suffocating fits beginning with a desire to cough and getting worse until he nearly despairs of getting over the paroxysm. . . . Stiffness of body with full consciousness; tetanic spasms of abdominal muscle" Lilienthal[36]

- "Moschus cures many hysterical [childen] who have come to adult age without ever learning what obedience means. They are **self-willed, obstinate** and **selfish**. When they have been encouraged to resort to **crafty cunning**, to have every whim gratified from infancy to eighteen years of age they become fit subjects for Mosch., Asaf., Ign. and Valer . . . they become adepts at producing at will a *kaleidoscopic complex of symptoms*, increasing in quantity and intensity until all their own desires are attained" Kent[37]

- "Musk is a well known perfume, which produces **fainting** in some by mere smelling of it; hence easy fainting in any diseased condition is its chief indication. . . . **Twitching; chokings**; globus hystericus, ending in unconsciousness . . . Nervous; shuddering, laughter, hiccough etc . . . Buzzing, squeezing, plug like sensation" Phatak[16]

Delusions

- Double – being
- Elevated – air; elevated in the – fall; and would
- **Faint; he would**
- Falling – height; from a *vs.* Floating – air; in
- *Figures – seeing figures – large black figures were about to spring on him*
- Hear; he cannot
- Hindered and opposed; he is – everyone; by
- *Identity – someone else; she is*
- Person – other person; she is some
- **Sick – being**
- Strange – familiar things seem strange

Rubrics

- *(K.J Muller)*
  - Ambition; ailments from, agg.; deceived
  - Ambitious
  - Mathematics, calculating; inept for
  - School, aversion to
  - Sympathetic, compassionate, too; animals, towards; only
  - Throws; things
  - Timidity; public, about appearing in

- *(F.J Master)*
  - Abusive – children
  - Ailments from – domination – father; by
  - Awkward
  - Chaotic / Destructive
  - Fearless
  - Fidgety
  - Laughing – immoderately
  - Malicious
  - Shameless
  - Striking
  - Talking – himself; to

Respiration (Bold type)
- Asthmatic – hysterical
- Asthmatic – *sudden* attacks
- Children; in
- Cold agg.; becoming
- Stridulous

Clinical _{Clarke}[17]

Italic type –
Catalepsy / Croup / Fainting / Heart – failure of / Hiccough / Hysteria / Hystero-epilepsy / Stings

Plain type-
Angina pectoris / Diabetes / Dyspnoea / Epilepsy / Herpes – mercurial and venereal / Hypochondriasis / Impotence / Laryngismus / Lungs – paralysis of / Pregnancy – complaints of / Rage – fits of / Typhoid fever / Vertigo / Whooping-cough

Other bold type particulars
- **Nose**
  - Congestion
- **Face**
  - Discolouration – red – one side – chill; during
- **Mouth**
  - Dryness – morning
- **Throat**
  - Lump; sensation of a – rising sensation
- **Stomach**
  - Thirstless – chill; during
- **Urine**
  - Copious
  - Odour – ammoniacal / strong
- **Larynx and trachea**
  - Laryngismus stridulus
  - Pain – Larynx – fever; during
  - Spasms – Larynx

- **Cough**
  - Morning
- **Chest**
  - Constriction – fever; during
- **Extremities**
  - Stiffness – convulsions – during
- **Chill**
  - One Side
  - Chilliness – headache – during
  - Coldness – External parts – sensation of
  - Descending – agg.
- **Fever**
  - Side – one side
  - Internal heat – external chill; with
  - Succession of stages – chill – External – heat; with internal
  - Uncovering – desire for
- **Skin**
  - Discolouration – pale – fever; during

Oryctolagus cuniculus sanguis (Rabbit's blood)

Phylum: Chordata.
Class: Mammalia.
Order: Lagomorpha.
Family: Leporidae.

Once classified as rodents, rabbits, hares and pikas are now ranked on their own as lagomorphs. *Oryctolagus cuniculus* is thought to be the descendant of early domestic rabbits released into the wild, and is now the subspecies that has been introduced throughout Europe and worldwide. Since speed and agility are a rabbit's main defences against predators, rabbits have large hind leg bones. These well-muscled hind legs allow for maximum force, manoeuvrability, and acceleration and are an exaggerated feature that are much longer than the forelimbs. Rabbits use their strong claws for digging and (along with their teeth) for defence. Constriction and dilation of blood vessels in the ears are used to control the core body temperature of a rabbit.

Rabbits are herbivores that feed by grazing on grass, forbs, and leafy weeds which means their diet contains large amounts of hard-to-digest cellulose. Rabbits solve this problem via a form of hindgut fermentation. They pass two distinct types of faeces: hard droppings and soft black viscous pellets. The average female rabbit becomes sexually mature at 3 to 8 months of age and can conceive at any time of the year for the duration of her life. The sexual encounter lasts only 20–40 seconds, and the rabbit gestation period is very short – ranging from 28 to 36 days with an average period of 31 days. They survive predation by burrowing, hopping away in a zig-zag motion, and, if captured, delivering powerful kicks with their hind legs. If confronted by a potential threat, a rabbit may freeze then warn others in the warren with powerful thumps on the ground.

Proving by: **Andrea Bartig, Nette Humphreys and the Sheffield Proving Collective, UK (2009).**[31]

Key Delusions

- *Ancestors – one with her ancestors; she is*
- Body – ugly; body looks – fat; too
- *Friend – surrounded by friends; being*
- Head
  - Heavy; his own head seemed too
  - Lift it off; can
  - Light; head is
- Intoxicated – is; he
- Meaningless; everything is
- Obstacles – in his way / Wrong – everything goes wrong
- *Pregnant; she is – distension of abdomen from flatus; with*
- Queen; she is an ice queen
- *Separated – world; from the – he is separated*

Mind

- Abrupt
- *Affectionate*
- Ailments from – mental shock; from
- Attracting others
- Awareness heightened – animal awareness – body; of – mammae
- Brotherhood; sensation of
- *Carefree*
- Change – desire for
- **Coition – amel.**
- Company – aversion to – desire for solitude
- *Company – desire for*
- *Contact; desire for*
- Emotions – loss of
- *Emotions – spontaneous and natural*
- *Emotions – strong; too*
- *Energised feeling*
- Ennui
- Estranged
- *Expansive*
- Expressing oneself – desire to express oneself
- Fear
  - ◦ *Attacked; fear of being*
  - ◦ Dogs; of
  - ◦ Gun; thunder of a
  - ◦ Noise; from – sudden, of
  - ◦ **Sudden** *(panic attacks)*
- *Fearless*
- *Firmness*
- Forsaken feeling – isolation; sensation of
- Freedom
- Grief
- *Grounded*
- Hatred – humankind; of
- Helplessness; feeling of
- *Hiding – himself*
- *Home – desires to go*
- Indifference – pleasure, to – things usually enjoyed
- Introspection
- *Intuitive*
- *Jesting*
- *Joy – spontaneous feelings of pleasure*
- Laughing
  - ◦ *Actions; at his own*
  - ◦ **Desire to laugh**
- Love
  - ◦ Exalted love
  - ◦ *Openness; and – friends; for*
- **Maternal instinct; exaggerated**
- *Mirth*
- *Mischievous*
- Mood – changeable – sudden
- *Naive*
- *Naked; wants to be*
- **Nymphomania**
- Playful
- *Positiveness*
- *Protected feeling*
- Quick to act
- *Responsibility –*
  - ◦ *Give up her responsibility; wanting to*
  - ◦ *Taking responsibility too seriously*
- Rest – desire for
- Satyriasis
- Senses – acute
- **Sociability**
- Space – desire for
- Sympathetic
- Talking – amel. the complaints
- Tough
- Tranquillity
- *Unification – sensation of unification – family; with his*
- *Vivacious*
- Yearning (Nostalgia)

Dreams

Amorous – fallen in love; has / Amorous – orgasm; with / Boyfriend – old boyfriend / Buildings / Children; about / Cities / Coition / *Coition – desire for, of* / Commune / Criticised; being / *Cutting – others; cutting or mutilating* / Dancing / *Danger – escaping from a danger* / *Dogs – bitten by dogs; being* / Escaping – danger; from / Family, own / Flood – house is in a / Groups / Hiding / House / Humiliation / Identity / Journeys – bus; by / Killing / Losing – family; his / Lost; being / Mother / *Mother – dead mother appearing* / Needles / Parties / *Prisoner – being taken a* / Pursued, being – man; by a / Rabbits / *Resolving – relationships; old* / Separated; being – relatives; from / Sexual / Shooting; about / Statue / *War – camp; being in a war* / Water / Wedding

Important Physicals

- *Stomach – Nausea – pregnancy – as if pregnant*
- *Abdomen – Distension – pregnancy – as from pregnancy*

Female

- *Conception – easy.* (One prover actually became unexpectedly pregnant during the proving due to ovulation starting earlier.)
- **Delivery** – during; complaints – delayed delivery. (*Clinical* – the remedy has been successfully prescribed to encourage waters to break.)
- **Menopause.** (One prover had her menses return 2 years after menopause. Another went into menopause shortly after the proving.)
- Menses – irregular
- *Menses – menopause – after*
- Menses – short; too
- *Ovulation – early*
- **Sexual desire – violent**
- *Sterility* (*Clinical* – The remedy has been used to treat infertility – *cf.* Salmon).
- *Tumors – Ovaries – cysts* (*Clinical* – a case is mentioned in the proving of a patient with polycystic ovaries becoming pregnant following successful treatment with the remedy).

Characteristic physicals

- **Chest – Pain**
  - Mammae – sore
- **Back – Pain**
  - Bending – amel.
  - Motion – agg.
  - Cervical region – lifting agg.
  - Coccyx – fall; as from a
  - Dorsal region – Scapulae – Between – extending to – Spine; down to
  - **Lumbar region**
    - Bending – amel.
    - Lying – amel.
    - Standing – agg.
    - Stooping – agg.
    - Walking – agg.
  - Sacrum
  - Stiffness – Lumbar region
- **Extremities**
  - Discolouration – Fingers – white
  - Numbness – Forearms
  - Pain
    - Lower limbs – stitching pain
    - Nates – right – shooting pain

- **Generals**
  - *Alternating states*
  - *Energy – excess of energy*
  - **Food and drinks**
    - § Bread – desire – toasted
    - § Cheese – desire
    - § Honey – desire
    - § Milk – desire
    - § Nuts – desire
    - § Oatmeal – desire
    - § Rice – desire
- **Pain**
  - Cutting pain – knife; as with a
  - Shooting pain
  - Sprained; as if
  - Stitching pain – needles; as from
  - Twinging
  - Stiffness – Muscles
  - Stretching out – Limbs – agg.
  - Sudden Manifestation
  - Tingling
  - Generals – warm – desire for warmth

Pantheris pardus sanguis (Blood of the leopard)

Phylum: Chordata.
Class: Mammalia.
Order: Carnivora.
Family: Felidae.

Compared to other wild cats, the leopard has relatively short legs and a long body with a large skull. Its fur is marked with rosettes. It is similar in appearance to the jaguar, but has a smaller, lighter physique. It is distinguished by its well-camouflaged fur, opportunistic hunting behaviour, broad diet, strength, and its ability to adapt to a variety of habitats ranging from rainforest to steppe, including arid and montane areas. It can run at speeds of up to 36 mph. The earliest known leopard fossils excavated in Europe are estimated 600,000 years old.

Proving by: **Olga Fatula, Russia (2005).**[34]

Themes

Having beautiful hair and the finest clothes were both very important features of the proving. A lot of attention was directed towards making oneself alluring, and being easily turned-on by the opposite sex, especially when well-groomed. Provers wanted to wear skin-tight clothing, so as to be at their most revealing.

> *The self-awareness was remarkable. I was satisfied with my appearance. The most distinctive feature was the hair. The desired hairdo was, all the hair collected in a long tail. I wore then an add-on wig – a long hair add-on. . . . I feel myself like something in between chocolate and a rose. As if everybody wants to scent me and lick me. . . . I want a dress of satin embossing, coffee-black, or a leopard colour, or a striped pattern. . . . All my clothes are skin-tight, stick to the body.*[34]

It was important to attract others, and there was a distinctly lascivious undertone to the proving.

I raised my eyes in the train today. Two men, as if on a cover page, pictures of beauty, elegant, in cashmere coats, expensive kid gloves, wonderful haircuts, pomaded hair. I could go crazy. They did not tally with others at all. Choose the one you want, the eyes go apart, one to the left, the other to the right. I want them both. I feel I can flare up a bit. . . . Have you been out today? Go, have a walk! There are so many men around.[34]

There was a good deal of malice, vengefulness and cruelty in the prover's diaries. They tended to become haughty, looking at others as if they were dirty or moronic. It appears to be a related remedy to Platina in these aspects. There was also a stripping away of morals, impulsively stealing and feeling no remorse; questioning why they had held back from such deeds until now.

The repertorisation I made of this succinct proving yields the following rubrics:

- **Delusions**
  - Beautiful – she is beautiful and wants to be
  - Dirty – everyone is
  - Great person; is a
  - Queen; she is a – *diva, a*

- **Hatred**
  - Revengeful; hatred and
  - Persons – offended him; hatred of persons who
  - *Vengeful* and *detached*

Mind

- Abusive
- Amorous
- Anger – **beside oneself; being**
- Anger – **cold and detached**
- Ardent
- *Attracting others*
- Audacity
- Awareness heightened – body; of – **face, her**
- Boaster – *squandering through* **ostentation**
- Clothes – *luxurious clothing,* **finery;** *wants*
- Company – aversion to – desire for solitude
- **Confident**
- *Contemptuous – humankind; of*
- Contradiction – disposition to contradict
- *Cruelty*
- Death – thoughts of
- *Deceitful*
- *Detached – calmness, ice-cold*
- Determination
- Dignified
- Diplomatic
- **Dress – indecently; dresses**
- Egotism
- Excitement – desire for
- **Extravagance**
- **Foppish**
- Gossiping
- Hard-hearted
- *Haughty – clothes – best clothes; likes to wear his*
- Kleptomania
- **Lascivious**
- Laziness
- *Love – opposite sex, for*
- Malicious
- *Moral feeling; want of*
- Pessimist
- **Plans – making many plans – revengeful plans**
- Pompous, important
- Purposeful
- Quarrelsome
- Reflecting
- Religious affections – too occupied with religion
- **Seduction – desire for**

- Selfishness
- **Self-satisfied**
- Sociability
- Striking
- *Suspicious – friends, his*
- Touched – aversion to be

- *Tranquillity – conflict; during*
- Tranquillity – settled, centred and grounded
- <u>***Vanity***</u>
- *Violent*
- Wrong; everything seems

Physicals
- **Eye – Pain**
  - Right – foreign body; as from a
  - Foreign body; as from a
  - Itching
- **Ear – Pain**
  - Night – midnight – after
  - Motion – amel.
  - Stopped sensation
- **Neck**
  - Pain
- **Stomach**
  - Appetite – increased
  - Appetite – increased – evening
  - Thirst

- **Abdomen**
  - Swollen sensation – Liver
- **Female genitalia/sex**
  - Sexual desire – increased
- **Back**
  - Bending – body – backward agg.
  - **Pain**
    - § Cervical region
    - § Dorsal region – Scapulae – Between
- **Sleep**
  - Sleepiness
- **Generals**
  - Food and drinks – wine – desire
  - Lie down – desire to
  - Rest – desire for

Dreams
"A brunette of an oriental appearance, with dark eyes, the hair is parted at one side. The idea is that we must look for men. She says, let's go for men, you can reckon on me. There is a wardrobe full of clothes, choose what you like . . . (desire) of *black dresses, close-fitting trousers* . . . Velvet and chiffon . . . I see myself with a new haircut, a fringe, large locks, curls, and long ringlets. It is a tall hairdo. **I am very much satisfied with myself**, with how much hair I have and what a nice wave they form. They gave me a small salary. Why so little? I call my boss crying 'I will not survive.' I sobbed a lot."[34]

Phascolarctos cinereus (Australian koala)

Class: Mammalia.
Infraclass: Marsupialia.
Order: Diprotodontia.
Family: Phascolarctidae.

Serum extract from the chest scent gland of an adult male Koala. This gland produces a pungent, orange-coloured secretion which they rub on the base of trees and along branches. Koalas typically inhabit open eucalypt woodlands, and the leaves of these trees make up most of their diet. Because this diet has limited nutritional and caloric content, koalas are largely sedentary and sleep up to 20 hours a day. Being marsupials, they give birth to underdeveloped young that crawl into their mothers' pouches, where they stay for the first six to seven months of their lives. These joeys are fully weaned at around a year old. Koalas have few natural predators and parasites, but are threatened by various pathogens, such as Chlamydiaceae bacteria and the koala retrovirus. They have one of the smallest brains in proportion to body weight of any mammal. This may be an adaptation to the energy restrictions imposed by its diet, which is insufficient to sustain a larger brain. They are hindgut fermenters and are asocial animals, spending just 15 minutes a day on social behaviours. It is one of the few mammals that has a face rather than a muzzle, a trait it shares with humans, which perhaps accounts for its popularity on the cuteness scale.

Proving by: **Phillip Robbins, Australia (1996).**[35]

Delusions
- **Despised – by everybody who loves him**
- Adrift; being
- Damage to mind and body; the proving caused irreparable
- Division between himself and others
- Forsaken; is
- **Friendless**; he is
- **Hostage**; being taken as a
- **Outsider**; being an

Mind
- Anxiety – *conscience; anxiety of –* **absent**
- Aversion – family; to members of / friends, to
- Company – aversion to – alone amel.
- Confidence – want of self-confidence – *failure, feels himself a*
- **Drugs**
  - Desire – heroin / psychotropic
  - Withdrawal; as if in
- Escape; attempts to – family and children; attempts to escape from her
- Estranged – family; from his
- Euphoria

- **Fear**
  - Captured; of being
  - Injury – being injured; of
  - Poverty; of
- Fight, wants to – space; for one's
- Forsaken feeling – isolation; sensation of
- Forsaking – children; his own
- Looked at; to be – cannot bear to be looked at
- Moral feeling; want of
- ***Secretive***
- Self-satisfied
- Suspicious
- Touched – aversion to be
- Water – loves – live closer to water; wants to

Dreams

Accidents / Amorous / Animals – cardboard boxes; in / Animals – slaughtered / Body – wrapped in newspapers / **Breast fed – guru; by one's** / **Burning things; are** – smoke screen; to hide behind a / Caesarean with a long scar / Closet – being on / Coloured – red / Coloured – yellow / Commune – country; in the / Disgusting / Dolphins – riding on / Fear – injuries / Fly eggs / **Gladiator**; being a / Hiding / **Homeless – being homeless** / House – facade; only a / Injuries / Insults / **Isolated**; of being – contact; can't make any / Leave; desire to / Lost; being – city; in a / **Men – breast; men's** / **Mummy; wrapped** up like a / Naked people – snow; small boy, naked in / Outsider – being an outsider / Poison; of – water; in / Quarrels / Repeating / Riding – train; on a / Shelter – warmth; for / Slap on the face / Soldier / Storms / Toxic orange cloud / Urinating – hide he is; tries / Vermin / Water – high waves / Women – breasts; with big

Physicals

- **Vertigo**
  - Accompanied by – staggering / Reeling
- **Vision**
  - Colours before the eyes – yellow – objects seem yellow
- **Face**
  - Saliva; sensation of – Mouth – Corner – left
  - Tension of skin – Forehead
- **Mouth**
  - Aphthae – Palate / Tongue
- **Abdomen**
  - Pain – Liver – lying – side; on – right – agg.
- **Rectum**
  - Constipation
  - Haemorrhoids – painful
  - Pain – pulsating pain
- **Extremities**
  - Eruptions – Nates – boils
- **Sleep**
  - Disturbed
- **Generals**
  - Wounds – painful – old wounds

Provers speaking as one

§ I can't stand to be in myself. I can't stand anyone looking at me. I can't get out of bed. . . . I think I **want to be on my own** – I can't deal with people, but I'm not self-contained either. **I don't like any of my friends**. Been **brutally honest**: 'how dare you!'. . .

§ **No sense of my centre** . . . I feel on the **edge of losing it; total ungroundedness**; just floating or cut adrift. . . . I am influenced by whatever comes in. I lose faith in myself and everyone else. In connections with people I feel really hurt. Nothing feels right. . . .

§ It is like the fuzzy feeling in one's head after a lot of acid trips – not down or up, but just wanting to be down. As if something extra in my brain. . . .

§ 'The best dream of my life'. In meditation with my Guru (a male) and other people. . . . I started to go into shocks and moans – a kind of chorea – from the spiritual energy in my body. **My guru leant over and uncovered his breast (a female breast) and fed me milk from it. I felt nurtured to my soul by God**. . . .

$ Dream: I **urinate** on a tray in a restaurant. Surprised at myself for doing it. I tried to hide the evidence. Waiter came to collect the tray. I looked at the ground rather than at him – hoped he wouldn't notice. . . .

$ I felt I **didn't belong** and that they were just inviting me to be nice. I felt an **outcast** – should go. Felt a lot more comfortable going . . . Dream: I had a cut in the sole of my right foot – inside the cut were two layers of spam – in between the spam was a rectangular **'nest' of flies eggs**. Completely **revolted** by dream all day. . . .

$ Intolerant of others, when it is different to my needs. . . . **It is not ok to be just me, I don't fit in**. . . . Felt like crying all day; felt sad and isolated. With friends, I didn't get the jokes, **felt different, isolated, stuck in self**.[35]

Rattus norvegicus / Sanguis soricis (Blood of the Norway Rat)

Phylum: Chordata.
Class: Mammalia.
Order: Rodentia.
Family: Muridae.

The brown rat's success has been to ride on the back of the rapid expansion of the human population. Their opportunistic lifestyle, agility and prolific breeding have helped them to colonise practically every part of the world. Rats have long been considered deadly pests; the rat flood in India occurs every fifty years, as armies of bamboo rats descend upon rural areas and devour everything in their path. They have also long been blamed as the chief villain in the spread of the Bubonic Plague. Rattus rattus, the black rat, is considered to be one of the world's worst invasive species – having been carried worldwide as a stowaway on sea-going vessels for millennia. Over the years, rats have been used in many experimental studies, adding to our understanding of genetics, diseases, the effects of drugs, and other topics that have provided a great benefit for the health and wellbeing of humankind. Their tail is used in thermoregulation – it is hairless and thin skinned but highly vascularised, thus allowing for efficient counter-current heat exchange with the environment.

Proving by: **Nancy Herrick, USA (1998).**[30]

Fundamental delusions
- *Black – gods.* (Dream – *"huge black woman with a really fierce face and long, curly, dark hair. She's wild"*)
- Bugs; sees – small, black bugs running across the floor; hundreds of
- *Dirty – he is* (*"can't bathe or wash my hands enough"*)
- Hunter, he is a
- Looking – everyone is looking at her (*paranoia*)
- *Man – old men – alone and lost after the death of their wives*

- Pursued; he was
- Small – he is (*cf. Insects and Snakes*)
- **Visions, has – goddess**; of a (*"Mother as universal, I am Mother, Everything is Mother."*)

Mind

- **Abrupt** (blunt, to the point)
- Antisocial
- Anxiety – conscience; anxiety of
- Clarity of mind
- Company – aversion to – desire for solitude
- Cursing
- **Darkness – desire for**
- Detached / Estranged – society, from
- Fear – observed; of her condition being
- *Femininity – increased sensation of*
- Hiding – himself
- Indifference – duties; to
- Industrious
- Laziness – heaviness of limbs; with
- **Light – aversion to – shuns**
- **Longing – anonymity**

- Looked at; to be – cannot bear to be looked at
- Meditating
- *Remorse – indiscretion; over past*
- Sensitive – odours, to
- Sitting – inclination to sit – stare; and
- Slowness – purpose; of
- Staring, thoughtless
- Wandering – desire to wander – night
- **Washing – desire to wash – hands; always** (*cf. Medorrhinum, Syphilinum*)
- *Watched; to be – desires to be watched – by men, in a woman (Sexuality)*
- Will – strong will power
- Woods – desire to be in the woods

Polarities (based on the above characteristic rubrics)

- Feminine, lightness, spiritual goddess *vs.* Black bugs, black gods, isolated old man. (*Fire-Air*)
- Industrious, impatience *vs.* Slowness of purpose
- Anonymous, hidden, estranged *vs.* Strong will power

Dreams

Anger / *Animals* / Anxious / Car / Car – find the car; cannot / *Cares, full of – children; about one's* / Children; about – *black* / Children; about – *neglecting her child* / *Clarity*; about / **Coition** / Coloured – white / Confused / *Dancing* (break-dancing) / **Danger** / Dirt / Floating / Flood / **Goddess**; of / Hell; of / Impatience; of / **Jealousy** / Light; of / **Men** / *Mother* / **Music – religious** – Middle Eastern music / Numbers; of / Numbers; of – seven / People / People – black / Robbers / Rooms – white / **Scorpions** / *Sexual* / *Shoes – high-heeled* / Singing / **Spiders** / Strange / **Violence** / Water – pools of water; of / Water – pools of water; of – *dark and murky* / Wild / **Women – huge, black with wild and fierce face**

Physicals
- **Vertigo**
  - Motion – agg. / Walking – agg.
- **Head**
  - Expanded sensation – Vertex – cone going upwards; like a
  - Pain – accompanied by – Eye – pain
- **Vision**
  - Acute – night – night vision
- **External Throat**
  - Pulsation – Carotids
- **Abdomen**
  - Conscious of the abdomen – Pelvis
  - Pain – flatus; passing – agg. – cramping
  - *Vibration and power; sensation of – Pelvis; in*
- **Female**
  - Itching – Vagina
  - Sexual desire – diminished
- **Cough**
  - Barking – night
- **Chest**
  - Constriction – Heart
    - § Grasping sensation
    - § Hand; like a hand around her heart
- **Sleep**
  - Interrupted
- **Skin**
  - Itching – bathing – amel.
  - Thick – sensation as if skin were thick
- **Generals**
  - Bathing – aversion to bathing
  - Expansion; sensation of
  - Food and drinks
    - § Farinaceous – desire
    - § Meat – desire
    - § Sweets – agg.
  - Heaviness – Externally
  - Sluggishness of the body

Provers speaking as one

§ Wishing for **anonymity** . . . wanting to be **separate**, not merged into regular society. . . . Didn't want to be seen, would stay in the **shadows**. . . . Thoughts of homeless people who sit all day looking out of their **secret** worlds. . . .

§ Feel like *I don't belong or fit in anywhere.* . . .

§ Dream – [crawling through] a long, low **tunnel**, glowing red. I am afraid to close the door behind me as I crawl in. . . .

§ Greater strength of my boundaries-feeling *solid, contracted, decisive, resolute.* . . .

§ Desire for a contemplative lifestyle. . . .

§ Dream: My husband is making love to another woman, but I don't mind . . . Foreign men in expensive cars trying to pick me up. One is a judge. "I am not a prostitute!". . . making **flirtatious** and **sexual** comments. Saying how handsome he was and wanting to go visit him in jail. . . .

§ **Goddess**, wanting to rock us in the cradle of loving kindness, but there is something **dark** and **evil** she fears, some force that **covets power** over us.[30]

Clinical

Since two of the major themes to emerge from this provings are regarding *Secrets* and *Sexuality*, Herrick suggests the possibility that this remedy may prove useful for those who have suffered from keeping a deep secret, perhaps involving an aspect of sexuality.

"Rat has a fighting quality. They may lose it, see red and arms would be flailing. People would run away from him. Family was really important but they let him down so he joined the crooks, thieves and robbers – *they became his surrogate family*. But he also abused his own family. Family cohesion is an important theme; not being betrayed / on the edge of betrayal." (M. Norland)

Rats in human consciousness
The rat pack. The rat race. Really cooperative – think lab rats! Abused by scientific research.

Despised / Gnawing / Chewing / Destroying / Vermin / Dirty / Gutter / Sewer / Underground / Survivor / Prolific breeding / Tough

Talpa europaea (European Mole)

Phylum: Chordata.
Class: Mammalia.
Order: Eulipotyphla.
Family: Talpidae.

The mole is a solitary creature that will fight to the death defending its territory except when female moles are on heat and the urge for a partner overcomes territorial issues. They are the only known mammal in which the female has been found to possess features of both female and male reproductive organs. The mole produces very high levels of testosterone, which may account for their aggressive nature and look-alike external features. High testosterone levels promote bone growth that link to the evolution and development of a 6th digit that is in fact, a modified wrist bone. The gestation period for female moles is 4–6 weeks and they will give birth to 3–6 young each year. After just a few months of growth, adolescent moles will be totally self-sufficient and will leave the adult home to find residence elsewhere, taking over unoccupied tunnel systems or digging their own. It is during this crucial time that they venture above ground and become vulnerable to predators such as stoats, owls, foxes and badgers. Moles have been known to live to the age of 6 years provided they are not picked off by predators or killed by humans, most live for 4 years.

Proving by: **Misha Norland and Mani Norland, UK (2012).**[32]

Keywords
Hated / Persecuted / Trapped / Dirty / **Intrusion** / **Invaded** / Bullied / Indignation / Industrious / Busy / **Loathing** – oneself / **Anxiety – conscience** / Violent / Confident / Content / Determination / Efficient, organised / Disturbed; averse to being / Childbirth / Digging / Dirt / **Pregnant** / Noble / Tunnel / Needles / Stitching / Diplopia / Hemiopia / Wandering, shifting pain / Neuralgic / Shooting pain / Energy – excess / Squeezed; as if / **Emotionally immune** / Feelings-fatigue

/ Rats / **Revulsion** / Worthless / **Disgusting** / Irked / Encroaching / Disconnected / Downward spiral / Suffocative / Kill people / Bloodbath / Lurch of revulsion / **Maternal** / Babies

- **Delusions**
  - Alone, being
  - Body – ugly; body looks
  - Crime – **committed a crime**; he had
  - Dirty – he is
  - Division between himself and others
  - Forsaken; is
  - *Hated; by others*
  - Hunted; he is
  - Invaded; one's space is being
  - *Persecuted* – he is persecuted
  - Space – small space; squeezed into, she is
  - Squeezed – small space; into, she is
  - *Squeezed – throat; being squeezed, is*
  - Trapped; he is
  - Worthless; he is
  - Wrong – done wrong; he has

- **Delusions (new)**
  - Bullied; being – decisions; into
  - Hole – *descending a hole in the middle of her being; rapid downward spiral*
  - Large – he himself seems too – people will look up to him, and
  - Nature – debased by man; is
- **New rubrics**
  - Aggression – others, of; directed towards him
  - Content – eating – during
  - *Omnipotence* – sensation of
  - Irritability – conversation, from – casual
  - Indignation – intrusion, about; personal space, of
  - Mirth – family; with
  - *Thoughts – babies*; about

Mind
- *Ailments from – anger – indignation; with*
- *Alert*
- *Anger*
- *Kill; with impulse to*
- Interruption; from
- Menses – before
- Throwing things around
- Violent
- Antagonism with herself
- *Anxiety – conscience; anxiety of*
- Biting
- *Buoyancy*
- Cheerful – eating – when
- Company – aversion to – desire for solitude
- Confident
- Content

- Despair
- *Detached*
- *Determination*
- *Disgust – oneself*
- *Disturbed; averse to being*
- *Efficient, organised*
- Escape, attempts to
- *Estranged*
- Fear – injury – being injured; of
- Frivolous
- Giggling
- Grounded
- Indifference – loved ones; to
- *Indignation*
- *Industrious | Busy*
- *Interruption – agg.*
- Irritability – company
- Irritability – conversation; from

- *Irritability – noise, from*
- Jesting
- Joy
- Kill; desire to
- Laughing
- Laughing – silly
- *Loathing – oneself*
- Mirth
- Positiveness
- Postponing everything to next day
- Responsibility – agg.
- Throwing things around
- Tranquillity – settled, centred and grounded
- Truth – desire for truthfulness
- Undertaking – things opposed to his intentions
- *Unfeeling*
- Vivacious

Dreams

Animals – wild / Annoying / Birds / **Childbirth** / Children; about – newborns / Children; about – **responsibility** for / Cut; being / Death – dying / **Digging** / **Dirt** / *Disabled people* / Dogs – bitten by dogs; being / Embarrassment / Escaping / Forsaken; being / Gambling / Guilt / Head – cut off / Helping – trying to help / Hiding / Injuries / Jealousy / Knives / Menses / Nakedness / Narrow place / **Noble**; she was / Outsider – being an outsider / Plants / **Pregnant** – being / Rooms – many / Stealing / **Trap** – being trapped / **Tunnel** / Unsuccessful efforts / Violence / Vomiting / Water – swimming in

Physicals

- **Head** – Pain
  - Sides – left – shooting pain
  - Temples
    - § Left – shooting pain
    - § Extending to – backward over ears
  - Vertex – extending to – Eye
- **Eye**
  - Ecchymosis
  - Pain
  - Foreign body; as from a
  - *Stitching pain – needles thrust into eyeball; as if*
  - Styes – Lid
  - Photophobia
- **Vision**
  - *Diplopia*
  - *Hemiopia* – left half lost
  - Loss of vision – headache – during
- **Nose**
  - Pain – Nostrils – right – cutting pain
- **Smell**
  - *Acute – urine*
- **Face**
  - Eruptions – Lips
- **Mouth**
  - Pain – Palate – cutting pain
- **Throat**
  - Pain
    - § Paroxysmal
    - § *Squeezed; as if*
- **Stomach**
  - Distension – eating – after – agg.
- **Abdomen**
  - Pain
  - Hypochondria – extending to – Ilium
  - Stitching pain – needles; as from
- **Female**
  - Menses – early; too
  - Ovulation – early
  - Pain – Ovaries – stitching pain – *needles; as from*

- **Chest**
  - Oppression – expiration – during
    – agg.
  - Pain
    - § Paroxysmal
    - § Mammae – stitching pain
- **Extremities**
  - Contraction of muscles and
    tendons –
  - Hands – Palm of
  - **Pain**
    - § Right – then left
    - § Neuralgic
    - § Pinching pain
    - § Shooting pain
    - § Stitching pain – needles; as from
- § Lower limbs – *shooting pain –
  upward and downward*
- § Wandering, shifting pain
- § Knees – blow; pain as from a
- **Skin**
  - Eruptions – elevated
- **Generals**
  - Morning – waking; on
  - Energy – excess of energy
  - **Pain**
    - § Cramping
    - § Cutting pain
    - § Intermittent
    - § Shooting pain
  - Pulse – slow
  - Wind – agg.

Provers speaking as one

ʄ I have enormous **industry** and **enthusiasm** for the **task**. I work all day, sort my children out and work again until bedtime. . . . The amount of **energy**, **industry** and **focus** is unusual as is the **detached** way I go about it without engaging myself emotionally in the fears and nerves that I had . . . I seem to have **endless energy** and enthusiasm to pour into my work. I am not tired . . . Very alert and efficient all day; getting many things done with a good amount of energy. . . .

ʄ I listen repeatedly to a recording I have taken of my son having a meltdown. I seem **emotionally immune** to it. Again and again I try to provoke a reaction in myself and it does not come. . . . *I have a sort of **feelings-fatigue**, I can't be bothered. I feel worn out on caring. I don't want to see friends . . . I just want stillness around me. I want to be apart from people. I feel indifference. It is an **absence of feeling**. . . . I don't want to sit down and talk to anyone, I'd just be going through the motions, I don't feel genuinely concerned. I'm irritable at small talk. It makes me feel "itchy" (restless), I want to leave, **I just want to get up and get out**. I just want stillness around me* (Common mammal themes). . . .

ʄ I don't want anything, I haven't made any plans for half term, it is just going to happen. I've usually got plenty of things I'm sinking my teeth into. I feel like I'm **switched off**. It is like being in a **holding pattern**. . . .

ʄ I have had more exposure than normal to **rats**, I am usually scared of them and feel **threatened** that they might attack but now it is more a sense of 'they are not interested in me'. I saw a seagull eating a dead rat and I found it absolutely fascinating whereas I would normally find it **disgusting**, it was picking the insides out from where the head use to be. It seems as if I **cannot empathise** with the dead rat, who has obviously met a very cruel fate . . . seen a large amount of road kill . . . and I find myself wanting to see more with none of the usual **revulsion** or **pity** I have when seeing dead animals. I feel distanced from their suffering. . . .

₰ **Feel dirty (unclean, need to wash), worthless, abandoned, miserable.** . . . (*Common Animal theme*) This guy is going to come at me at the gym. I feel like saying, "how dare you! **Get away from me**!" The prospect of having someone get that close to me. . . . It seems the grossest sort of **intrusion**. I'll either burst into tears or **bite his head off** and shout at him. I feel really really angry and I feel like crying. I find it difficult to think that I'll be able to *tolerate having him right in my face*. My reaction is extreme. . . .

₰ Now it feels like something's **got me by the throat** . . . like a **squeezing sensation**, an internal sensation inside my throat. It feels like a rubber ball being squeezed. . . . Stronger sense of people and things **intruding** and **encroaching** on me. I am starting to feel like the space of freedom, solitude and calm that I have in my centre is being squeezed or invaded. . . .

₰ I am **irked** by people turning up on the doorstep unannounced. . . . I wake up feeling annoyed with people and life encroaching. I feel *squeezed into a smaller space than I would like by my responsibilities*. . . .

₰ I feel very **lonely** and **disconnected** from everyone. It is making me feel **desperate**. I have **gone down a hole in the middle of me unexpectedly fast**. It is a **rapid downward spiral**. The walls of the hole have smooth edges – you couldn't climb out, it is inexorable. It is a bit like you are 'waving not drowning'. I felt like I wouldn't be able to articulate how I'm feeling, and there is **nobody around** *who would hear it, nobody would understand* . . . all I can see is a **tight**, **suffocative** press of bodies around me in the **dark**, shuffling and pressing. I feel like I want to **escape, urgently**. . . .

₰ Dream – I don't want to be part of the group. I don't really want to be there but feel some sort of obligation to be present. It is a confined space and I don't enjoy being there . . . my family insisted that I was keeping to myself and they felt I was **isolating** myself. . . .

₰ I want to **kill people on the street** when driving. They are not even in my way, I **just want to run them over**. Same goes for the dogs, I want to **kill** them, **stab** them create a **bloodbath**, get rid of them and my anger. I know being "red" or even "white" with anger but usually I turn against myself, act in a self-destructive way, but would never harm anyone or even think about it. . . .

₰ My husband asked me to pass the iPhone charger and as I passed it, a thought flashed into my head that the wire is most probably thin enough to **garrotte him**. I have absolutely no malice towards him and the last thing I want is for him to die. . . .

₰ There are very **graphic thoughts on the best ways to kill animals**; slitting their throats would cause them to bleed and die slowly and be completely aware of the pain whereas severing the spinal cord would eliminate the pain but instil fear . . . as I come into conscious awareness of my body **I feel a lurch of revulsion at how disgusting my body is**. It feels like my stomach lurches. I want to get out of myself again. . . .

₰ I feel **bullied** into decisions or into having to do things I would rather not must. . . . People have been *disproportionately aggressive towards me*. Where the level of aggression has not been warranted. . . .

◊ **Feel everyone hates me**, people I work with, family members, people in community. . . . **Self-loathing**, what am I doing, is it all worth it. . . . Every situation that comes up makes me question if I have done it right, or if **I have wronged the person**. . . .

◊ There are many **babies in my thoughts**, both in my dreams and in daily life at the moment. My sister, and several of my friends are having babies and there seem to be many babies around. . . . Lots of **maternal** issues around birth, breastfeeding and nurturing from my own past have been brought up birth in my dreams. . . .

◊ Pain in region of my left ovary. Feels like it is being needled. Intermittent for 3 hours. It seems like I'm ovulating early. I'm sure this is the same ovary as last month too. . . .

◊ Dream that I am pregnant, 4th month maybe. I see my belly expanding and I feel the child in my womb. It is a mystery to me as I never had sex with a guy, but of course everyone just laughs that off, not believing me. I worry about all the practical things like buying new clothes etc. . . .

◊ Sexual desire is still strong. Once is not enough. I wake my husband in the middle of the night. It is definitely on my terms. I am more keen and more dominant than usual. He is delighted.[32]

REPERTORY ADDITIONS FOR THE MILKS / MAMMALS
(to existing rubrics in Synthesis[11]):

- **MIND**
  - ACTIVITY – desires activity – creative activity
  - ADDICTED; TENDENCY TO BECOME
  - AFFECTION – yearning for affection
  - AFFECTIONATE
  - AILMENTS FROM
    - § abused; after being
    - § anger – suppressed
    - § disappointment
    - § domination
    - § neglected; being – mother; by one's
    - § position; loss of
    - § shame
    - § suppression
    - § violence
  - AMBITION – increased – competitive
  - AMUSEMENT – desire for
  - ANGER – authority; against
  - ANIMALS – love for animals
  - ANTAGONISM WITH HERSELF
  - ANXIETY – family; about his
  - ATTACHED
  - ATTRACTING OTHERS
  - BENEVOLENCE
  - CARES, FULL OF
    - § others, about
    - § relatives, about
  - CARING
  - CLAIRVOYANCE
  - CLARITY OF MIND
  - COMPANY
  - desire for – group together; desire to keep
  - COMPETITIVE
  - COMPLY TO THE WISHES OF OTHERS; FEELING OBLIGED TO
  - CONCENTRATION – difficult
  - CONFIDENCE
    - § want of self-confidence
    - § inferior; feels
    - § self-depreciation

- CONFLICT – within oneself
- CONFUSION OF MIND – identity; as to his
  - boundaries; and personal
  - duality; sense of
- CONNECTION; SENSE OF
- CONSCIENTIOUS ABOUT TRIFLES
- CONTACT; DESIRE FOR
- CONTEMPTUOUS
  - self; of
- CONTENT
- CUDDLE – desire to be cuddled
- DELUSIONS
  - alone; being
  - betrayed; that she is
  - body – out of the body
  - body – ugly; body looks
  - despised; is
  - dirty – he is
  - divided – two parts; into
  - emptiness; of
  - faces; sees
  - fail; everything will
  - family; does not belong to her own
  - floating – air; in
  - forsaken; is
  - laughed at and mocked at; being
  - light = low weight – – float; he was so light he could
  - light = low weight – – is light; he
  - looked down upon; she is
  - neglected – he or she is neglected
  - outcast; she were an
  - separated – group; he is separated from the
  - separated – world; from the – he is separated
  - superiority; of
  - unreal – everything seems unreal
  - victim; she is a
- worthless; he is
- wrong – suffered wrong; he has
- DEPENDENT OF OTHERS
- DESIRES
  - group together; to keep
  - suppressing his desires
- DETACHED
- DICTATORIAL
- DIRTY
- DISCONNECTED FEELING
- DISGUST
  - oneself
- DUTY
  - too much sense of duty
- EMOTIONS – suppressed
- ESCAPE, ATTEMPTS TO
- ESTRANGED
  - family; from his
  - friends and relatives
- FASTIDIOUS
- FEAR
  - authority; of
  - cancer; of
  - control; losing
  - crowd; in a
  - failure; of
  - narrow place; in
  - self-control; of losing
  - snakes; of
- FIGHT, WANTS TO
- FORSAKEN FEELING
  - beloved by his parents, wife, friends; feeling of not being
  - friends or group; by
  - isolation; sensation of
- FRATERNISED WITH THE WHOLE WORLD
- FRIENDSHIP – maintain; need to
- GROUNDED – not grounded
- HARMONY – desire for
- HELD – desire to be held
- INSECURITY; MENTAL
- INTOLERANCE
- LOATHING – oneself
- LOVE
  - children; for

§ exalted love
§ family; for
§ friends; for
○ MALICIOUS
○ MATERNAL INSTINCT;
EXAGGERATED
○ MEMORY – weakness of memory
– read; for what he has
○ MOOD – changeable
○ MOTHER COMPLEX
○ MOTHER FIXATION
○ NURSING OTHERS
○ PLAYFUL
○ PLEASING – desire to please
others
○ RAGE
○ REPROACHING ONESELF
§ sexual thoughts; about
○ RESPONSIBILITY – taking
responsibility too seriously
○ SADNESS – menses – during
○ SELF-CONTROL – loss of self-
control
○ SERVILE
○ SHAMEFUL
○ SOCIABILITY
○ SPACED-OUT FEELING
○ SUBMISSIVE
○ SUCKING – objects into the
mouth; sucking
○ SUICIDAL DISPOSITION –
thoughts
○ SYMPATHETIC
○ TIMIDITY
○ TRANQUILLITY
○ TRIFLES – important; seem
○ UNDERTAKING – things opposed
to his intentions
○ UNIFICATION – sensation of
unification
○ VIOLENCE
○ WATER – loves
○ YIELDING DISPOSITION
• VERTIGO
○ ACCOMPANIED BY – Head – pain
in head

○ FLOATING; AS IF
• HEAD
○ CONSTRICTION – Forehead
○ HEAT
○ HEAVINESS
○ PAIN
§ accompanied by
▪ nausea
▪ vomiting
§ jar agg.
§ pressure – amel.
§ Forehead – Eyes – Above
§ Occiput
§ Sides – left
§ Temples – pressing pain
§ Vertex – pressing pain
○ PULSATING
§ Forehead
§ Temples
• EYE – TIRED SENSATION
• FACE – ERUPTIONS – herpes
• MOUTH
○ APHTHAE
○ BLEEDING – Gums
○ ODOUR – offensive
• THROAT
○ LUMP; SENSATION OF A
○ PAIN – swallowing – agg.
• STOMACH
○ APPETITE
○ increased
○ wanting
○ DISORDERED
○ DISTENSION
○ EMPTINESS
○ ERUCTATIONS
○ NAUSEA – morning
○ PAIN
○ burning
○ cramping
○ eating – after – agg.
○ THIRST – large quantities; for –
often; and
○ VOMITING; TYPE OF – food
• ABDOMEN
○ DISTENSION

- ○ FLATULENCE
- ○ HEAVINESS
- ○ PAIN
- ○ cramping
- ○ dragging, bearing down
- ○ Hypogastrium
- ○ Inguinal region
- **FEMALE GENITALIA/SEX**
  - ○ LEUKORRHEA – yellow
  - ○ MENSES
  - ○ clotted
  - ○ copious
  - ○ early; too
  - ○ frequent; too – day – two days too early
  - ○ frequent; too – week – one week
  - ○ painful
  - ○ scanty
  - ○ PAIN – Ovaries
  - ○ SEXUAL DESIRE
  - ○ diminished
  - ○ increased
- **CHEST** – SWELLING – Mammae – menses – before – agg.
- **SLEEP** – WAKING – dreams, by
- **DREAMS**
  - ○ ACCIDENTS
  - ○ ACCUSATIONS
  - ○ AIRPLANES
  - ○ ANGER
  - ○ ANIMALS – wild
  - ○ ATTACKED; OF BEING
  - ○ CAR
  - ○ CHILDREN; ABOUT
  - ○ DANGER – death, of
  - ○ DEAD; OF THE
  - ○ DEATH
  - ○ DISEASE
  - ○ DISGUSTING
  - ○ DOGS
  - ○ DROWNING
  - ○ FAMILY; OWN
- ○ FIGHTS
- ○ FOOD
- ○ FORSAKEN; being
- ○ FRIENDS – old
- ○ GROUPS
- ○ GUILT
- ○ HIDING – danger; from
- ○ HORSES
- ○ HOUSE
- ○ INSECTS
- ○ JOURNEYS
- ○ LIONS
- ○ MONEY
- ○ MOTHER
- ○ MURDER
- ○ MUSIC
- ○ NAKEDNESS
- ○ PARTIES
- ○ PEOPLE
- ○ PURSUED; being – man; by / police; by
- ○ QUARRELS
- ○ RATS
- ○ ROBBERS
- ○ SNAKES
- ○ TEACHING
- ○ TIGERS
- ○ UNREMEMBERED
- ○ UNSUCCESSFUL EFFORTS
- ○ WEDDING
- ○ WEEPING; ABOUT
- ○ WOMEN
- **GENERALS**
  - ○ ALTERNATING STATES
  - ○ CONTRADICTORY AND ALTERNATING STATES
  - ○ EMPTINESS; SENSATION OF
  - ○ FLOWING
  - ○ FOOD AND DRINKS – milk – aversion
  - ○ HEAVINESS
  - ○ WARM – desire for warmth

References

1 Artemis Greek Goddess of the Hunt and the Moon. MammaliaGreek Mythology. Available online at: *https://www.greekmythology.com/Olympians/Artemis/artemis.html* (Accessed 23rd April 2020.)

2 Kalathia G, Hristova Z. Mammal general themes and classification *Interhomeopathy*; August 2016. Available online at: *http://www.interhomeopathy.org/mammal-general-themes-and-classification* (Accessed 18th September 2020.)

3 Hatherly P. *C4 Trituration of Lac humanum*. Brisbane, 2005. (Accessed in RadarOpus.)

4 Sankaran R. *Provings – Similia similibus curentur – Lac humanum*. Mumbai: Homeopathic Educational Services; 1998.

5 Houghton J. *The Homeopathic Proving of Lac humanum*. (Accessed in RadarOpus.)

6 Herrick N. *Animal Mind Human Voices – Lac delphinum*. Grass Valley CA: Hahnemann Clinic Publishing; 1998.

7 Herrick N. *Animal Mind Human Voices – Lac lupinum*. Grass Valley CA: Hahnemann Clinic Publishing; 1998.

8 Robbins P. *Phascolarctos cinereus (Australian Koala secretion)*. Australia, 1996. (Accessed in RadarOpus.)

9 Schulz E. *Lac humanum proving (vol. 1 and 2)*, 1996. (Accessed in RadarOpus.)

10 Sankaran R. *Provings – Similia similibus curentur – Lac Leoninum*. Mumbai: Homeopathic Educational Services; 1998.

11 Schroyens F. *Synthesis 9.1* (Treasure edn). Ghent: Homeopathic Book Publishers; 2009 (plus author's own additions).

12 Bailey P. *Lac Remedies in Practice*. Perth, Australia: Emryss Publishers; 2010.

13 Norland M, Fraser P. *Meles meles – The Homeopathic proving of Badger – School of Homeopathy*. Stroud; 2009. Available online at: *https://www.homeopathyschool.com/the-school/provings/badger/* (Accessed 23rd April 2020.)

14 Herrick N. *Animal Mind Human Voices – Lac loxodontum africana*. Grass Valley CA: Hahnemann Clinic Publishing. Unabridged edition; 1998.

15 Hardy J. *Lac medicines*. Havant: Available online at: (Accessed 23rd April 2020.)

16 Phatak SR. *Materia Medica of Homeopathic Medicines*. Maharashtra. (Accessed in RadarOpus.)

17 Clarke J.H. *Dictionary of Practical Materia Medica* (Vols 1–3). Mumbai: B Jain; 2005. (Work originally published in 1900.) (Accessed in RadarOpus.)

18 Ward J. *Unabridged Dictionary of the Sensations "as If"*. Noida UP: B Jain Publishers; 1995.

19 Smits T. *Inspiring Homeopathy – Lac maternum*. The Netherlands. (Accessed in RadarOpus.) Available online at: *http://www.tinussmits.com/3871/lac-maternum.aspx* (Accessed 21st April 2020.)

20 Herrick N. *Animal Mind Human Voices – Lac Equinum*. Grass Valley CA: Hahnemann Clinic Publishing; 1998.

21 Herrick N. *Animal Mind Human Voices – Lac Leoninum*. Grass Valley CA: Hahnemann Clinic Publishing; 1998.

22 Sankaran R. *Provings – Similia similibus curentur – Proving of Lac vaccinum defloratum – Skimmed cow's milk*. Mumbai: Homeopathic Educational Services; 1998.

23 Master F. *Lacs in Homeopathy*. Mumbai: Lutra; 2002.

24 Herrick N. *Animal Mind Human Voices – Lac loxodontum africanum.* Grass Valley CA: Hahnemann Clinic Publishing; 1998.

25 Hatherly P. *The Lacs – A Materia Medica.* Brisbane, 2010. (Accessed in RadarOpus.)

26 Chabra D. Proving of Lac felinum – Cat's milk. *Homeopathic Links*, Spring edition 1995.

27 Sommerman E. *Proving of Lac ovinum.* St Lukes Part MN: Northwestern Academy of Homeopathy; 2002. Available online at: *http://www.interhomeopathy.org/sheeps-milk-proving-sacrifice-without-reward* (Accessed 23rd April 2020.)

28 Sankaran R. *Provings – Similia similibus curentur – Lac caprinum – Goat's milk.* Berkeley CA: Homeopathic Educational Services; 1998.

29 Dam K. Proving of Lac caprinum – Goat's milk. *Homeopathic Links.* Autum 2000.

30 Herrick N. *Animal Mind Human Voices – Proving of Rattus norvegicus sanguis (Sanguis soricis).* Grass Valley CA: Hahnemann Clinic Publishing; 1998.

31 Bartig A, Humphreys N. *Proving of Oryctolagus cuniculus sanguis – Rabbit's blood – The Proving Collective.* Sheffield; 2009. Available online at: *http://www.hominf.org/remedy/oryctola.htm* (Accessed 23rd April 2020.)

32 Norland M, Norland M. *Talpa europea – The Homeopathic Proving of Mole.* Stroud, 2012. Available online at: *https://www.homeopathyschool.com/the-school/provings/mole/* (Accessed 23rd April 2020.)

33 Norland M, Fraser P. *Meles meles – The Homeopathic Proving of Badger.* Stroud, 2009. Available online at: *https://www.homeopathyschool.com/the-school/provings/badger* (Accessed 23rd April 2020.)

34 Fatula O. *The Homeopathic Proving of Pantheris pardus sanguis – Blood of the leopard.* Russia, 2005. (Accessed in RadarOpus.)

35 Robbins P. *Phascolarctos cinereus (Australian Koala secretion).* Australia, 1996. (Accessed in RadarOpus.)

36 Fraser P. *Personal communications* (August, 2020).

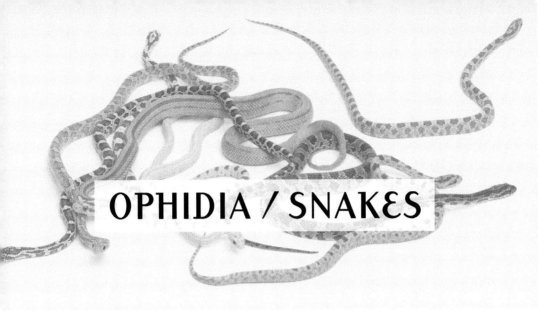

OPHIDIA / SNAKES

MYTHOLOGY

The serpent's role in the bible is to tempt Eve into transgressing God's wishes leading to separation and the beginning of psoric suffering. The serpent is a potent symbol of death and rebirth; the snake eating its own head. "In the Judeo-Christian creation myth the snake is portrayed as the evil tempter and seducer, the very personification of deception and intrigue, premeditating and perpetrating the downfall of mankind. Aptly it is coiled round the Tree of Knowledge, or of Intellect, and induces Adam, via Eve, to partake of the fruit and lose his innocence." [Lilley][1] Biting of the fruit takes you out of paradise into a world of ambiguity and division – noticing the difference between opposites. Male and female, good and evil. Coming out of the dream world into the trappings of dualism. Snake influence gives us the knowledge that makes suffering known to humanity.

Pluto / Hades

Dissolution of form. Syphilitic. Destruction – end of struggle, go out fighting. Custodian of the underworld. This is the realm of total transformation, of death and rebirth; the power can feel absolutely immense (*cf. Actinides*). The lens of Pluto is to see a world of extreme forces; the theme of subconscious power is very strong and there is an urge to transform the outgrown compulsions of the self in order to access the hidden magic of the mystical, occult or taboo.

Qualities

Tyranny, Destructiveness, Chaos.
Transformation, Rebirth. Taboo, Occult.
Obsessive-compulsive, Perversion, Depth.
Suicidal, Psychosis, Criminal, Genius.
Underworld, Death, Annihilation.
Rapes Persephone. Crisis. Survival or death.

Mars – Pluto

Fighting to the death. Compulsive winning. Assertion of power from the underworld. Sexual power. Buried rage. Subconscious rage.

Affinities / pathologies for Scorpio (ruled by Pluto)

Syphilis, rupture, scurvy, fistula, piles, disease – womb and uterus, reproductive system, prostate, nasal catarrh, mucous membranes, nasal cartilage.

SNAKES IN HOMEOPATHY

The Snakes resurfaced from the caverns of the underworld having undergone some major physiological changes during the reign of the dinosaurs. For example, their eyes are always open and they lost their limbs to slither into ever smaller cracks and crevices. Some people bestow the quality of wisdom upon the snakes, because they never shut their eyes – they are always seeing everything. In their underground environment, they wouldn't have needed their eyes. In order to find prey, they will track you down by the vibrations of your heartbeat and then suddenly strike, without you even knowing you were in danger. It is a venom that kills you through your blood stream; your borders are penetrated at a very deep level. Snake venom gets into your system and poisons you, making you toxic. At a psychological level, this leads to a state of suspiciousness and paranoia; the delusion that you're about to receive an injury. There is also the feeling of being under superhuman control; you've been taken over and it is controlling you. The venom has entered your blood stream – it digests you from within, dissolving your form, eating into you.

Injured, vulnerable and withdrawn vs. self-aggrandisement, one-upmanship and rivalry

Competitive; feels disadvantaged, injured by their surroundings; need to be cunning to survive. Conspiratorial, calculating, scheming and manipulating. These qualities may all be projected onto others and denied within themselves. The snake patient may feel 'injured by their surroundings' in the sense that the problem comes from those they surround themselves with. So long as the energy in the case corresponds closely with the theme, it matters not whether the patient denies or accepts these qualities as part of their own psyche; only that the feeling is of being manipulated and injured.

Repressed, suspicious, brooding *vs.* Loquacity, boastful, attention-seeking

"One of the first parts of the body to be affected by some snake venoms is the tongue." Fraser[2]

This theme expresses a tension of opposites between the melancholic and sanguine temperaments. When decompensated, the closed, brooding type may suddenly become loquacious and attention-seeking or vice versa. If left untreated, this tension of opposites can progress to bipolar states, or manic-depression as it used to be known. It is interesting that one of the single remedy delusions of Black mamba is that she is not understood. So, whilst on the one hand we have the famous loquacity of Lachesis, other snake remedies can express the feeling that they are not heard, that their opinions do not count; and that their manner of conveying themselves is not accepted or understood.

Purity and goodness *vs.* Jealousy and desire

Kundalini energy, religiosity and spirituality *vs.* Perversity and sexual power.
Split in the mind, or antagonism with himself. Religious / spiritual interest.

Clairvoyance, under a powerful influence / superhuman control

Instinctive and intuitive understanding of hidden motives.
Awareness of or infatuation with their own and others' subconscious desires.
Attracted to the taboo, occult and mysticism. Dreams about dead people / spirits.
When unaware of these impulses, they are channelled instead through physical / mental pathology (somatisation).

General symptoms

- Sensation of a lump in the throat (*Prey is swallowed whole*). Swallowing agg.
- Symptoms often take effect at the throat (where slightest restriction <)
- Restriction agg. Tight clothing < *"feeling restricted pushes me to the limit. . . . I cannot be dictated to."*
- Cyclical release of inhibitions – shedding the skin. Periodicity. amel. after menses.
- Spasm – 'sensation of a ball' amel. by eating solids.
- Complaints of nervous system and circulation.
- High blood pressure, left / right-sided ailments, depression, apoplexy, suicidal disposition.
- Congestion; swollen sensation, ulceration, erysipelas, necrosis, haemorrhage, paralysis.
- In mannerisms, dress sense and speech they can be vivid, imaginative and colourful.

- Strong fear of water and drowning. Strong fear and dreams of snakes.
- Sensitive to temperature. Worse after sleep. Sleeps into an aggravation.
- One sided symptoms. Lachesis is left sided, Crotalus right sided.
- Dissolution of form / necrosis; mainly syphilitic miasm.
- Ailments from blood loss.

MAPPA MUNDI

Melancholic – Sanguine

Constriction *vs.* Haemorrhagic tendency.
Injured, vulnerable, withdrawn *vs.* Self-aggrandisement, one-upmanship, rivalry.
Purity and goodness *vs.* Jealousy and desire.
Repressed, suspicious, silently brooding *vs.* Loquacity, boastful, attention seeking.

Air – Fire

Delusion-divided into two parts, antagonism with oneself;
vs. Delusion – under a powerful influence.
Neurotoxic.

Mappa Mundi themes

Melancholic

Clothes feel too restrictive.
Throat – cannot bear any pressure; constant swallowing when suppressed.

Sanguine

Discharges amel., After menses amel.
Haemorrhagic Poison.

Fire

Increased flow of ideas.
Powerful imagination.
Clairvoyance.
Increased amorousness.
Cyclical release of inhibitions.
Originality.
Sensitive to music.
Ecstatic.
Religious / spiritual inclinations – particularly in Hindu mythology.
Naja has more of this theme than Lachesis.

Air

Indifference, loses train of thought.
Suicidal disposition.
Neurotoxic.

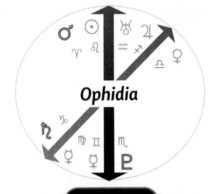

Fire/ Sky Realm

AMBITION - increased
CLAIRVOYANCE
DANCING
DELUSIONS - great person /
superiority
ECSTASY
FEAR - high places, of
IMPULSIVE

INSIGHTFUL
LASCIVIOUS
RELIGIOUS AFFECTIONS - too
occupied with religion
DREAMS - FIRE
DREAMS - VIVID
CIRCULATION; COMPLAINTS OF
THE BLOOD

Sanguine

AMOROUS
COMPANY - desire for
DANCING
DELUSIONS - enlarged
IMPULSIVE
LOQUACITY
MIRTH
DISCHARGES - amel.
HEMORRHAGE

Ophidia

Melancholic

BROODING
DECEITFUL
DELUSIONS - forsaken /
poisoned - he - has been /
wrong - suffered wrong
HATRED
HIDING - himself
JEALOUSY
LOATHING - life
MANIPULATIVE
MUTTERING
SUSPICIOUS
CONSTRICTION

Air / Underworld

ANTAGONISM WITH HERSELF
ANXIETY - conscience; anxiety of
CONFUSION OF MIND - identity, as to
his - duality, sense of
CRUELTY
DEATH - thoughts of
DECEITFUL
DELUSIONS - injury - being injured; is /
people - behind him; someone is /
persecuted - he is persecuted /
pursued; he was / pursued; he was -
enemies, by
specters, ghosts, spirits / wrong - done
wrong; he has
DESTRUCTIVENESS
FEAR - evil; fear of
FORSAKEN FEELING - isolation

HATRED
LOATHING - life
MALICIOUS
MANIPULATIVE
MORAL FEELING; WANT OF
STRIKING
SUICIDAL DISPOSITION
TRANCE
UNFEELING
WICKED DISPOSITION
WILL - two wills; sensation as if he had
DREAMS
DEAD BODIES / DEAD; OF THE / DEATH /
FALLING / FRIGHTFUL / GHOSTS /
MURDER / NIGHTMARES / PURSUED,
BEING / SNAKES
GENERALS - APOPLEXY

Figure 6.1 *Mappa Mundi dynamics for the Snakes*

THEMES

Shedding the skin; outgrowing the past

- Snakes are forever in clothes that are too tight.
- Feeling of being constricted and hating it. Any restriction aggravates snake patients.
- They are much relieved by discharge / release.
- Marked Periodicity – once a year they can change their clothes, shedding layers that come to feel restrictive. Cyclical waves (for example, menstrual and digestive problems).

The main sensation is of being strangled in their own skin. This is also related to the theme of *overstimulation seeking an outlet.* Vithoulkas[8] The famed serpentine loquacity is an important expression of this; everything that has been held-in eventually comes flooding out in gushing torrents. Snakes are better for expression, which is why they are often interesting and insightful people with an intense personality. They like learning, probing and investigating the hidden or deeper aspects of a subject – *bringing buried underworld treasure out into the open.*

Shedding the skin is a metaphor for the powerful urge to transform outgrown compulsions of the self; in order to 'grow' on a deeper level. This involves leaving the past behind; shedding one's earthbound, materialistic nature to explore the inner realm of understanding subconscious motivations – exploring their underworld power. *cf. Insects – they seek to escape their grubby earthbound nature to become airborne, experiencing the freedom and exhilaration of the sky realm.* Fraser[2]

Pluto in Astrology is a symbol for the deepest transitions in a person's life (where the old self is cast aside and that layer is shed). These upheavals sweep away attachments and give rise to a deeper understanding of one's life purpose. When an individual is unconscious of their own inner motives, a difficult aspect to Pluto is expressed as a compulsive need for power, often gained by underhand means.

Rubrics
External throat – Clothing agg. | Neck – Constriction or band | Pressure – clothes; of – agg. | Generals – Clothes – tight; too | Clothing – intolerance of | Clothing – pressure of clothing | Discharges – amel. | Fullness; feeling of – internally | Periodicity – year – every | Pressure – agg.

Intuition, inner conviction

Their gift of penetrating insight comes directly from the tree of knowledge. They want to get to the roots, which descend downwards into the underworld; the richest kingdom – where you bury your gold, and precious jewels. Hades is the wealthiest of the gods – all our resources are mined from the underworld. By over-using these resources, we risk destroying our planet (*Syphilitic*). The snake's mythological connection to the underworld equates to a dwelling in the subconscious realm of the psyche. Patients responding to Snake potencies can sense the motivations of others and are able to read into the undertones of what someone says or does. They can see the subconscious / hidden desires of others even if the other can't see it themselves (*clairvoyance*). This can be both a gift of penetrating insight or when failing, can lead to suspicion, paranoia and reading too much into everything.

> *I can sense what they're trying to do rather than taking the words at face value. They tried to pull the wool over my eyes. Feels really unjust. They react in a way that denies they were thinking in that way. . . . Instead of having to process thoughts, you just have this feeling. It is an inner compass that gives you a lot of conviction; there is no manoeuvring on it and that is the truth.* _{crot-c.}

They feel as though they are **under a powerful influence**, able to penetrate to the heart of any matter with their sharp senses. Because they are so finely attuned to the subterranean motives in themselves, they can sense it in others too. They have the guile and wit to expose others' shortcomings and won't hesitate to do so if they feel they have been wronged or unfairly treated.

Rubrics
Clairvoyance | Delusions – influence; one is under a powerful | Insightful | Intense personality | Unconsciousness – conduct; automatic

Competitive advantage and one-upmanship

- Threatening, competitive, cunning, self-preserving.
- Conspiratorial, calculating, brooding and scheming.
- Manipulative, jealous, suspicious.

These qualities may be disavowed within the psyche and projected onto others / society as a whole. Highly competitive, with the feeling that they are **disadvantaged** or **small**; leading to an inner conviction that they will require cunning or devious manoeuvres to survive. Alternatively, the patient may become **brooding** and **silent**; dwelling on the feeling of being **wronged** and **misunderstood**. Certain snakes can hold-in their anger leading to the rubric; ailments from suppressed anger, which contains both Black mamba (denr-pol.) and the Rattlesnake (crot-c.). Naja has the delusion – **wrong – suffered wrong** he has.

> *Feel that I am being fooled, cheated. Feel that I should take revenge, do to others what they have done to me. . . . Felt like retaliating at any opportunity, at interference. . . . If I was in this state (of mind) any longer, I should take up a martial art or fighting skill to survive street fights, or take the first strike.* _{crot-c.}[4] *Find myself frequently brooding over past incidents or over whatever happened in the day.* _{bit-ar.}[5] *Very, very upset [at the smallest hurt] . . . irritable; very angry; wanted to take revenge on everyone; was remembering past events and was giving it back; didn't want to interact with anyone. . . . At home I was being reprimanded for my snappish behaviour, for which I retaliated. Repentance for my emotional outburst. . . . They feel hurt and want others to experience the same painful feeling. Past offences are recalled with a lot of anger and resentment.* _{oxyurn-sc.}[6]

Rubrics

Brooding | Competitive | Cunning | Deceitful | Delusions – misunderstood; he is | Delusions – persecuted – he is persecuted | Delusions – small – he is | Delusions – wrong – suffered wrong; he has | Impulse; morbid – violence; to do | Jealousy | Malicious | Manipulative | Striking

Power games

The Snake is a powerful predator, so the world out there is seen as powerful and predatory. They lie in wait and take down much larger prey when they least expect it. This is why Sankaran mentions the phrase "caught off guard" as being central to the way an ophidian patient may express their vital sensation. *"Felt it could be anywhere, and that it might come when I am **off-guard** and do something horrible to me."* crot-c.[4]

The theme of power is strong in Snake cases, they will want to **retaliate** against those who have wronged them (although duty-conscious Naja might suppress their desire for retribution until much later). There may be a core feeling of having been taken advantage of, **exploited** or **manipulated** by others. Conversely, this may be how the patient themselves treats others. As always, what one perceives in other people is often a projection of one's own sensitivities; we attract that quality in other people especially if we suppress it in ourselves.

> According to the Joshis[7], Lachesis correlates to Row 7 of the Periodic Table as it shares *the feeling of powerlessness, manipulation and destructiveness . . . crocodiles and snakes give the appearance of victims, but when we come to the deeper pattern we see the need to be in the topmost position, a need to have so much power they can destroy others.* This destructive tendency also relates to the syphilitic miasm as well as the Actinides. One Black mamba patient explained that they could *get so angry I could explode and destroy you [partner] and everything.* dendr-pol. One prover of Crotalus cascavella puts it in the following way; *A feeling of being tremendously exploited by my landlords; I felt that they were taking maximum advantage without giving me anything in return. Was angry; felt violent, near explosion. Wanted to destroy, smash up the building, set it on fire; could not hold it anymore.* crot-c.[4]

Rubrics

Destructiveness | Power – love of / sensation of power | Delusions – conspiracies | Fight; wants to

Clairvoyance, superstition; magic, occult, taboo

The clairvoyance of Snake remedies is well known in Homeopathy. These patients can have an interest in the spiritual world, or feel a connection to their ancestors, spirits or ghosts. They may have a fascination with the occult or shamanic practices or like to explore taboo sexual practices. In extreme cases, the workings of the subconscious may be played out in sexual power games such as sadomasochism.

Knowledge is power; the positive aspects of Snake energy bring you in touch with a sense of the divine by harnessing the subconscious power of the Underworld. This is expressed especially in Indian culture where the Snake is revered and upheld as a symbol of divinity. It has both creative and destructive power.

While in a clairvoyant state, he speaks to someone who does not answer. crot-c.[9] *Woke up in the night with the feeling that I had heard a loud noise, like a cow's moo. Then felt it could be a ghost. Was afraid to go back to sleep, to switch off the lights, to shut the window. Felt it could be anywhere, and that it might come when I am off-guard and do something horrible to me. . . . More religiously inclined. Totally dependent on God with the feeling that he will do everything to help me.* crot-c.[4] *Desire to read spiritual books.* ancis-p.[10]

Rubrics
Clairvoyance | Delusions – trapped; he is – underworld; in the | Religious affections | Superstitious

Ambush, deception and manipulation; surprise attacks

Snakes lie in wait, attacking suddenly, swiftly, ruthlessly and precisely from a concealed position; squeezing, crushing, choking, and closing in on you.

Snake are insidious, we do not see them as they slide silently into our world and often the first we know of them is when they bite us. . . . They also tend to be deceptive . . . they are unable to really control [their animal instincts, which] makes them appear predatory, violent and sexually aggressive. Fraser[2] *(cf. Mercurius and Stage 12)*

Like the snake itself, there is a singularity of purpose about the ophidian patient – once they have caught the scent of their 'prey', they are tuned in to every little vibration of its movement with heightened awareness. Yet the *unsuspecting prey has no idea they are being sized up for a meal.* In human terms, this may be expressed in **venomous (abusive) remarks** that cut right to the core of the other person. In a snake case, the patient may explain that they are the victim of such remarks rather than the perpetrator. However, the important aspect in terms of seeing an overall pattern of the snakes, is that the patient seems to attract this energy and is sensitive to it.

Abusive for 4–5 days without cause. Became argumentative. Desire to hit and strike somebody during an argument. Became unreasonable and did not listen to people in the family. ancis-p.[10] *Abusive – insulting – calls everyone a dog.* dendr-pol.[11]

Snake patients use their highly-tuned awareness of the subconscious to observe the other's inner weakness (or they feel that others are doing this to them). Because they can recognise other people's weak spots, they know how to strike where it hurts the most. They might take advantage of others through their knowledge of how to manipulate the hidden world of the subconscious and when they feel unfairly treated, they may be remorseless about injecting a venom that invades, stupefies, immobilises and destroys their competitor.

Rubrics

Abusive | Cursing | Malicious | Remorse – want of | Rudeness | Sensitive – weakness; to other people's | Striking

Bringer of death

Hades is the Greek god of the Underworld; the undertaker who takes you to your death. When Hades comes for you, there is no escape. *cf. Syphilitic miasm.* Snake pathology involves necrosis, ulceration, haemorrhage, neurological poisoning, suffocation, cyanosis, swelling, thrombosis, septicaemia, gangrene, fistulae, convulsions. In other words; serious, end stage pathology that can bring you to your death. An individual whose disease requires a snake remedy may not have progressed to such a level (and indeed one hopes not!). But, the manner in which their life unfolds and the way they express their experience will reveal a sense of despair or little hope of survival.

> *They are charming and frightening at the same time. They draw us towards them and they repel us. . . . The snake is not merely dangerous, it is a bringer of* [silent and remorseless death] Fraser[2]

Rubrics

Suicidal disposition | Wicked disposition | Apoplexy | Catalepsy | Cyanosis | Haemorrhage | Necrosis | Septicaemia, blood poisoning | Syphilis

Underworld; wielding subconscious power

The Mafia connection is also part of the underworld theme. *Crotalus cascavella* has the symptom – Sympathetic – Mafia leader; towards. Mafia power is corrupt, uncompromising and absolute, yet it goes largely unseen by the general public. It is hidden until you come into contact with it, at which point you have no choice but to submit or face a cruel death. Stage 12 has an affinity with the snakes, so it is interesting to see that Scholten's published case of Dysprosium nitricum (a *Stage 12 remedy*) had a dream of being fatally shot in the head by the mafia.

> *Because the snake remedies are so connected to the underworld, they understand what is going on in people's minds* [in a clairvoyant way]. Fraser[2] Alligator mississippiensis (another reptilian remedy – proving by Todd Rowe) has the following dream which expresses the themes of sexual power, mafia and underworld forces: *I was dressed all in black robes and my head was wound in black; I looked up and saw Donald Trump watching me through his window; he picked me up and began making love to me; then I had been taken by an Aboriginal looking man in his car; he was threatening me and I was fearful; next I was sitting on his lap and having sex; I knew that I would have two children with this man. . . . I headed upstairs as he was leaving and saw a good place to hide with the children; some men (Mafia or soldiers) were after Donald Trump.* allig-mi.[12]

Interestingly, Donald Trump's presidential rule in America does have ophidian undertones. He comes from the world of the hidden corporation (*Actinides, row 7*) and accuses the media of publishing 'fake news' whilst he himself rules through policies that divide and lead to malice. He does this through the medium of Twitter, where he seems to vent without any filter!

Antagonism with oneself, poor integration of instincts

It is like having an argument with yourself. I hear that voice in my head and start engaging with it, playing out what I would've wanted to say (after clashing with a friend). Think about it from every angle, giving my retaliation. The other person retaliates too. crot-c. *His mind wandered, but at last he got better, and was able to go out again; a short time after, having an axe in his hand, going, as he said, to cut wood, he suddenly split his own head in two; he had become insane.* naja[13] *Losing one's own identity being sucked in by the other gender . . . for women, they feel sucked in by the father . . . [Or there is a] release of what has been confined or cut off.* pyth-re.[14] *Was terribly frightened that some strange animal side of me would surface when I felt attracted to a bar dancer. Wanted the sexual indulgence but was afraid that it would spoil the image I had of myself. Had the fear that I would lose my self-control and indulge in sex.* crot-c.[4]

Rubrics
Antagonism with herself | Confusion of mind – identity, as to his – duality, sense of | Delusions – influence; one is under a powerful | Delusions – superhuman; is – control; is under superhuman

Loquacity; the forked tongue

Snake patients can writhe from one point to another like the animal itself weaving its way through the undergrowth towards its prey. Lachesis types are famed for their exaggerated mannerisms; vocal undulations illustrating their points with arcing hand gestures delineating the somewhat erratic train of thought. The excited manner of speech reveals an unabashed enthusiasm for the subject of interest; it can be a torrent of speech overflowing with vivid, imaginative and colourful explanations. Suppressed sexuality can be channelled into these loquacious soliloquies.

Rubrics
Loquacity – changing quickly from one subject to another

Kundalini energy and spirituality *vs.* Perversity and sexual power

Purity and goodness vs. *Jealousy and desire.*
Tantra is an art-form which elevates sexual practices to a spiritual level and can be a way to transcend the trappings of the ego, attaining a higher state of awareness by awakening the energy of the serpent, transcending material origins into higher chakras and Spirit. Astrological Pluto is an important symbol for all kinds of death and transmutation. One of the ways we 'die' is by losing our sense of isolated "I" through merging in sexual union.

The game Snakes and Ladders was *"associated with traditional Hindu and Jain philos-ophy contrasting karma and kama, or destiny and desire. The board was covered with symbolic images, the top featuring gods, angels, and majestic beings, while the rest of the board was covered with pictures of animals, flowers and people. The ladders represented virtues such as generosity, faith, and humility, while the* **snakes represented vices such as lust, anger, murder, and theft.** *The morality lesson of the game was that a person can attain salvation (Moksha) through doing good, whereas by doing evil one will inherit rebirth to lower forms of life."* (Wikipedia).

Dissolution of form, digesting things whole

Snakes swallow their prey whole – dissolving the entire form. In Snakes, the organs are one-sided and moveable to allow for digesting big prey. There are strong rhythmic waves and muscular spasms; winding and coiling motions. Snake types also have an innate ability to digest mental concepts whole without even having to chew. Their mind is the type that can grasp inner meaning without having to grapple with all of the basics first; there is a leap of faith and the knowledge is felt with an internal sense of conviction. Perhaps this is why it is hard for the more logically-minded to follow the multiple trains of thought as they spontaneously depart? (*Loquacity – changing quickly from one subject to another*). This can also equate to the precocity of children requiring snake remedies – it is as if they are born with an older nature, ready to tackle the adult world from an early age. From the moment snakes are hatched, they are ready to survive independently – in stark contrast to the experience of most mammals who require an extended period of parental nurturing and learning from their tribe.

Mental overstimulation

Snakes have internalised their organs of movement; one can extrapolate that physical movement is internalised resulting in overstimulation of mental processes and lethargy on the physical plane. Vithoulkas' essence for Lachesis (the type remedy for the group) is over-stimulation seeking an outlet.

The way a snake moves is often one of the things that humans dislike about them; the slithering and writhing is so starkly different to the way mammals move about. They have evolved to lose their limbs, gaining a powerful venom that renders prey immobile. This immobility could be said to represent the chemical opposite to the biological function of physical limbs which drive movement, resulting in paralysis of all movement. Gutman[15]

Touch / vibration

Snakes have a highly developed sense of touch, sensitive to even the slightest vibration. *cf. Spiders*

Venomous

The venom of the bushmaster is a potent cocktail of virulent enzymes, which are primarily destructive to the blood (haemotoxic) and the soft tissues (proteolytic and cytolitic), thus causing haemorrhage and necrosis. By contrast the venom of Naja, the cobra, which belongs to the family Elapidae, is primarily poisonous to the nervous system (neurotoxic) and the heart (cardiotoxic). These differences in venom action assist the homeopath in his choice of snake remedy. Lilley[1]

Snakes in human language

- Cunning, Deceit, Poison, Constriction, Slyness.
- Wisdom, Kundalini, Direct spiritual path, Revered or Reviled.
- Strike, Mesmerism, Sneak, Snake in the grass.
- Shedding your skin, A Snake in your pocket.
- Forked Tongue, Pit of vipers.
- Writhing, Coiling and Uncoiling.
- Reptilian – Cold blooded; someone without emotion. Only the reptilian brain is functioning.

Differential Diagnosis

Predominantly Syphilitic Miasm
Actinides
Stage 10–12 (Periodic table)
Solanaceae (underworld)

Umbelliferae (violence, fury)
Rutaceae (choking, strangling)
Dioscoreacae (coil / uncoil)
Papaveraceae (war, violence)

Snakes (Ophidia) - Remedies

adeps-boa-co. ancis-p. **bit-ar.** bit-cd. bit-ga. bit-ns. boa-co. boa-dum. **both.** both-a. both-ap. both-ax. both-bz. both-cr. both-in. both-jaca. both-jasu. both-n-ur. bung-cd. bung-cl. **bung-fa. cench.** ceras-ce. cloth. crot-ad. crot-ax. **crot-c.** crot-cr-cr. crot-d-t. crot-ey. **crot-h.** crot-lp. crot-v-v. dendr-ang. **dendr-pol.** dendr-vir. **elaps** hydroph. **LACH. NAJA** naja-ac. naja-an. naja-hj. naja-ko. naja-ml. naja-mo. naja-n. naja-nv. naja-pl. ophioph-hn. oxyurn-sc. pyth-re. toxi. **vip.** vip-a. vip-a-c. vip-a-m. vip-b. vip-d. vip-l-f. vip-l-l. vip-pl. vip-r-s. vip-ser. vip-t. vip-xt.

Bitis arietans (Clotho arietans / Puff adder)

Phylum: Chordata.
Class: Reptilia.
Order: Squamata.
Family: Viperidae.
Subfamily: Viperinae.

The puff adder is a venomous viper species found in savannah and grasslands throughout much of Africa. They are responsible for more snakebite fatalities than any other African snake due to their wide distribution, common occurrence, large size, potent (& copious) venom, long fangs, and their habit of basking by footpaths – sitting quietly when approached. They can be sluggish – relying on camouflage for protection – but when agitated, they move with surprising speed in a typical serpentine movement. Although mainly terrestrial, they are also proficient swimmers and climbers; often to be found basking in low bushes. If disturbed, they will hiss loudly and continuously, adopting a tightly coiled defensive posture. Their strike is deadly, fast and sudden – the force of the impact is so strong, and the penetration of the fangs so deep, that prey can be killed by the physical trauma alone. The venom is toxic to cells. Effects of bites are divided into two categories: those with little or no surface extravasation, and those with haemorrhages evident as ecchymoses, bleeding and swelling. Both cause severe pain and tenderness but in the latter, there is also widespread necrosis and compartment syndrome. Females produce a pheromone to attract males, which engage in neck-wrestling combat dances.

Provings by: **Farokh Master, India (2000)**[5] **and Craig Wright, South Africa (1998).**[29]

Themes
- *Detached, spaciness, left-out, disconnected vs. Excitable, hyperactive, manic, overstimulated.*
- Sentimentality.

- **Depression, explosive** – *"feel morbid, apathetic, despairing and unable to cope. Feeling of greyness; heavy in my being. Had a sensation all day that people were struggling. . . . Felt drained by lectures – wondering how long I can keep all this work up. The depression was consuming and all-encompassing . . . depressed at the pointlessness of a lot of life. It is a hard, often joyless existence."*[29]
- **Split / divided** – *"I feel also an amazing split in me. I feel split between two images. As I lie in bed, my body is split longitudinally. Superimposed on the left side is a grainy black-and-white image of a woman; on the right hand side is a grainy black-and-white image of a man. Both images are equal in size and have indistinct features. I feel a physical pull between the two halves. I am aware of a conflict between the two – the one wants something from the other, but what it is, I am not sure."*[29]
- **Laziness** *vs.* **Cleaning and tidying.**

Dreams
- *Gambling* and getting things which are not really yours.
- **Shooting**, pursuit, impending danger, detached and helpless.
- **Ambiguous sexuality** – *"I dreamt that I had just made love to my girlfriend and I said that I wanted her to make love to me. Somehow she turned into a man – a friend of mine – and we were just about to make love when something interrupted. I was left with a strange ambiguous feeling about love and making love."*[29]

Perceptions
- ∮ Feeling of having *deep spiritual insights* into my world – a sense of *profundity*.
- ∮ Image of a *reptile coiled at the base of my skull*. . . .
- ∮ As if inside my body there is light which escapes through pinholes giving me a *tingly, buzzy feeling* where the light leaves. Specific areas have been my left earlobe and pinna and left eyebrow.
- ∮ I felt bloated and thought of myself as 'fat'.[29]

Rubrics
- **Mind**[29]
  - ○ Awkward – drops things
  - ○ *Brooding*
  - ○ Conversation – aversion to
  - ○ *Dancing*
  - ○ **Delusions**
    - § Body – out of the body
    - § Buzzing; everything seems to be
    - § ***Enlarged – body is – fat; feeling***
    - § Far off; as if
    - § Seeing – physicality of the world; through
    - § *Separated – body and mind are separated*
    - § Separated – world; from the – he is separated
  - § Snakes – in and around her
  - § Space – large space in the head; having a
  - § Unreal – everything seems unreal
  - § ***Veil – mind and reality; between***
  - ○ Detached
  - ○ Dream; as if in a
  - ○ Drugs – taken drugs; as if one had
  - ○ *Energised* feeling
  - ○ *Exhilaration*
  - ○ Fastidious
  - ○ Fear – accidents; of
  - ○ Fear – attacked; fear of being

- Forsaken feeling – *isolation*; sensation of
- Homesickness
- Hurry – occupation; in
- Sensitive – opinion of others; to the
- *Sentimental*
- Spaced-out feeling
- Stupefaction
- Thoughts – *two trains of thought*
- Untidy
- **Mind**[5]
  - *Ambition; loss of*
  - Anger; alternating with; repentance; quick
  - Contradiction; from
  - Violent
  - ***Approached; aversion of being***
  - Brooding
  - Confusion of mind; identity, as to his; sexual
  - *Contemptuous; oneself; of*
  - Debauchery; as after
  - Delusions; robbed; going to be
- Detached
- Emptiness of mind; sensation of
- Ennui, boredom
- *Envy*
- *Estranged*
- Fear; impulses; of his own
- Fear; self-control; losing
- Frivolous
- ***Greed, cupidity***; desires, greater than her needs; are
- Industrious, mania for work; frantic, hurried
- music; amel.
- Postponing everything to next day
- ***Reality; flight from***
- *Remorse*, repentance; quick
- *Shame*
- *Striking*
- Stupefaction, as if intoxicated; marijuana; as from
- Time; fritters away his
- *Violence, vehemence; rage leading to deeds of, agg.*

Clinical

"I had a small theme that indicated to me that the person who requires Clotho is: a very **lonely** man. **Unloved** by the family, society and world. **Mild.** Suffers from severe **depression** with poor concentration. These features are often seen in *old persons living all alone and who have been deserted by their family members. . . .*"[5]

Dreams[29]

Aggressive / Amorous / Anger / Boat / Boat – foundering / **Cheating** / Children; about – newborns / **Coition – girlfriend who turns into a man; with** / Dead bodies / Death / Escaping – unable to / Family; own / Father / **Gambling** / Guns / Helpless feeling / Horrible / Jumping – height; from a – landing easily; and / Kissed / Lift / Lottery / *Mother – hitting her daughter* / *Mother – **strangled** by her daughter* / Murder / Nightmares / Observing – as if, although in the dream / People – escape; attempting to / Pursued; being / Sea / Ship / *Shooting*; about / Shopping / Snakes / Teeth / Teeth – cleaning / ***Triumph*** / Unremembered / Water / Waves – **tidal wave** / Window – jumping from window

Dreams[5]

Animals, of; biting him / Calling out / Care taking; lady, old / Dead; bodies; lying on railway lines and roads / Examinations; failing an examination / **Failures** /

Gambling / *Mammae; bare, naked* / *Nakedness, about; man and woman, brought up on stage and beaten* / People, of; old people; old lady / **Pursued; of being; murderers; by** / **Religious**; discourses; listening to / **Riots** / Shoes / Shooting / Snakes; bitten by; of being / Urinating; of / Violence / Water

- **Physicals**[29]
  - **Respiration**
    - § Asthmatic – night
    - § Deep – desire to breathe
    - § Difficult – fanned; wants to be
    - § Sighing
    - § Superficial
  - **Chest**
    - § Oppression – respiration
    - § Conscious of heart's action – slower; as if beating
    - § Constriction – inspiration agg.
    - § Oppression – cough – during – amel.
  - **Ear**
    - § Equalising of pressure is difficult
    - § Stopped sensation – Eustachian tubes
  - **Generals**
    - § Anemia – haemorrhage; after
    - § Blackness of external parts
    - § Buzzing
    - § Electricity; sensation of static
    - § Heat – lack of vital heat – warm covering does not amel.
    - § Heat – sensation of – layer around body

  - § *Haemorrhage – blood – non-coagulable*
  - § Leukocytosis
  - § Necrosis
  - § Periodicity – week – every
  - § Thrombosis
  - § Wounds – bleeding freely
- **Physicals**[5]
  - **Head**
    - § Falling out; hair, alopecia; spots; in, alopecia areata
  - **Ears**
    - § Inflammation; labyrinth; inside
  - **Abdomen**
    - § Clothing – sensitive to
    - § Distension – constipation; with
  - **Heart and circulation**
    - § Palpitation heart – waking; on
  - **Blood**
    - § Coagulation – difficult, absent, hemophilia (*toxicological*)
  - **Skin**
    - § Ecchymosis
  - **Generals**
    - § Energy – lots of
    - § Fasting, hunger – amel.
    - § Sleep – loss of; from

Bothrops lanceolatus (Martinican pit viper)

Phylum: Chordata.
Class: Reptilia.
Order: Squamata.
Family: Viperidae.
Subfamily: Crotalinae.

Bothrops lanceolatus is generally considered endemic to the island of Martinique in the Lesser Antilles. As ambush predators, they wait patiently somewhere for unsuspecting prey to wander by. With few exceptions, crotalines are ovoviviparous, meaning that the embryos develop within eggs that remain inside the mother's body until the offspring are ready to hatch, at which time the hatchlings emerge as functionally free-living young. The venom has toxins that can cause clotting, and bleeding in humans, as well as muscle damage and swelling.

Proving by: **Matheus Marim, Argentina (1996–8).**[27]

Delusions
- Alone; being – world; alone in the
- Body – out of the body – observe herself; can
- Consciousness – outside of his body; his consciousness were

Mind
- Ailments from – ***indignation***
- Ailments from – ***mortification***
- Answering – aversion to answer
- Anxiety – causeless
- Aphasia – paralysis; with – right side; of
- Company – *aversion to – bear anybody; cannot*
- Contradiction – intolerant of contradiction
- **Egotism**
- ***Emotions – loss of***
- Fight; wants to
- Forgetful – words while speaking; of
- Independent
- Injustice; cannot support
- Mistakes; making – speaking; in – words – wrong words; using
- Mocking – sarcasm
- ***Pessimist***
- ***Respected*** – desire to be
- Sensitive – want of sensitiveness
- Slowness
- Talking – others agg.; talk of
- ***Unfeeling***
- Yearning (nostalgia)

Physicals
- **Head**
  - ***Cerebral haemorrhage***
  - Empty, ***hollow*** sensation
  - Lightness; sensation of
  - Motions of head – ***swaying*** – to and fro – sensation as if
- **Eye**
  - Bleeding from eyes – Retinal haemorrhage
  - Paralysis – Optic nerve – accompanied by – Retinal haemorrhage
- **Ear**
  - Discharges – blood
- **Face**
  - Discolouration – cyanotic
  - ***Erysipelas***
  - Lockjaw
- **Mouth**
  - Speech – stammering
- **Rectum**
  - Fistula
- **Urine**
  - Bloody
- **Female**
  - Metrorrhagia – fluid
- **Larynx and trachea**
  - Paralysis – Vocal cord
  - Voice – lost – accompanied by – Tongue; without complaints of
- **Chest**
  - Embolism – Lungs; of
- **Back**
  - Opisthotonos
- **Fever**
  - ***Fever, heat in general***

- **Extremities**
  - Gangrene – threatened with blue parts
  - Milk leg
  - Paralysis – *hemiplegia*
  - Paralysis – Legs – sensation of
  - Suppuration – Legs
  - Thrombosis
- **Skin**
  - Cicatrices
  - Bleeding
  - Break open
  - Gangrene
  - Purpura – haemorrhagica
- **Generals**
  - Side – crosswise
    - § Right upper and left lower
    - § Left upper and right lower
  - Convulsions – *tetanic rigidity*
  - Faintness – frequent
  - Haemorrhage – orifices of the body; from
  - Hypotension
  - Injuries – extravasations; with
  - Necrosis – Bone
  - Sluggishness of the body
  - *Thrombocytopenia; idiopathic*
  - Wounds – heal; tendency to – slowly

Clinical _{Clarke}[22]

- Blindness – day / Bone – **necrosis** of / **Gangrene** / **Haemorrhage** / Lungs – congestion of /
- Tongue – paralysis of
- "Bothrops suffers from general confusion. Everything seems **foggy**. He cannot really grasp anything, has problems with expressing himself and articulating clearly. He may develop into a specialist of murky and unclear intellectual effusions." _{Neesgard}[21]

Cenchris contortrix (Eastern Copperhead Snake)

Phylum: Chordata.
Class: Reptilia.
Order: Squamata.
Family: Viperidae.
Subfamily: Crotalinae.

Like all pit vipers, copperheads are primarily ambush predators; taking up a promising position and waiting for suitable prey to arrive – although when hunting insects they actively pursue their prey. When lying on dead leaves or red clay, they can be almost impossible to notice; with such effective camouflage, they often freeze instead of slithering away. They exhibit defensive tail vibration behaviour when closely approached and are capable of vibrating their tail in excess of 40 times per second – faster than almost any other non-rattlesnake snake species. Bite symptoms include extreme pain, tingling, throbbing, swelling, and severe nausea. Damage can occur to muscle and bone tissue, however copperheads often employ a "warning bite" when stepped on or agitated – injecting only a small amount of venom, if any at all.

Historical proving by: **J.T. Kent, USA (1888).**

Fundamental delusions

- Asylum – she will be sent to (*cf. Lach*)
- Die – about to die; one was (*cf. Acon, Arg-n, Chel, Solanaceae, Thuj*)
- Enlarged – body is (*cf. Bovista, Snakes, Kali-br, Cicuta, Opium*)
- Intoxicated – he is (*cf. Python, Falcon, Limulus, Gelsemium, Nux-v, Nux-m*)
- People – beside him; people are (*cf. Ars, Med*)
- Persecuted – he is persecuted (*cf. China, Drosera, Kali-br, Spiders, Snakes*)
- Person – present; someone is
- Place – two places at the same time; of being in
- Suspicion: *that he is being* **plotted against**; her husband is going to put her in an insane asylum.

Dreams

Affecting the mind / **Animals – copulating** / Animals – wild / *Continuation – dreams; of – waking; after* / Dead; of the – children – infants / **Dissecting** – dead bodies / Dissecting – people / Exciting – starting; with / **Indecent behaviour of men and women** / Injuries / Lions / *Men – following to violate her* / Men – naked / Naked people / Nakedness / People – drunken / *Pursued; being – animals; by – wild* / Pursued; being – man; by a – violate her; to / **Rape – threats of rape** / Snakes – biting him / *Suffocation* / *Teeth – pulled out; being* / Terrapin / Walking

Clinical _{Clarke}[22]

Amaurosis / Catarrh / Diarrhoea / Eyes – swelling over / Headache / **Heart – affections of** / Leucorrhoea / **Menorrhagia** / Nightmare / Ovaries – pain in / **Throat – affections of** / *Vulva – eruption on* / *Vulva – throbbing in*

Clinical _{Ward}[25]

Abdomen not expanded / Aching nasal bones / Aching nose / Biting fly / Biting temple / Bloated intoxicated / ***Blood ooze*** / Bottle hypochondrium / Bursting body / **Chest distended** / Chest filling / Contracted abdomen / Contracted umbilicus / Cord hip / Cramping stomach / **Crawling** cheek / **Crick back** / **Die suddenly** / **Distended heart** / Dyspnoea dying / Edgy teeth / *Electricity scalp* / Emptiness stools / Fallen heart / Flushed body / Fluttering thigh / Fly crawling / **Formication** cheek / Heart fell / Heart sore / **Heart swelled** / Helpless cough / Helpless mentality / Hopeless mind / Intoxicated bloating / Liver warmth / *Rectum prolapsed* / Red hands / Sinuses aching / Stool complete / Suffocating sensation / Teeth edgy / Throbbing thigh / Umbilicus not expanded / Weakness eye

Characteristic physicals

- **Face**
  - Discolouration – ***mottled***
- **Throat**
  - Choking – sleep – going to sleep; on – agg.
- **External Throat**
  - clothing agg. (*Snakes*)
- **Rectum**
  - Diarrhoea – morning – waking with urging
- **Female**
  - Pain – Ovaries – motion – agg.
- **Larynx and trachea**
  - Constriction – Larynx – sleep – during – agg.

- **Respiration**
  - Arrested – sleep – during – agg.
  - Difficult
    - § Bending – forward – amel.
    - § Sleep – falling asleep; when
- **Chest**
  - ***Fullness – Heart***
  - Pain – Heart – extending to – Back
- **Extremities**
  - Coldness – Nates – night – bed agg.; in
- **Skin**
  - Ulcers – Spring; in
- **Generals**
  - Seasons – spring – agg.

Sexuality

"**Cenchris rejects man's normal sexuality and reproductive function. He rejects sexuality, as he does not want to reproduce.** He experiences sexuality as a violent infringement, as he is forced to reproduce against his Will … sexuality, and the circumstances around sexuality are experienced as punishment" Neesgard[21]

CASE 6.1 Post traumatic stress disorder

Patient: Male, age 60

Prescription: **Cenchris contortrix 200c**

Important expressions

∫ ***Bayonet first, ask questions later!*** (Animals).

∫ A lesser man would've committed suicide 7 times by now (syphilitic miasm).

∫ I've got more mental power, I am on the verge here of losing the plot and **ripping my limb off** so the mental power takes over and stops it (snakes have no limbs).

∫ I've had the ability to master pain all my life; it is there to tell you you're alive.

∫ My brain is trying to play games with me; verging on the ludicrous or the **fatal** (antagonism with himself).

∫ Gasping for air (suffocation).

∫ Stop breathing, put the pillow over my bloody head and finish it, get it over with (syphilitic miasm).

∫ Wake up as you've **lashed out. Sheer violence of lashing out** (Animals).

∫ **Used to dream in serial episodes** as a boy; of pageantry, castles and princesses. (SRP)
∫ Parents **destroyed each other** (syphilitic miasm).
∫ Life starts **falling apart** (syphilitic miasm).
∫ Unable to feel emotion / sentiment. Become promiscuous because you can't have intimacy anymore.
∫ There's **volatility, unpredictable, aggressive, threatening and violent behaviour** (Animals).

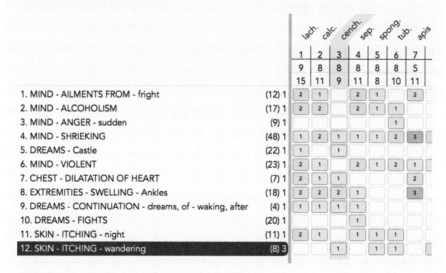

	lach.	calc.	cench.	sep.	spong.	tub.	apis
	1	2	3	4	5	6	7
	9	8	8	8	8	8	5
	15	11	9	11	8	10	11
1. MIND - AILMENTS FROM - fright (12) 1	2	1		2	1		2
2. MIND - ALCOHOLISM (17) 1	2	2		2	1	1	
3. MIND - ANGER - sudden (9) 1						1	
4. MIND - SHRIEKING (48) 1	1	2	1	1	1	2	3
5. DREAMS - Castle (22) 1	1		1				
6. MIND - VIOLENT (23) 1	2	1		2	1	2	1
7. CHEST - DILATATION OF HEART (7) 1	2	1	1				2
8. EXTREMITIES - SWELLING - Ankles (18) 1	2	2	2	1			3
9. DREAMS - CONTINUATION - dreams, of - waking, after (4) 1	1	1	1	1			
10. DREAMS - FIGHTS (20) 1				1			
11. SKIN - ITCHING - night (11) 1	2	1		1	1	1	
12. SKIN - ITCHING - wandering (8) 3			1		1	1	

Figure 6.2 *Analysis (limited to animal remedies)*

Crotalus cascavella (Brazilian Rattlesnake)

Phylum: Chordata.
Class: Reptilia.
Order: Squamata.
Family: Viperidae.
Subfamily: Crotalinae.

Crotalus cascavella is a species of venomous neurotoxic pit viper. Bites are almost devoid of localised symptoms and instead follow the pattern more expected from the bite of an elapid – with potential blindness, paralysis of the peripheral muscles, especially of the neck, which becomes so limp as to appear broken, and eventually life-threatening respiratory paralysis.

Proving by: **Rajan Sankaran, Mumbai, India (1995).**[4]

Fundamental delusions

• *Contaminated – being contaminated; she is* • **Deceived; being** • **Insulted; he is – looked down upon** • Voices – hearing – follow; that he must • Talking – people talk about her • People – conversing with absent people • Footsteps; hearing – behind him	*These delusions reveal the paranoia and suspiciousness of the remedy which, like other snakes, can descend into psychoses or full-blown schizophrenic states. The feeling of being under control by another is also expressed in that he must do as the voices say despite being deceived by them.*

SRP rubrics

- **Delusions**
  - Forced; that she is
  - Groans – hears
  - Great person; is a
  - *Outcast*; she were an
  - *Neglected* – he or she is neglected
  - *Small* – body is smaller
  - Skeletons; sees
  - Wrong – done wrong; he has

- **Fear**
  - Attacked; fear of being
  - Caught; of being
  - Coition – *rape*
  - *Falling*; of
  - High places; of
  - *Injury* – being injured; of
  - *Punishment; of – divine (single remedy)*
  - Robbers; of (*Ars.*)

Provers speaking as one

§ Feel others are wrong while I am right. Feel that others should listen to me . . . Feel **insulted**, *looked down upon*, treated as if I am **nothing, of no importance**. Was very angry, but didn't express it. Was disrespectful . . . Felt **inferior** in comparison to others. Felt that others laughed at me. . . .

§ Feel that I am being fooled, **cheated**. Feel that I should take **revenge**, do to others what they have done to me. . . . A feeling of being **tremendously exploited** by my landlords; I felt that they were taking maximum advantage without giving me anything in return. Was angry; felt **violent**, near **explosion**. Wanted to **destroy**, smash up the building, set it on fire; could not hold it anymore. . . .

§ Felt **sympathetic** towards unclothed, helpless **beggars**. At the same time felt **contaminated**, and reacted violently if they tried to touch me. . . . Felt tremendously **attacked** by beggars, and nearly started a street fight with them. . . .

§ Wanted to "**finish off**" the offenders with words and enjoy my **superiority**. . . . Felt like **retaliating** at any opportunity, at interference. Had the fear that I would lose my self-control and **indulge in sex**. . . .[4]

Other important expressions in rubrics

- Abusive
- Ailments from – *anger – suppressed* (dendr-pol, Staph, Stage-11, Germanium, Ign)
- Ambition – increased – *competitive*
- Answering – unable to answer – hurt emotionally; when
- Anxiety – conscience; anxiety of (Guilt)
- Censorious
- Cruelty
- Cut, mutilate or slit; desire to – knife; with a sharp
- Death – thoughts of – alone; when
- Deceitful
- Deja vu
- *Destructiveness – alternating with – fear of being harmed*
- Grief – silent
- Hatred – revengeful; hatred and
- Helplessness; feeling of
- Insightful
- Kill; desire to – *sudden impulse to kill – disturb him; those who*
- Mocking – *sarcasm*
- Orphans
- Plans – making many plans – *revengeful plans*
- Self-control – loss of self-control
- *Sympathetic – Mafia leader; towards*
- Talking – war; of
- Unfeeling
- Violent – *deeds of violence*; rage leading to
- Will – two wills; sensation as if he had

Dreams

Amorous – homosexuality – disgusted by / Astray; going / Attacked; of being – knife; with a / *Battles* / **Betrayed; having been – friends; by** / Brakes – function any more; do not / Caught; of being / Climbing – ladders – broken ladder; a / Coffins / Danger – boat capsizing / Dead bodies / Dogs / **Escaping – Mafia; from the** / *Falling – height; from a – pushed off from behind / Falling – ladder; from a* / *Fights – rights; for her* / Fleeing / **Forsaken; being – mountain; on a huge** / *Ghosts* / Helping – people – unable to help others / Home – away far from; being taken / Horses – drowning / Hyperthyroidism; having / *Indecent proposal* / **Jaws – stuck together** / Killing / **Lions – bite; which do not** / Lizards / *Neglected being – friends; by* / Peaceful / Pursued, being – Mafia; by the / Riots / Sailing / Sexual – *anal intercourse* / **Shameless** / Snakes – biting him / Snow / *Spiders – enormous, hairy spiders* / Teeth – *breaking off* / **Threatening** – professor; he is threatening his / *Thrown; being – high place; from a* / Twins / **Unimportant – being** / **Unsuccessful efforts – harm other; to** / War

Important physicals

- **Head**
  - Constriction – *armour*; as if in
  - Pain – Brain – pressing pain – ***bound*** up; as if / ***helmet; as if by an iron***
- **Nose**
  - Epistaxis – blood – bright
- **Face**
  - Expression – besotted
  - *Lockjaw*
- **Mouth**
  - Froth, foam from mouth – bloody
  - Paralysis – Tongue
  - Speech – difficult – heaviness of tongue
- **Throat**
  - Foreign body; sensation of a – swallowing – not amel.
- **External Throat**
  - Clothing agg.
  - Constriction – ***Thyroid gland***
  - Fullness – Jugular; in
  - **Goitre** – constriction
- **Abdomen**
  - Clothing; sensitive to
- **Female**
  - *Menopause*

- **Respiration**
  - Anxious
- **Chest**
  - Anxiety in – Heart; region of
  - ***Constriction – armour; as if from an***
  - Pain – Axillae – right – cutting pain
- **Back**
  - Coldness – Spine
  - Spasms
- **Extremities**
  - Coldness – Feet – icy cold
  - Paralysis – hemiplegia
- **Fever**
  - Septic fever
- **Skin**
  - Eruptions – ***urticaria*** – burning
  - ***Erysipelas*** – gangrenous
  - Formication
- **Generals**
  - Haemorrhage – blood – non-coagulable
  - ***Paralysis – right***
  - Prickling – Externally

Crotalus horridus (Timber Rattlesnake)

Phylum: Chordata.
Class: Reptilia.
Order: Squamata.
Family: Viperida.
Subfamily: Crotalinae.

The *Timber rattlesnake* is one of North America's most dangerous vipers due to its long fangs, impressive size, and high venom yield. They are reputed to have a relatively mild disposition, a long dormant period in the life cycle and often perform a good deal of preliminary rattling and feinting before striking. This snake became a prominent symbol of anger and resolve during the American Revolution due to its fearsome reputation. Different venom patterns have been described for this species: Type A is largely neurotoxic. Type B is haemorrhagic and proteolytic.

Historical proving by: **Constantine Hering, USA (1836).**

Delusions
- Animals – surrounded by ugly animals
- Brain – intoxicated; brain is – **blood; by degraded**
- Brain – softening
- Enemy – surrounded by enemies
- *Old* – feels old
- *Outcast*; she were an
- Specters, ghosts, spirits – **death appears as a gigantic black skeleton**
- These delusions portray a very syphilitic state indeed! The remedy is mostly indicated in cases of sepsis, haemorrhage and malignant states.

Mind
- Ailments from – *grief*
- Alcoholism
- Ambition – increased – *competitive*
- Anguish – pain; from – Stomach
- Answering – disconnected
- Anticipation – *stage fright*
- Anxiety – driving from place to place
- Aphasia – apoplexy – after
- *Coma* – septicaemia; with
- Decomposition of shape – rapidly
- Delirium – sepsis; from
- Delirium tremens – face; with red, bloated
- *Disgust* – oneself
- Fear – *failure*, of
- Indifference – *quiet*
- Memory – weakness of memory - expressing oneself; for
- *Misanthropy*
- Orphans
- Pain – head agg.; pain in
- *Senses – vanishing of*
- Speech – bombast
- Stupor – apoplectic
- Suicidal disposition – throwing – height; himself from a

Dreams
Anger / Animals – fighting – with animals / Anxious / Churchyard / Dead bodies – smell of dead bodies / Father / Frightful / Horses – drowning / Journeys / Murder / Quarrels – father; with his

Clinical Clarke[22]
Amblyopia / Apoplexy / Appendicitis / Bilious affections – fever / Boils / Cancer / Carbuncle / Cerebrospinal meningitis / Chancre / Ciliary – neuralgia / Convulsions / Delirium tremens / Dementia / Diphtheria / Dysmenia, or dysmenorrhea / Dyspepsia / Ear – discharge from / Ecchymosis / Epilepsy / **Erysipelas** / Eyes – affections of / Face – distortion of / Face – eruption on / Haematuria / **Haemorrhagic diathesis** / Headache / Heart – affections of / Herpes / Hydrophobia / Intestinal – haemorrhage / **Jaundice** / Keratitis / Liver – disorders of / **Lungs – affections of** / Mastitis / Measles / **Meningitis** / Milk-leg / Ovaries – affections of / Ozaena / Palpitation / Peritonitis / Perityphlitis / Phlebitis /

Psoriasis – palmaris / **Purpura** / Pyaemia / **Remittent fever** / Rheumatism /
Scarlatina / Sleeplessness / Smallpox / Stings / Sunstroke / Syphilis / Tetanus /
Thirst / Tongue – cancer of / Tongue – inflammation of / **Ulcers** / Urticaria /
Vaccination – effects of / Varicocele / Varicosis / Vomiting – bilious / White-leg
/ Whooping-cough / **Yellow fever**

Important physicals

- **Head**
  - *Apoplexy*
  - Inflammation – Brain – *Cerebrospinal*
  - Pain
    - § Unconsciousness; with
    - § Occiput – extending to – Spine and arms; down
- **Eye**
  - Bleeding from eyes – Retinal haemorrhage
  - *Ecchymosis*
  - Photophobia – light; from – artificial light – agg.
  - Inflammation
    - § *Erysipelatous*
    - § Media – followed by – *meningitis*
- **Nose**
  - Epistaxis
    - § *Diphtheria*; in
    - § *Whooping cough*
- **Face**
  - *Erysipelas* – periodical
  - Veins Distended – nets as if marbled
- **Mouth**
  - Discolouration – Gums – red – Margins
- **Throat**
  - *Gangrene*
- **External Throat**
  - Clothing agg.
- **Stomach**
  - Nausea – deathly
- **Bladder**
  - Tenesmus – vomiting, purging and micturition

- **Female**
  - Menses – late; too – six to eight weeks
  - Metrorrhagia – fluid / menopause – during
- **Respiration**
  - Difficult – constriction – Larynx; of (*Snakes*)
- **Chest**
  - Discolouration – spots – mottled
  - Pain – Mammae – Nipples – touch of clothes agg. – sore
- **Fever**
  - Remittent
  - Typhoid fever – haemorrhagic
- **Skin**
  - *Cicatrices* – break open
  - *Eruptions*
    - § Pemphigus
    - § Petechiae
    - § Pustules – malignant
    - § Vesicular – cracked, breaking

Ulcers
    - § Gangrenous
    - § Phagedenic
- **Generals**
  - Anemia – pernicious
  - *Blood – disorganisation*
  - *Cancerous affections – sarcoma*
  - Convulsions – apoplectic
  - *Haemorrhage* – tendency to
  - *History; personal – erysipelas; of recurrent*
  - *Thrombosis*
  - Weakness – diphtheria; in
  - Weather – hot – agg.
  - Wounds
    - § Injection, from painful
    - § Reopening of old

Natural behaviour

The rattle is a warning before they attack; to keep you away from the group. They defend their territory and their gang. An important point of differentiation from other more assertive snakes. Their smell is really strong (similar to Tiger urine). Used as a territorial marker.

CASE 6.2 Post traumatic stress disorder, blood-loss, trauma

Patient: Male, age 50

Prescription: Crotalus horridus 1M

Presenting symptoms
- Banging headache (as if struck on the occiput), and the sound of my pulse beating in my head so loudly. Swimmy, discoordination. Very ungrounded. Dizzy, floaty. **Concussed, hit at back of head.** *Feeling of not being of significance.*

Experience of losing blood after 3rd serious motorbike accident
∫ I've been going on for years about this feeling of **concussion**. Now it seems so clearly that it is the feeling before fainting. . . . I'm heading towards losing consciousness in a **drug-like feeling**. Intoxicating light headedness . . . yet a heavy feeling in the back of my head . . . as if I've been bashed . . . so its not concussion but the feeling I'm going to faint/pass out . . . this is also the seat of the headaches I've been getting. The horror, the horror (Apocalypse Now quote) **now I'm having to relive the horror** I experienced in the hospital after the accident. Fatally concerned for my wellbeing . . . taking it like a man at the time to be **trampled** by it 4 years later. So it is very apt for me to be feeling this so much . . . biting my nails . . . give it a bite. . . . WHERES MY FUCKING REMEDY?!

∫ Going through the **blood transfusion** thing. **Fucking vile**, the whole fucking hospital experience. Bad enough being run over . . . but . . . Been recording my descriptions of the incident. And must listen to them. For memory . . . Listening back – it knots my stomach. **I am still very alert** to the issue. **It is still very alive. Perpetually a bit jumpy and susceptible to people talking about horrible things. Repulses me – makes me . . . shy away.** . . . The sight of your own blood makes me go wonky and light headed. **The blood transfusion was like being invaded.** Half of the feeling was my body's joy of taking up so much needed blood. The other half was **utter disgust at invasion of a substance that wasn't mine.** Just letting a load of something into me that was foreign. **I had visions of places I had never been, as if from the other person's blood.** Very very unpleasant and unnatural. Like having a party, leaving the doors open and allowing anyone to come in to me. **Like biological rape. But life-saving** at the same time. . . . I hate the way the insurance company treats you. You think you are safe in the hospital to then find out you are not safe, not of any significance. It is just profit not people.

∫ I had a banging headache, with the sound of my **pulse beating in my head so loudly**. Massive. **Throbbing, burning** heat in my head. Hot and dry – **2/3rds of my blood missing**. Could see eyes moving away from mine. They were sorry or ashamed about the fuck up. The catheter bag overflowed on the floor. Nobody bothered emptying it. Did I ever raise my voice or say anything nasty to anybody? **I was in a state of needing. Being as needy as I was after you've been bashed.**

∫ **I expect care.** Is it asking too much to treat anybody with care / respect? People are busy. When in hospital, or been **injured** and can't earn any money. They leave you skint as well. When the cheque turns up on Xmas eve with your name misspelt on it. **It says; I don't care about you, that is 'fuck you'!** The machine is responsible, there's not a person on the end of it. Do unto others as you would like that done to your relative. Solicitors – they're not interested that **you're injured and broke** as result of their responsibility. Bitter, bad taste about the whole shebang. Very negative perception. Fuck you. Fuck it, fuck the whole thing.

		ars.	crot-h.	ign.	nat-m.	nux-v.	phos.	acon.	alum.	
		1	2	3	4	5	6	7	8	9
		5	5	5	5	5	5	4	4	4
INTOXICATED; AS IF etc...*	(164) 1	1	1	1	1	3	1	2	2	1
MIND - SUICIDAL DISPOSITION	(219) 1	2	1	2	2	2	1	1	2	2
MIND - UNCONSCIOUSNESS	(364) 1	2	2	3	2	2	2	3	2	1
Clinical - BLOOD, general - loss, of blood, ailments from	(45) 1	2	1	1	2	2	2			1
HEAD - PAIN - blow; pain as from a	(56) 1	1	1	1	1	1	1	1	1	

Figure 6.3 Repertorisation

Dendroaspis polylepsis (Black mamba)

Phylum: Chordata.
Class: Reptilia.
Order: Squamata.
Family: Elapidae.

The black mamba is the most feared snake in Africa because of its size, speed, aggression and sudden onset of symptoms following envenomation. Unlike many venomous snake species, their venom does not contain protease enzymes. Therefore, bites do not generally cause local swelling or necrosis, and the only initial symptom may be a tingling sensation in the bitten area. They tend to bite repeatedly and let go so there can be multiple puncture wounds. The venom is neurotoxic, with symptoms becoming apparent within ten minutes. Early neurological signs of poisoning include metallic taste, drooping eyelids (ptosis), gradual symptoms of bulbar palsy, myosis, blurred or diminished vision, paresthesia, dysarthria, dysphagia, dyspnea, an absent gag reflex, fasciculations, ataxia, vertigo, drowsiness, loss of consciousness and respiratory paralysis.

Black mambas are diurnal; basking between 7 and 10 am and again from 2 to 4 pm, returning daily to the same basking site. Reputedly unpredictable, they are also extremely agile – moving quickly with head and neck raised, allowing them to strike upwards at their prey. Their threat display involves gaping to expose their black mouth, flicking of the tongue, hissing and spreading of the neck into a hood similar to that of the Cobra. During this display, any sudden movement by the intruder may provoke the snake into performing a series of rapid strikes, leading to severe envenomation.

Proving by: **Rajan Sankaran, Mumbai, India (1994).**[23]

Fundamental delusions
- **Understand – being understood; she was not** (Single remedy rubric)
- Clouds – black cloud enveloped her; a heavy (*cf. Lac-c., Cimic., Adam.*)
- Injury – about to receive injury; is (*Theme of the Snakes as a group*)
- Persecuted – he is persecuted (*cf. Cench., China., Cycl., Dros., Kali-br.*)
- Strong; he is (*cf. Lac-leo., Hydrog., Androc., Plat.*)
- Tormented; he is (*cf. China., Lyssin.*)

SRP rubrics
- **Deceitful – blame; avoids**
- Abusive – **insulting** – dog; calls everyone a
- Answering – violently
- Delusions – penis – two penises; he had (*Syphilitic – perversion*)
- Fight, wants to – helpless people; for
- Impulse; morbid – tease; to – women – sexually
- Impulse; morbid – climb out of running train; to
- Impulse; morbid – hurt others; to
- Reproaching oneself – sexual thoughts; about

- **Other important expressions:**
  - Ailments from – anger – suppressed
  - Cruelty
  - Kill; desire to – contradicts her; the person that
  - Mirth – wretched; simulating hilarity while he feels
  - Quarrelsome – family; with her
  - Threatening

- **Contrasted by the following symptoms which reveal a more vulnerable side:**
  - Anxiety – family; about his
  - Delusions – forsaken; is
  - Delusions – worthless; he is
  - Estranged – cut-off; feels
  - Fear – high places; of
  - Sympathetic – black persons; for (*those who have been treated unfairly*)

Dreams that express the syphilitic miasm
- Beaten; being
- Drowning – man is drowning
- Murdered – being
- Pursued; being – murderers; by
- Stabbed; being

Characteristic physicals
- **Head**
  - *Heaviness* – Temples
  - *Numbness*; sensation of
  - Pain
    - § *Bursting* pain
    - § *Fever – during – agg. – bursting pain*
    - § Temples – talking – agg.
    - § Pulsating – accompanied by – Eye – pain
- **Eye**
  - Closing the eyes – desire to
- **Face**
  - Pain
    - § *Neuralgic*
    - § Jaws – Joints
- **Mouth**
  - Thick; sensation as if – Tongue was
- **Teeth**
  - Sensitive, tender – Incisors
- **Throat**
  - Pain
    - § *Swallowing – empty – agg.*
    - § Extending to – Ear

- **Male**
  - Masturbation; disposition to
- **Vertigo**
  - *High – places*
- **Larynx and trachea**
  - Pain – sore
- **Extremities**
  - Awkwardness – Hands – drops things
  - Perspiration – Leg – cold
- **Generals**
  - *Exertion; physical – ability for – increased*
  - *Hypotension*
  - Pain
    - § Appears suddenly
    - § Shooting pain
  - *Paralysis* – Muscles
  - *Pulsation* – Internally
  - *Trembling* – Externally
  - Weakness – paralytic – sliding down in bed from a half sitting position

CASE 6.3 Partner problems

Patient: Male, age 45

Prescription: Dendr-pol. 200C

Presentation
- Doesn't look at me throughout the consult and talks mostly about family situation and relationship problems with partner, rather than about himself. Cursing a lot. Head in hands.

Chief complaint
- Vertigo in high places – feels off-balance.
- Stressful family situation – 3 children with behavioural problems.

Suppressed anger
- "She starts laying into me – about my fucking job. You're aggressive, controlling, job is shit. I am absolutely fucking furious. She can throw all this shit at me but I can't say anything back. . . . She never said sorry – how the fuck dare you say these things and accuse me of not caring. . . . How dare you!! Emotional trauma – tit for tat."
- "She misunderstands me all the time. I cannot speak. Piles the weight on me – all my fault. Only thing making me angry – feel like my opinions don't matter."
- "I love my fucking children, how dare you think I don't feel anything, or I don't care. Huge massive emotional drain – afterwards I am fucked, could go to sleep, need to lie down . . . I don't want to go there – so I might not want to talk openly about things. Just want to walk away – curl up in a corner . . . Life just not worth bothering with. . . . Children's meltdowns lead to verbal abuse. . . ."
- "Eventually – I get so angry I could explode and destroy you and everything. How dare you put this tonne of weight on me. . . . Suddenly when things getting better – there's light at end of tunnel – you release a tonne of shit on me. . . . Can't see a release – there is no good option." (Syphilitic)
- "I am not a manipulative person – I am not intelligent enough." (Spontaneous denial)
- "Some bloody-minded person is telling me my failings but I can't reciprocate. The kids' behaviour – he pushes you – you want to squeeze his neck until he stops."

Analysis
Animals
- *Who* is the problem not *what* is the problem.

Snakes

- I am not a manipulative person. I cannot speak. I could destroy you and everything. Some bloody-minded person is telling me my failings but I can't reciprocate.
- Problem projected onto the partner.
- Squeeze his neck.

Miasm – Syphilitic

- Just when there is light at the end of the tunnel, a tonne of shit is released on him.

Synthesis

- Off-balance, misunderstood, accused & cannot reciprocate. He could explode and destroy everything.

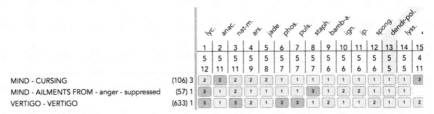

		lyc.	anac.	nat-m.	ars.	jade	phos.	puls.	staph.	bamb-a.	ign.	ip.	spong.	dendr-pol.	lyss.
		1	2	3	4	5	6	7	8	9	10	11	12	13	14	15
		5	5	5	5	5	5	5	5	5	5	5	5	5	5	4
		12	11	11	9	8	7	7	7	6	6	6	6	5	5	11
MIND - CURSING	(106) 3	2	3	2	2	2	1	1	1	1	1	1	1	1	1	3
MIND - AILMENTS FROM - anger - suppressed	(57) 1	3	1	2	1	1	1	1	3	1	2	2	1	1	1	
VERTIGO - VERTIGO	(633) 1	3	1	3	2	1	3	3	1	2	1	1	2	1	1	2

Figure 6.4 *Repertorisation*

		dendr-pol.
		1
		1
		2
1. MIND - ABUSIVE - insulting	(24) 1	1
2. MIND - AILMENTS FROM - anger - suppressed	(57) 1	1
3. MIND - ANXIETY - family; about his	(42) 1	1
4. MIND - CONCENTRATION - difficult	(466) 1	1
5. MIND - DELUSIONS - understand - being understood; she was not	(1) 1	1
6. MIND - FEAR - high places, of	(130) 1	1
7. MIND - IMPULSE; MORBID - violence, to do	(21) 1	2
8. MIND - LOQUACITY	(237) 1	1
9. MIND - QUARRELSOME - family, with her	(17) 1	1
10. VERTIGO - HIGH - places	(20) 1	1
11. HEAD - HEAVINESS	(452) 1	1
12. EXTREMITIES - AWKWARDNESS	(172) 1	1
13. GENERALS - EXERTION; PHYSICAL - ability for - increased	(3) 1	1

Figure 6.5 *Reverse repertorisation – Black mamba*

- Forsaken feeling; cannot depend/rely upon others, must do everything oneself.
- Black depression, as if surrounded by a black cloud, **as if going into tunnel that is getting narrower and narrower, blacker and blacker.** Overwhelmed by thoughts of death and accidents, esp. of relatives. Nothing can be done; nothing is left; no one understands; no point to try.
- Demanding that others listen and agree, but refusing to listen to anyone himself. (PARTNER)
- Deceitful, lying; avoids blame, or feels wrongly accused.
- The person tries to act maliciously by trying to torment and destroy the offending person's happiness. (PARTNER)

Elaps corallinus (Coral Snake)

Phylum: Chordata.
Class: Reptilia.
Order: Squamata.
Family: Elapidae.

Coral snakes are elusive, burrowing snakes who spend most of their time buried beneath the ground or in the leaf litter of a rainforest floor – coming to the surface only when it rains or during breeding season. Like all elapids, they possess a pair of small hollow fangs to deliver their venom, although they are not aggressive or prone to biting. When confronted by humans, they almost always attempt to flee, biting only as a last resort. Their venom, a powerful neurotoxin that paralyzes the breathing muscles, is one of the most potent of any North American snake.

Historical provings by: **Benoit Jules Mure, Brazil (1845); Lippe, USA (1859).**
Modern proving by: **Reinhard Flick, Austria (1991).**

- **Delusions**
  - Beaten; he is being
  - Injury – being injured; is
  - *Rowdies would break in if she was alone*
  - Talking – hears talking; he

- **Ailments from**
  - Abused; after being
  - Death of loved ones – child; of a
  - Grief

Mind

- *Anger – himself; with* – spoken to; does not wish to be (*Aurum*)
- Anger – violent
- Company – aversion to – *fear of being alone; yet* / *sight of people; avoids the*
- Desires – full of desires – *cavern*; desire to be in a
- Dream; as if in a – daytime
- *Forebodings*
- Nature – loves
- Playing – *desire to play – grass; in the*
- Sitting – inclination to sit – wrapped in deep, sad thoughts and notices nothing; as if
- Striking – desire – strike; to
- Talking – others agg.; talk of
- Timidity – *bashful*
- Unconsciousness – *conduct, automatic*

Dreams

Dead bodies – *embracing* / Dead bodies – *knife into wounds of; digging* / Dead bodies – *shroud; putting dead body in* / Dead; of the – relatives / Events – previous – day; of the previous / Exciting / <u>Falling – abyss; into an</u> / Falling – pit; into a / Fights / Frightful / Heavy / Journeys / Nightmares / Remorse / Vexatious / War / Weeping; about

Pathogenetic Ward[25]

Air pharynx / Alone apprehension / **Anus formication** / Audible swallowing / Bar loins / Blood streamed / Blue hand / **Bones coldness** / Boring eyes / Carried weight / Constricts abdomen / Contraction shoulder / Corset chest / Fever eyes / Fingers blood / **Fly ear** / **Heart tearing** / Ilium swollen / Instep fatigue / Iron bar / Lancinations toe / **Lung ice-water** / **Lungs torn** / Numb side / Peppermint larynx / Periostitis ilium / Plaster throat / Pleurae pulled / Pulled sternum / Pullings trachea / Raw occiput / Rising tibia / **Rolled intestines** / **Sink colic** / Sinking cerebellum / Sponge oesophagus / Temple body / Tube abdomen / Valve trachea / Valve tube / Vision moving

Clinical Ward[25]

Abdomen blood flowing / *Alone fearful* / *Anxiety alone* / *Anxiety horrible* / Backward blood flowing / Blood collected / Burst intra-uterine / **Carried weight** / Chill bones / Coldness lung / Constriction elbow / Cord intestines / Corkscrew swallowing / Crampy elbow / Deglutition arrested / Fear alone / **Fly meatus** / Food turns / Horrible happenings / **Intestinal strangulation** / **Laceration heart region** / Lung water / Restless head / Rough lids / **Rumbling ear** / Soreness hypogastrium / Sponge oesophagus / Spraining knee-joint / Sticky eyeballs / Stiffness knee-joint / Stomach sink / **Strangulating intestines** / **Tearing heart** / **Tearing precordial** / Thunder ear / Torn lungs / **Twisted bowels** / Weight arm / **Womb burst**

The up and down snake – Edited case by Gabriella Serban[26]

∫ Dreams falling, dreams falling into the abyss, dreams falling into the pit. From my Indian teachers I have learned that Elaps is a playful, rhythmic snake close to Palladium in its feeling: '**I must be perfect. I mustn't fall from the pedestal, everybody expects me to be there**'. (A hint of the cancer miasm – striving for perfection.) . . .

∫ How could she tell me something like that, when I put her on such a **high pedestal**, when she was my sister? I had such high expectations of her and now my expectations have fallen down totally. She does not respect me, does not feel solidarity with me in gardening, she quarrelled with me, she stuck me (sic!).

∫ I feel so humiliated, so mortified. If somebody has a quality I appreciate, I have great faith in her and if she lets me down, the whole castle falls down. I can never forget and never forgive, never. . . .

∫ I was the best of 500 students at school, I love competition, I put everything I had into my studies, always on the top, I escalated, I think high. Later on I went down in my studies, because relationships became more important, so I put everything I had into relationships. I want them to be perfect. **When this friend destroyed our solidarity, <u>I fell into the black abyss</u>.**[26]

Important physicals

- **Ear**
  - ○ Noises in – cracking – swallowing agg.
  - ○ *Perforation – Tympanum*
  - ○ Wax – increased
  - ○ Hearing – *Impaired – increasing – suddenly*
- **Nose**
  - ○ Discharge – offensive – putrid
  - ○ *Epistaxis – blow; from a*
- **Throat**
  - ○ Gurgling; esophagus is
  - ○ Mucus – drawn from posterior nares (*Cor-r.*)
  - ○ Pain – extending to – Ear – swallowing agg.
  - ○ *Spasms – Esophagus*
  - ○ External Throat – clothing agg. (*snakes*)
- **Stomach**
  - ○ Coldness – ice, with pain; like

- **Prostate Gland**
  - ○ Emission of prostatic fluid
- **Urethra**
  - ○ Discharge – mucous
- **Female**
  - ○ Metrorrhagia – black / fluid
- **Expectoration**
  - ○ Bloody – black
- **Chest**
  - ○ Pain – Axillae – right – extending to – left – cutting pain
- **Back**
  - ○ Pain – Lumbar region – lancinating – downward
  - ○ Pain – *Spine – whole – cutting pain*
- **Extremities**
  - ○ Paralysis – *hemiplegia – left*
- **Generals**
  - ○ Aids
  - ○ Food and drinks – ice – desire
  - ○ Weather – windy and stormy weather – before

Lachesis muta (Bushmaster snake)

Phylum: Chordata.
Class: Reptilia.
Order: Squamata.
Family: Viperidae.
Subfamily: Crotalinae.

Lachesis muta is a venomous pit viper species found in South America. Lachesis is one of the three Fates in Greek mythology and was supposed to assign to man his term of life – something this species is more than capable of doing. They are similar in appearance to rattlesnakes and vibrate their tail vigorously when alarmed, but owing to a lack of rattle, they were termed *mutus* (meaning mute). They are the third longest venomous snake in the world and are badly affected by stress – rarely living long in captivity. Their venom is both haemotoxic and neurotoxic, containing potent protein-dissolving enzymes. Envenomation causes intense pain, swelling, and extensive necrosis at the bite site, sometimes followed by gangrene.

Historical proving by: **C. Hering**, USA (1834–35).

Fundamental delusions
- **Injury – being injured; is – surroundings; by his**
- Crime – about to commit a
- Superhuman; is – control; is under superhuman
- Charmed and cannot break the spell
- Lost; she is – salvation; for

SRP delusions
- Persecution in delirium; delusions of
- Animals – being an animal right through
- Asylum – mental asylum; sent to
- Bed – sinking – she is sinking – with the bed
- Conspiracies – against him; there are conspiracies
- Friendless; he is – morning – waking; on
- Murdering; he is – has to murder someone; he
- Someone else – she were someone else – power; and in their
- Spied; being
- Talking – friends are talking about her
- Voices – hearing – commit crime; voice commands him to
- Voices – hearing – confess things she never did; she must
- Walking – behind him; someone walks

Key themes
- Suppression leads to a need to burst out
- Cannot be restricted or opposed in any way

- Clothing feels too tight
- Jealousy at somebody else taking the spotlight
- Jealousy at partner who has been unfaithful to her
- Suppressed sexuality leads to aggravation from loquacity – thoughts spew out disconnectedly, jumping from one topic to the other whilst others are unable to follow what are her normally lucid perceptions
- Feeling of being torn / divided into two selves
- Under superhuman control – is able to channel information gleaned from intuition
- Clairvoyance, able to impress people with gifts of insight into their nature
- In health – abundance of ideas, quick witted, charming (able to deceive and disarm others)
- Agg. from heat – hot flushes
- Sleep into aggravation / fear of sleep

Naja tripudians (Indian Cobra)

Phylum: Chordata.
Class: Reptilia.
Order: Squamata.
Family: Elapidae.

Naja is native to the Indian subcontinent and revered in Indian mythology and culture; often to be seen with snake charmers. The cobra's dramatic threat posture gives the appearance of a swaying motion to the tune of the charmer's flute. The Hindu god Shiva can be depicted with a cobra coiled around his neck, symbolizing his mastery over "maya" – the illusory world of form. Vishnu is usually portrayed as reclining on the coiled body of a giant snake deity with multiple cobra heads. Cobras are oviparous and lay their eggs between the months of April and July. The hatchlings are independent from birth and have fully functional venom glands. The venom acts on the synaptic gaps of the nerves – paralyzing muscles – which in severe bites leads to respiratory failure or cardiac arrest. The components include enzymes such as hyaluronidase that cause lysis and increase the spread of the venom. Envenomation symptoms may manifest between 15 minutes and 2 hours following the bite.

Historical provings by: **William Stokes, UK (1852–53)** and by **Russell, UK (1853)**.

No high potency provings so most symptoms derive from crude doses or clinical observations.

Fundamental delusions
- **Neglected – duty; he has neglected his** (*cf. aurum*)
- *Wasting away / Starve – being starved*

- Succeed; *he does everything wrong*; he cannot (*cf. aurum., bar-c., anac.*)
- Deceived; being (*cf. Crot-c., Drosera, Ozonum*)

SRP delusions
- Drawn – organs seem to be drawn together
- Rainstorm; she is in a

Common ophidian delusions
- Injury – being injured; is – surroundings; by his
- Superhuman; is – control; is under superhuman
- Wrong – suffered wrong; he has

Characteristic rubrics
Ailments from
- Abused; after being – marriage; in
- Abused; after being – sexually
- Domination – children; in – parental control; long history of excessive

Mind
- Antagonism with herself (*cf. anac, milks, gems*)
- Answering – *unable to answer – hurt emotionally; when*
- Benevolence
- Brooding – suicidal disposition; with
- *Bulimia* – nervosa
- Confidence – want of self-confidence – *failure*; feels himself a
- Self-depreciation (children; in)
- Consciousness – paralysis; with
- *Duty* – too much sense of duty – *children; in*
- Fear – death, of – pain, from – heart; around
- Impulse; morbid – *reckless* things; impelled to do
- *Insanity – split his head in two with an axe; suddenly wants to*
- Love – *perversity*; sexual
- *Rebellious*
- *Secretive*
- Sadness – *wrong way, as if having done everything in*
- *Sadness – superfluous, feeling*
- Speech – inarticulate
- Suicidal disposition – axe; with an
- Weary of life – unworthy of the gift of life
- Will – *two wills*; sensation as if he had
- Wrong; everything seems

Dreams
- Business – day; of the / Fire / Killing / Murder / Shameful / Suicide

Important physicals

- **Head**
  - Pain – Occiput – **blow; pain as from a / stunning pain**
- **Throat**
  - Discolouration – redness – Pharynx – dark red
  - Paralysis – post diphtheritic
  - Spasms – Esophagus / Stricture of esophagus
- **Female**
  - Ovaries; complaints of – left – extending to – Heart
  - Pain – Vagina – coition – during – sore
- **Larynx and trachea**
  - Paralysis – Larynx
- **Cough**
  - *Heart affections; with*
  - Sympathetic

- **Chest**
  - *Fatty degeneration of heart*
  - **Hypertrophy** – Heart; of
  - **Infarction**; Myocardial
  - **Murmurs** – cardiac murmurs – valvular
  - Palpitation of heart – speak; unable to
  - Weakness – Heart – About the heart; sensation of weakness
- **Extremities**
  - Cramps – Shoulders
- **Generals**
  - Complaints – extending to – Upward
  - Cyanosis – children; in – infants
  - Riding – streetcar; on a – amel.

A perusal of the characteristic Mind rubrics for Naja reveal the sensitivity of the remedy, and the **capacity for feeling as though one has failed**, not only to stand up for oneself, but also if one does give in to the temptation to fight back against aggressors that one will have failed in a higher sense of their spiritual desire to transcend such acts of vengeance. There is a need for tolerance rather than violence.

Rajan Sankaran writes that "Lachesis comes from South America where people are extroverted, expressive, communicative and have a strong ego – whereas Naja comes from India where people are subdued, suppressed and wronged, but yet are known to be spiritual, responsible and duty conscious."[16] This seems to relate to the Cobra as a god in Hindu Mythology, and so there is an idea of nobility, perhaps similar to Aurum where the urge to strike back is suppressed due to a feeling of spirituality or heightened responsibility (especially for the family, which came through in the proving) – as Sankaran describes – "Its unique feature is its feeling of duty consciousness. Naja people have a certain quality of nobility about them, of morality, of responsibility. Often this feeling is in conflict with the feeling of having suffered wrong and neglect, with intense feelings of malice and impulse to neglect or harm the offending person."[17]

However, there is a kind of duality inherent in the remedy, in that the Indian Cobra is used by the snake charmer, presumably not only for its mesmerising movements but also because this is a snake that really does not like to attack. It can put up with a lot of abuse before it will, and even then it usually only feigns to strike or uses a small amount of poison so that it isn't a fatal dose. Naja appears to be very different in essence to Lachesis and many other snakes, as observed by Farokh Master – "the species is very reluctant to bite, and even when it does, it fails to inject venom in more than half of the bites . . . it will make every attempt to escape or may feign death. . . . The temperament is completely different from Lachesis. Not the intensity, hatefulness, and aggressiveness. . . . It can be understood that these people have a lot of tolerance and do not easily retaliate. There is a lot of grief inside, which becomes the most important causative factor, they may want to retaliate after a lot of harassment but they are so duty bound that on one side they want to get back with the person (i.e. take revenge) but on the other side want to perform their work dutifully."[18]

Fear of failure naturally springs from a place where a person has a sense that they are of importance – (Delusion – great person he is / Ailments from Egotism), indeed the snake family have a theme of Superior / Inferior according to Sankaran.[19] This importance is of a spiritual nature in Cobra, given its place in Hindu scripture as representing Kundalini energy which ascends the chakras to reach towards enlightenment.

Python regius (Ball python)

Phylum: Chordata.
Class: Reptilia.
Order: Squamata.
Family: Pythonidae.

This terrestrial species is known for its defence strategy that involves coiling into a tight ball when threatened, with its head and neck tucked away in the middle. In this state, it can literally be rolled around. Favoured retreats include mammal burrows and other underground burrows. In captivity, they are considered good pets, with their relatively small size and placid nature making them easy to handle. The ball python is particularly revered by the Igbo people in southeastern Nigeria, who consider it symbolic of the earth, being an animal that travels so close to the ground. They let them roam or pick them up gently and return them to a forest or field away from houses.

Proving by: **Brigitte Klotzsch, Germany (2001).**[14]

Key words
Betrayed / Old / Forced / Paralysed / Animal consciousness / Confident / Control; losing / Strangled / Suicidal / Trance / Recognition / Burden / Ugly / As if under a blanket / Vortex / Whirlpool

G. Johnson[14]
"The essence of Python regia is that the powerful and the powerless exist in a mutually dependent relationship where the former smothers the latter. The python is dependent on her rodent prey, but in order to use them she must smother them. There is a state of clinging to / being addicted to their partner and in the relationship one is powerful and one is powerless (*cf.* Adamas). The

partners may lose their own feelings and take on those of the other. The powerful feels as bracketed together and dependent as the powerless, so it is a remedy to consider giving to both partners. The child may feel totally addicted to the parents and must visit them frequently. There is also a male / female power struggle. There may be too much responsibility expected at a young age, or a refusal to accept responsibility."

Delusions

- Alone; being
- Betrayed; that she is
- Body – ugly; body looks – fat; too
- *Divided* – two parts; into (*as if his body had a life of its own*)
- Experiences everything as if *under a blanket* (*transfixed under the bedclothes*)
- Floating – air; in (Hovering)
- *Forced*; that she is
- Influence; one is under a powerful
- Insane – he is insane
- Intoxicated – she will be; taking the remedy; by
- *Move – not move; he could* (As if *rooted to the spot*)
- *Old* – feels old
- *Paralysed; he is* (*arms and legs; of being*)
- Poor; he is
- Pulled – he was – downward
- Separated – body – mind are separated; body and
- *Sucked up; she is being* (*Into a whirlpool or vortex*)
- Superhuman; is – control; is under superhuman
- Woman will force men to have sex
- *Young*; she is again

Mind

- Activity – desires activity / Busy
- **Animal consciousness** (Snake; she is a)
- Ardent
- Clairvoyance
- *Cleanness – mania for / Order – desire for*
- Company – desire for – family; of his
- Concentration – difficult – studying
- **Confident**
- Egotism
- Emotions – strong; too
- Emotions – suppressed
- *Estranged – family; from his*

Fear

- **Control; losing** / *Self-control; of losing*
- Happen; something will – terrible is going to happen; something
- *Malicious, being – hurting other people's feelings*
- Starving; of
- *Strangled; to be*
- *Suffocation, of*
- Water; of – running water; of (*Whirlpool*)

Mind (continued)

- Forgetful – possessions; leaves behind
- Forsaken feeling – isolation; sensation
- Hysteria
- Industrious
- Late – too late; always
- **Laughing**
  - *Causeless*
  - *Embarrassing situations; in*
  - *Hysterical*
  - *Mocking*
  - *Sardonic*
- Marriage – unendurable; idea of marriage seemed
- Mistakes; making – speaking; in – words – misplacing words
- Mocking
- Prophesying
- ***Recognition***; *desire for*
- Reproaching oneself – poor; for being / fat; for being / crazy for being
- *Sadness – **burden**; as from a*
- Sadness – causeless
- Self-control – loss of self-control
- Self-esteem – high
- Sociability
- ***Staring, thoughtless***
- Suicidal disposition – thoughts – ***restrains himself because of his duties to his family*** (*Nat-s.*)
- Suspicious – medicine; will not take
- Timidity – bashful
- Touched – aversion to be
- Trance
- Work – impossible

Dreams

"I left my house to go and get something. My husband came after me, all concerned. I ended up in a **sex hell**. All the people were pale and naked. I watched them from a distance as if they were on TV. They were painted white. The woman had two rivulets of blood which ran down the front of the abdomen to the right and to the left. The woman screamed and he fucked her standing up and I got a close up as he entered her with his penis. She seemed to sort of hover in front of him. I wasn't bothered much by it. I seemed to keep an emotional distance. . . ."[14]

Clinical

Case of obesity reported in the proving, prescribed Python 200c on the following symptoms:

"Embarrassment/shame about her weight / Defense of others but not of self / Fear of suffocation / Heavy bleeding in uterine region with / Fear of bleeding to death / Neck stiffness / Willingness to show enthusiasm"[14]

Physicals (a selection of the more characteristic / more frequent
proving symptoms)

- **Head**
  - Pressing above nose
  - Pressing against top of skull
  - As if a wave of heat
  - Numbness
  - Head pain, with pain in neck
  - Pulling on temples
  - Pulsating scalp
- **Vertigo**
  - Dizzy, everything goes black
  - Heat sweeps over from bottom to top
  - Ice-cold feet
  - Sensation of to-ing and fro-ing
  - Spinning around
  - Waves from nausea, from stomach to head
- **Stomach and bowels**
  - Eructations
  - Foreign bodies in stomach (*stitches, stones lurching from side to side*)
  - Heartburn in oesophagus
  - Heat in stomach
  - Nausea
  - Retching and vomiting in car
  - Sensation of retching, *as in bulimia*
  - Stomach feels bigger
  - Wants to vomit to feel better
- **Chest and Lungs**
  - Pressure on sternum or lungs
  - Hard to get breath, as if stone pressing
  - ***Feels as if corseted when taking deep breath***
  - *Suffocative* feelings
  - *Senses piercing of heart*
  - Heart rhythm problem
  - Heart needs space
  - Dry cough
  - For fresh air, need to be able to breathe

- **Ears**
  - Cramping; left ear in
  - Pressing; ears of
  - Roaring in ears
  - Tinnitus shifts from right to left
- **Teeth and jaw**
  - Battery, sensation as if
  - *Reduced saliva in times of conflict*
  - *Intense salivation*
  - Looseness of – sensation
  - Teeth clenched tight
  - Release of locked jaw during panic attack. . . .
- **Intestines and abdomen**
  - Cramps like a clenched fist, pulling sensation
  - Debility
  - Diarrhoea
  - Digestion incomplete; lettuce
  - Haemorrhoids
  - Sheep-droppings
  - Violent movement of bowels
- **Hands**
  - Finger injured by cut: *bleeding stopped*
  - Fingernails suddenly soft and break
  - Hands feel as if in a freezer
  - Numb feeling in fingers
  - Sensation of electrical impulses
  - Slowly crawling or pulsating
  - Stiff fingers
- **Back**
  - Waves of chilliness from L to R
  - Rhythmically or just one-sided
  - Pain in small of back extends to hips
- **Pelvis**
  - Wonderfully soft and warm, as if
  - Enveloped and cradled
  - Prickling like needles in pelvis

- **Legs**
  - *Deep wound in right thigh: bleeding stopped* (curative)
  - Numbness and twitching
  - Right leg as if anaesthetised
- **Eyes**
  - Eyes stuck together with pus, mornings
  - Eyes water for no reason
  - Field of vision increased
  - Restless eyelids
  - Rolling of eyes
  - Sensations as if eyes are turned
- **Nape of neck; throat; shoulders**
  - Weight down on shoulders; sensation
  - As if shoulders pulled out of sockets
  - Breathes easy, deeper than usual (curative)
  - Nape of neck hot
  - Neck, radiate to shoulders
  - Of a yoke on shoulder
  - Sensation of lump in throat
- Stabbing
- Stiffness
- **Arms**
  - As if right arm were longer than the left one
  - **Hands and arms numb; as if paralyzed**
  - Twitching in the right upper arm
  - Vibration and itching in the arms
  - Stone lying on the right elbow; as if
  - Crawling in right elbow
  - Heaviness in the elbow
- **Female**
  - Menses one week too early
  - Lump, clear, sticky jelly
  - ***Sensation as if uterus were turned inside-and she were losing all her blood***
  - *Very heavy menses, as if pouring out*
  - *Failure to reach orgasm / orgasm absent*
  - Pelvis and genitalia, as if stimulated

ANGUIMORPHA (closely related to the Ophidia)

Anguimorphs include alligators, lizards, glass lizards, galliwasps and legless lizards. Together, they constitute the proposed "venom clade" Toxicofera of all venomous reptiles. There are 9 genera found within the Anguidae family. They are characterised by their heavy armouring with non-overlapping scales. They have pterygoid teeth, and many members have tail autotomy (the casting-off of a part of the body by an animal under threat).

Alligator mississipiensis (American alligator)

Phylum: Chordata.
Class: Reptilia.
Order: Crocodilia.
Family: Alligatoridae.

The American alligator is a relatively large species of crocodilian. The teeth number 74–80. Juveniles have small needle-like teeth that become more robust, and narrow snouts that broaden as they develop. When on land, they move by sprawling or walking – the latter involving the reptile lifting its belly off the ground. In water they swim like fish, moving their pelvic regions and tails from side to side. They inhabit swamps, streams, rivers, ponds and lakes – primarily basking on shore, but also climbing onto tree limbs. The teeth are designed to grip prey, but cannot rip or chew flesh like canids and felids – they depend instead on their gizzard to masticate food. Both males and females bellow loudly by sucking air into their lungs and blowing it out in intermittent, deep-toned roars to declare territory or attract mates. The female remains near the nest throughout the 65-day incubation period, protecting it from intruders. Hatchlings gather into pods and are guarded by their mother and keep in contact with her through their "yelping" vocalisations. They are tiny replicas of adults, with a series of yellow bands around their bodies that serve as camouflage.

Proving by: **Todd Rowe, USA (2001).**[12]

Theme of being confident, being the hero; "the issue of power, self-confidence and self-assertion was one of the strongest themes in the proving. . . . Crocodilians are symbolically associated with darkness and the greedy moon, which devours the sun each night. They are also associated with the cycle of **death and rebirth**."[12]

Mind

- Alert
- Ambition – increased – *competitive*
- *Anger*
- Beside oneself; being
- *Destroy things; with tendency to*
- Noise; at
- Sudden
- Violent
- Anxiety – sudden (Panic attacks)
- Carefree
- Confident
- *Death – thoughts of*
- *Delusions – attacked;* being
- *Destructiveness*
- Estranged
- *Fear*
  - Control; losing
  - Sudden
  - Terror
- Fearless
- Forsaken feeling – *isolation*; sensation

- Freedom
- *Greed*, cupidity
- Impatience
- Indifference – joyless
- Intolerance
- Irritability
- Jesting – *joke; cannot take a*
- Lascivious
- Mania – alternating with – depression (*Bipolar*)
- Mood – changeable – sudden
- Morose
- Offended, easily
- *Pessimist*
- *Power – sensation of*
- Religious affections
- Sensitive – noise; to
- *Snappish*
- *Suicidal disposition – thoughts*
- Thoughts – sexual
- Violent

Dreams

Animals – dead / Beautiful dreams / Cats / Crimes / Crocodiles, alligators / Danger / Darkness / Dead; of the – friends – talking with deceased friends / Death / Dinosaurs / **Drug dealers** / Helping – people / <u>Hero; of being the</u> / Insects / Police / Powerful / Religious / **Resolving – relationships; old** / Robbers / Water – diving in / Water – irrigation

Generals

amel. Exertion / agg. Afternoon / Icy coldness / Stitching pains / Left sidedness / Craving for fish / Metallic sensation in the body / Hypertension / Paralysis from fright / Appetite amel. during the day / Appetite agg. at night / Explosive frontal headaches accompanied by nausea / Dryness, throat / Throat, pain / Nausea / Diarrhoea / Neck, pain / Increased sex drive / Deep sleep / Itching of lower extremities / Acid reflux / Sprain of left groin muscle / Pinching hip pain, amel. sitting / Sensation of dislocation in left thumb / Difficulty falling asleep / Restless sleeplessness[12]

Provers speaking as one

∮ "Dream – I was a cop; inside a gang of **drug dealers**; I can arrest the boss; but my partner left the situation because it was too **dangerous**; feeling of [being the] **hero** because I can do this operation alone (friend had too much **fear**); felt more **powerful** because I really had the situation in hand. . . . I had a **conflict** with a close friend; I allowed myself to be totally **present** and be myself. . .

∮ My **terror** was that I could not control my anger. If I did not everything would **explode**. It was a feeling of **infinite anger** – so angry that I could **destroy everything around me**. . . .

∮ Strong connection to **death** . . . [Deceased partner] filled my entire dream – as if he was the only thing that existed. We talked all night and . . . covered [areas] that I wanted to say and never said before. He soothed away all my pain – *it was more real than anything I ever experienced while I was awake*. It was beautiful beyond comparison and there was a feeling of **peace** and **joy**. What allowed me to do this was that I **felt much closer to death than before** – life and death were much closer. Now I feel much more at peace with my fiancée. . . . I woke up **paralysed with fear and total terror**. I was **frozen and could not move**. It was the most fearful that I have ever been in my life. . . .

∮ Dream: I was in a cave in the sea with another friend and we were ready to make a scuba dive. . . . All the other friends were not prepared like me. **I can save the situation** and go without oxygen tanks to bring back the oxygen tank and **no one else can help me. I was the best and could help the others**. . . . [There was a] feeling of **cocooning (being safely protected)** – Dream: Monarch butterfly that . . . enlarged to the point that the butterfly just *wrapped his wings around my son and me and I knew that he would be OK and that we would be connected forever on some level*. . . .

∮ **Intolerant** of people right now; irritable if people are not considerate. *Someone presenting themselves as a victim makes me want to tear my hair out*. . . . I felt a lessening of my **grip** on life. The sense of adventure, of excitement was gone. Most importantly, I rarely if ever felt joy . . . mental **confusion, disconnection** with a feeling of not being able to handle simple events . . . a building sense of **pessimism**, negativity, and despondency. I lost my feeling of confidence and competence . . .

§ **Itching** and **stinging** sensations. I felt my physical *body became an impediment to the enjoyment of life* with all the sore muscles that limited walking. . . . Sexually, I felt as if **drained of any sexual feelings** or identity . . . very sensitive; anything like scolding the inner child triggered it; terribly **hurt** and **snappish; touchy;** easily triggered; Feeling **defensive** and touchy; **attacking. . . .**"[12]

Geochelone sulcata (African spurred tortoise)

Phylum: Chordata.
Class: Reptilia.
Order: Testudines.
Family: Testudinidae.

The *African spurred tortoise* is a species of tortoise inhabiting the southern edge of the Sahara desert. It is the third-largest species of tortoise in the world. In the wild, they can burrow very deep, tending to plants such as grasses and succulents which grow around their burrows if kept moist with their own faeces. Copulation takes place right after the rainy season. Males combat each other for breeding rights with the females and are vocal during copulation.

Proving by: **Todd Rowe, USA (2010).**[3]

"Reptile themes present in this remedy include constriction and compression, attack and defence, violence, conspiracy, suspicion, antagonism with himself, sexuality, loquacity, sudden unpredictable attack, fear of death, and desire to kill. There was a strong theme of killing, particularly around cutting off the head. Tortoises are particularly vulnerable in the head area. There was a strong theme of being split and divided that came out during the proving. This is a common animal theme, which is particularly strong in the reptile family."[3]

Delusions
- Body – out of the body – observe herself; can
- Caged – tiger; he is a / Trapped
- **Dirty – he is**
- Knives

Mind

- Ambition – increased
- Anger – beside oneself; being
- Anxiety – conscience; anxiety of
- **Benevolence**
- Cleanness – desire for cleaning
- Confidence – want of self-confidence
  - **Failure**; feels himself a
  - **Self-depreciation**
- *Contemptuous – self; of*
- Darkness – desire for
- Dirty
- **Disgust**

- Helping others
- Helplessness; feeling of
- *Loathing – oneself*
- <u>**Love – love-sick**</u>
- <u>**Snappish**</u>
- Sociability
- ***Suicidal*** *disposition – knife – sight of a knife; at the*
- Talking – desire to talk to someone
- *Tormenting – himself (leprosy miasm)*
- *Verses – making (love poems)*
- Will – loss of will power

Characteristic physicals

- **Head**
  - Constriction – ***Armor***; as if in (*carb-v, choc, coc-c, crot-c, geoc-ca*)
  - ***Band*** or hoop – iron
  - ***Swashing*** sensation
  - *Water*; sensation as of
  - *Waving* sensation
  - *Vertigo – Rising – agg.*
- **Generals**
  - Pain
  - ***Burning*** / Neuralgic / Stitching pain / ***Wandering pain*** / ***Prickling*** / ***Tingling***

- **Generals**
  - *Emptiness*; sensation of
  - *Flabby feeling – Internal*
  - Formication
  - Fullness; feeling of – Internal
  - Heat – flushes of – night
  - ***Knotted sensation – internal***
  - Lightness; sensation of
  - Motion – downward motion agg.
  - Obesity
  - Riding – car; in a – agg.
  - Swelling – general; in

Provers speaking as one[3]

§ *Suicidal from pains.* Wanted to shoot myself. Wanted to **cut my head off with a knife** or machete. It was crazy; felt like my world had been flipped upside down; every day walking around with headache; extremely **debilitating**. . . . Every word my partner said felt like a **knife piercing my heart**. . . .

§ **Life has no purpose**. Depressed and sad. Feel like the world is falling apart. Feeling of *giving up*. Regrets about choices that I have made. . . . Feel **empty** and unwanted – *like someone passed away*. . . .

§ I want him to quit putting restrictions on me; that issue came to a head. **Restriction** is not able to move or deep breathe; being **confined**; like the same feeling with the belly. . . .

§ Feels like my stomach is too big and in the way. Feels bruised and sore to the touch. Fat like I am going to burst. Liver hurts. Worse laying on back. Sensation of being an upside-down turtle. Like I am on my back and cannot turn over. Like I am **contained in a shell**. Like it is contained and **bloated**. . . .

§ Feels constricted and **contained**. Feels **stuck**. . . . Beside myself with worry about my son. Feel **gripped** by this. Felt like I wanted to *crawl out of my skin*. High anxiety . . . **crushing pressure** radiating down to my breastbone. . . .

§ Irritable and **bitchy** . . . I finally **snapped** and yelled – raised voice and the works – that she had to stop **browbeating** me, had to **respect** me and not assume that I was totally at her beck and call. . . . I had no tolerance; would snap at people . . . snap at things like a dog; *take a little nip out of them*; be quiet; snappy; like I was being annoyed or getting **poked**; like the rational part of me knew that people were not going out of their way to bug me and annoy; poking **prodding**. . . .

§ I could face the **confrontations** with people with more **precision** of action rather than coming from a place of anger or insecurity; *Like a duel*; come on let's go. . . . I started thinking about sex all the time. I started attracting younger men and a number of them asked me out. . . .

§ Dream: Penis inside of my vagina. It was just there and felt full. No movement. Warm feeling. . . .

§ **Romantic love**; fell in love with someone 16 years younger . . . suddenly I started writing poetry again; writing poems to him; the whole process was stupid; the attention was flattering. . . . Felt like I was going through a **mid-life crisis**. Later I saw him and wondered why I was interested after that; I turned into this psycho. . . .

§ **Compassionate** and confessional. This is not like me! **Benevolent**. . . . Wanting to help people. **Altruism**. I get a rush of energy in my chest area thinking about it. . . .

§ Felt **spacy**. Difficulty connecting to work. More of a **scattered** feeling; my thoughts are in so many places; cannot collect them to have a coherent thought. . . . Feel as if something/someone bad is approaching or will **jump out at me**. . . .

§ *Dream about penguins. Sense of incarnating into one with human consciousness and how that would be.* Would you help the other penguins or would they ostracise you as being different. Scary feeling. Looking out into empty whiteness. . . .

§ **Dream**: I broke the arm of the clock and it started ticking. The priest started laughing and said it was a **bomb**. I ran to the back with the clock and threw it and it hit an apartment complex and I heard a big **explosion**. I felt horrible and thought of all the people who will be out of a home. **Torturing myself with my regrets**. The voodoo priest went home saying "I have no time to waste, I have clients to see". I shouted back at him *"you will never be a healer, a teacher, nor a doctor, you will always be a **voodoo** priest causing harm to others; you will never be good enough."*. . .

§ Dream of **cockroaches**. I was at this house and it was full of roaches. There was a young girl there. I asked her to help watch my kids. She was afraid and said that I will never let her go. She felt that I would "keep her forever". . . .

§ Dream of a man masturbating in front of me and making noises. Feeling **shocked, devastated** and **dirty**. Felt **violated** . . . Lice and parasites everywhere. Feels gross . . . I dreamt that I sat down in the dark on my own toilet.

I discovered it was filled up with someone else's shit and was so full of shit that it got all over my ass. . . .

Heloderma suspectum (Gila monster)

Phylum: Chordata.
Class: Reptilia.
Order: Squamata.
Family: Helodermatidae.

The Gila monster is the largest extant lizard native to North America. They have one close living relative, the beaded lizard (*H. horridum*), as well as many extinct relatives – the evolutionary history of which may be traced back to the Cretaceous period. They are reported to spend 90% of their time underground in burrows or rocky shelters. They feed primarily on bird and reptile eggs, and only eat infrequently (five to ten times a year in the wild). When they do feed, they may eat up to one-third of their body mass. Prey can be crushed to death if large, or eaten alive if small – swallowed head-first and helped down by muscular contractions and neck flexing. After finishing their meal, they immediately resume tongue-flicking and search behaviour, perhaps resulting from a history of finding prey clumped-together; such as eggs and young in nests. The Gila monster produces venom in modified salivary glands in its lower jaw, unlike snakes, whose venom is produced in the upper jaw. They lack the musculature to forcibly inject their venom, so it is propelled from the gland to the tooth by chewing. *H. suspectum* produces only small amounts of venom and therefore the bite is not fatal to healthy adult humans. In 2005, the FDA approved the drug exenatide for the management of type 2 diabetes. It is a synthetic version of a protein, exendin-4, derived from the Gila monster's saliva.

Provings by: **Todd Rowe, USA (1996)**[30] and by **Robert Bocock, USA (1892–3).**

Mind

- *Alert*
- Ambition – loss of – evening
- Anger – cold and detached
- Busy
- *Carefulness*
- *Cautious*
- Communicative
- Company – aversion to – desire for solitude
- Concentration – difficult – one subject; on
- Content
- *Contrary*
- *Courageous*
- *Delusions – possessed; being*
- Delirium – raging
- *Detached*
- *Dictatorial*
- *Disturbed; averse to being*
- *Dogmatic*
- *Destructiveness*
- Emotions – loss of / strong; too
- Estranged
- Expansive
- *Fight; wants to*
- Forgetful – words while speaking; of

- *Idiocy*
- Joy
- Laziness
- Laziness – work – *harm; he thinks the work will do* him
- Mistakes; making
  - Speaking; in – spelling; in
  - Speaking; in – words
  - Writing; in
- Obstinate
- Remorse – want of
- Striking – desire – strike; to

- Taciturn
- *Talking – slow learning to talk*
- Theorizing
- Thoughts – intrude and crowd around each other
- *Tranquillity*
  - *Conflict; during*
  - Settled, centred and grounded
- Unconsciousness – sudden
- Unification – sensation of unification
- Violent

Dreams
Alien from outer **space** / Animals / Animals – tails / Battles / **Bound**; being / Buildings / Cats / Churches / Circus / Coloured – black, red, white, yellow / Computers / **Constructing**; about / Conversations / Country – foreign / Desert / Dogs / Driving – car; a / Father / **Feeding – people** / Fights / Fire / Flying / Flying – airplane / **Forest** / Friends – old / Head – cut off / Hospitals / Hotels / **Journeys** – airplane; by | bus; by | train / Mother – dead mother appearing / Motion; of – fast / Murder / Nakedness / Ocean / Palaces / **Poisoned**; being / **Punching** / Rain / **Resolving – relationships; old** / Restaurant / *Scorpions* / Sexual / Speeding / **Speeding** – dry dusty roads / Swimming / **Teacher – spiritual; of a** / Telephones / Violence / Water / Water – under water

Prover #4
§ Irritable with people; **wanted people away from me**; sense of well-being; thinking felt sharp and clear; could see things well laid out; felt **possessed**; felt **crazy**; mind was **racing**; talked **fast**; *people could not wait to get away from me* in my environment; could not find centre or get centred; feeling the need to get things done and **accomplished**; wanted to be by myself; rankled feeling; no one come and bother me as I have work to do; irritability; feeling of great centredness and being herself; things shifting in head and finally feeling balanced; feel **welcoming** to others; feeling of **quiet joy** and **connection** to everything; need to do and not be interrupted; have found a **balance** point like a geographical place in my mind. . . .

§ I dreamt that I was auditioning for *Les Miserables*, I was so good in the dream that they gave me the lead role and it seemed the answer to my fondest dream, until pieces of the show began to be cut and **my role didn't seem special anymore**.[30]

Pathogenetic
"**Ferocious coldness pervading any part.** The coldness is described as an **arctic feeling, freezing, the cold breath of death, deadly cold**, a cold frosty wind, frozen to death and that as if the feet and hands are lumps of ice."[31]

Self-proving by Bocock _{Johnston}[32]

"Severe feeling of **internal coldness, so intense as to cause me to fear being frozen to death**, ensued . . . awakened suddenly with a **jerking** in my head. Central part of frontal bone so queer as to awaken me. When my office bell rang it threw me into a **startled** and **trembling** condition, something new to me."

Physicals

- **Vertigo**
  - Accompanied by – staggering
  - *Continuous*
  - Fall; tendency to
    - § Right; to
    - § Backward
  - Lying – must lie down
  - Motion – head; of – agg. – rapid motion
  - *Sudden*
  - Swaying – right; to
  - Turning; as if – he turns in a circle
  - *Walking on a sponge; as if*
  - Waves; in
- **Head**
  - Bores head in pillow
  - Brain; complaints of – base
  - Cerebellar diseases
  - *Coldness, chilliness*
  - *Hand; as if touched by an icy cold*
  - *Extending to – Brain; base of*
  - Occiput – extending to – Feet – waves; in cold
  - Constriction – band or hoop – cold agg.
  - Falling – sideways of head – right side; to
  - *Inflammation*
    - § *Brain – Cerebrospinal*
    - § *Meninges*
  - Lightness; sensation of – lying down – amel.
  - Numbness; sensation of – Brain
  - **Pain**
    - § Come off; as if top of head would
    - § Pressing pain – *band*; as from a
    - § Pressing pain – *cap*; as from a
    - § *Spots; in* – sore
    - § Paralysis of brain
    - § Shocks – waking him or her from sleep
    - § Skullcap; sensation of a
- **Eye**
  - *Bleeding from eyes* – Conjunctiva
  - Discolouration – red – Cornea
  - Falling – Lids; of
  - Opacity – Cornea
  - Opening the lids – difficult – keep the eyes open; hard to
  - Protrusion – *exophthalmos*
- **Ear**
  - Catarrh – Eustachian tubes
  - Noises in – ringing – right
  - Pain – pressing pain – outward
  - Wax – increased
- **Face**
  - *Coldness – icy coldness*
  - Discolouration – mottled
  - *Formication*
  - Heat – sensation of
  - Haemorrhage – Eyes – orbits – around
  - Stiffness – Jaws – lower
- **Mouth**
  - Discolouration – Tongue – blue
  - Paralysis – Tongue
  - Speech – thick
  - Taste – bitter – morning – waking; on
- **External throat**
  - Sensitive – touch; to slightest
- **Stomach**
  - Nausea – waves; in
  - Pain
    - § Radiating
    - § Epigastrium – sore

○ Vomiting – paroxysmal / persisting
- **Abdomen**
  ○ Contraction – Intestines
  ○ Rigidity of muscles
- **Chest**

- **Respiration**
  ○ *Difficult – breathing – last; as if the next would be the*
  ○ Forcible
  ○ Superficial
- **Extremities**
  ○ Discolouration – Hand – blueness
  ○ *Ecchymoses*
  ○ Gangrene
  ○ Heat – alternating with cold
  ○ Heat – Feet – Soles
  ○ *Haemorrhage – easily*
  ○ Milk leg
  ○ Pain – Feet – Soles – bed – in bed – agg. – burning
  ○ *Shaking*
  ○ Soft – Feet – Soles – sensation of
  ○ Sponge; as if walking on a
  ○ Tingling – Feet – Soles
  ○ Walking – lift feet higher than usual – down hard; and brings them
  ○ Wool; as if stepping on
- **Generals**
  ○ Air; draft of – sensation of a draft – fanned; as if

○ *Coldness* – Heart – sensation as if heart were cold
○ Pain – respiration
○ *Trembling* – Heart
○ *Weakness* – Heart – about the heart; sensation of weakness

○ Bathing – affected part; bathing the – ice cold water; in – amel.
○ Cold – spots
○ Energy – excess of energy
○ Food and drinks – eggs – desire
○ *Hypotension – sudden*
○ *Pain*
  § *Agonising*
  § *Disappear suddenly*
  § *Neuralgic – excruciating*
  § *Radiating*
  § *Shooting pain*
  § *Stabbing pain*
  § *Touch – agg. – sore*
  § *Violent*
○ *Paralysed* parts
○ Paralysis – painful
○ Paralysis agitans
○ *Prickling* – externally
○ Pulse – thready
○ Stretching – amel.
○ *Wavelike sensations*
○ Wounds
  § Bites – poisonous animals; of
  § Bleeding freely
  § Heal; tendency to – slowly

Maiasaura lapidea Good mother lizard (Dinosaur fossil)

Phylum: Chordata.
Class: Reptilia.
Order: Ornithischia.
Family: Hadrosauridae.

Hadrosaurs are extinct dinosaurs that are commonly called the 'duck-billed dinosaurs' due to their distinctive bill-like mouth shaped similar to those possessed by many waterfowl. They lived in herds – raising their young in nesting colonies in which individuals were packed closely together, like those of modern seabirds. Upon hatching, fossils of baby Maiasaura show that their legs were not fully developed and that they were incapable of walking. Fossils also show that their teeth were partly worn, which means that adults brought food to the nest.

Proving by: **Nancy Herrick, USA (1997).**[33]

- **Delusions**
  - ○ *Accidents – fatal; he will have a*
  - ○ *Animals – devoured by* – being
  - ○ *Assaulted; is going to be*
  - ○ **Danger; impression of** – life; to his
  - ○ Faces; sees – closing eyes; on
  - ○ Hole – digging a big
  - ○ *Insane – become insane; one will*
  - ○ Mutilated bodies; sees

  - ○ *Repulsive* fantastic
  - ○ Robbed; is going to be
- **Fear**
  - ○ Evil; fear of – forebodings; of evil
  - ○ Free-floating
  - ○ Poisoned – being poisoned; fear of
  - ○ Terror – causeless
- **Mania**
  - ○ Laughing and gaiety; with
  - ○ Spasmodic sensation; with

Mind
- Adventurous
- Anticipation – impending evil; sensation of
- Anticipation – *stage fright* – unusual ordeal; of any
- Anxiety – duty; as if he had not done his
- *Cursing* – desire to curse
- Joy – *fits of joy with bursts of laughter*
- Magic – *rainbow* feels like
- Sadness – conscious of *unnatural state of mind*; because

Dreams
Abused; being / Accidents – **mutilated** body in mangled car / **Attacked**; of being – above; from / Bitten; being – animals; by – rear; from – heads bitten off / Body; parts of – dead / **Brakes – function any more; do not** / Bus – wrong place; bus takes him/her to the / Children; about – newborns – **found a living premature baby** on city street / **Climbing** – ladders – **tall ladders** / Coition / Dead bodies – searching for / Desert – seashells and cacti like seaweed / **Disgusting** / Eating / Ecstasy; of / **Eulogy for man died of aids** / **Excrements** / **Eyes – three; having** / **Face – two faces** – having two faces / Family; own / Fights – men; with – no one hurt / God; of – word of **God; talking about one's love for** / Hostages – **taken as – sexual torture; for** / *House – sexual liaisons; for* / *Lascivious – smutty* / **Manure** / Men – rough – unshaven / *Men – staring; a man is – women in shower though eyeglass; at* / Money – disputing about money / Monsters / *Nakedness – unashamed* / Prisoner – being taken a / Pursued; being – animals; by / Restaurant – pay for meal; cannot – expensive / Restaurant – venison; eating / Sexual – **captivity; of** / **Sexual – disgust – sex and death with** / Sexual – **seduced** wife's sister / Sexual – sleeping bag; in a – **quick** and **rough** / Stones / Weeping; about – love of the word of God / Women – clothing; without much

Characteristic Physicals

- Vertigo – Floating; as if – body feels
- **Face**
  - Itching – Whiskers
  - Pain – Submaxillary glands – prickling
  - Veins distended – spider nevi
- **Mouth**
  - Pain – Sublingual glands – prickling
  - Pain – Submaxillary glands – prickling
- Speech – stammering – fast; when talking
- Throat – Pain – extending to – Ear – swallowing agg.
- Stomach – Eructations; type of – food – sensation of
- Larynx and trachea – Constriction – Vocal cords
- Chest – Itching – Axillae – left

Provers speaking as one

"It came, I opened the bottle, felt I had opened Pandora's box, and I had a strong feeling I shouldn't take it. It felt, **dark, evil, sinister, powerful**. . . . I felt a huge **sadness** in my heart. I felt an overwhelming sense of sadness. Intellectually, I thought I'd get a lot of **pain in my limbs**. . . . I inhaled the remedy. It felt safe to do it this way. I felt an immediate **flush** over my face. An hour later I was reading, and I got **fasciculations** all over my face. I wondered if it was a **neurotoxin** . . . increased hunger and an irritability. I wanted to **gnaw** on things, like gnaw on people (irritability with the headache). . . . Dream: Next night more **sex** and **death**. **Murder** and **disgust**. There was a **mutilated** body in a mangled car at the roadside. Then there was some **sexy** sex in a sleeping bag. **Quick** and **rough** sex. Some woman roughly examined the **dead body**. There was a **hacksaw** blade . . . I was in a park climbing over ladders, very tall ladders and piles of manure."[33]

REPERTORY ADDITIONS FOR THE SNAKE FAMILY
(to existing rubrics in Synthesis[11]):

MIND

- ABUSIVE
- AMBITION – increased
- **AMBITION – increased – competitive**
- AMOROUS
- ANGER – contradiction; from
- ANGER – violent
- **ANTAGONISM WITH HERSELF**
- ANXIETY – conscience; anxiety of
- APHASIA
- BOASTER
- BROODING
- CLAIRVOYANCE
- COMPANY – desire for
- COMPETITIVE
- CONFUSION OF MIND – identity; as to his – duality; sense of
- CRUELTY
- CUNNING
- DANCING
- DEATH – thoughts of
- DECEITFUL
- DELIRIUM – sepsis; from
- DELUSIONS
  - § choked
  - § **conspiracies**

§ **divided – two parts; into**
§ enlarged
§ enlarged – body is
§ fancy, illusions of
§ forsaken; is
§ great person; is a
§ images, phantoms; sees
§ influence; one is under a
　　powerful
§ injury
§ about to receive injury; is
§ being injured; is
§ **being injured; is –**
　　surroundings; by his
§ people – behind him; someone
　　is
§ **persecuted – he is persecuted**
§ poisoned – he – has been
§ poisoning people; she is
§ pursued; he was
§ pursued; he was – enemies; by
§ small – he is
§ snakes
§ snakes – in and around her
§ specters, ghosts, spirits
§ **superhuman; is – control; is**
　　under superhuman
§ superiority; of
§ trapped; he is – underworld; in
　　the
§ visions; has
§ voices – hearing
§ wrong – done wrong; he has
○ DREAM; AS IF IN A
○ ECSTASY
○ ESCAPE; ATTEMPTS TO
○ FEAR
　　§ evil; fear of
　　§ high places; of
　　§ robbers; of
　　§ snakes; of
○ FIGHT; WANTS TO
○ FORGETFUL – words while
　　speaking; of
○ FORSAKEN FEELING
　　§ isolation; sensation of

○ GESTURES; MAKES
○ GRIEF
○ HATRED
　　§ revengeful; hatred and
○ HIDING – himself
○ IDEAS – abundant
○ IMPULSE; MORBID
○ VIOLENCE; to do
○ IMPULSIVE
○ INSIGHTFUL
○ INTENSE PERSONALITY
○ INTUITIVE
○ JEALOUSY
○ KILL; DESIRE TO
○ LASCIVIOUS
○ LOATHING – life
○ LOQUACITY
○ MALICIOUS
○ MANIPULATIVE
○ MENSES – before
○ MIRTH
○ MISTAKES; MAKING – speaking,
　　in
○ MORAL FEELING; WANT OF
○ MUTTERING
○ ORPHANS
○ POWER – sensation of
○ RAGE
○ RELIGIOUS AFFECTIONS – too
　　occupied with religion
○ RUDENESS
○ SENSITIVE – weakness; to other
　　people's
○ SLY
○ SPEECH – incoherent
○ STRIKING
○ STUPOR
○ SUICIDAL DISPOSITION
○ SUSPICIOUS
○ THREATENING
○ TIME – slowly; appears longer;
　　passes too
○ TORPOR
○ TRANCE
○ UNCONSCIOUSNESS – conduct;
　　automatic

- UNFEELING
- VIOLENCE
- VULNERABLE
- WICKED DISPOSITION
- WILL – two wills; sensation as if he had
- **HEAD** – LOOSENESS OF BRAIN; SENSATION OF
- **THROAT**
  - CHOKING
  - LUMP; SENSATION OF A
  - SWALLOW, CONSTANT DISPOSITION TO
  - SWALLOWING – difficult
- **EXTERNAL THROAT** – CLOTHING AGG.
- **NECK**
  - CONSTRICTION OR BAND
  - PRESSURE
  - clothes; of – agg.
- **MALE GENITALIA/SEX** – SEXUAL DESIRE – increased
- **FEMALE GENITALIA/SEX** – SEXUAL DESIRE – increased
- **SLEEP** – WAKING – dreams; by
- **DREAMS**
  - AMOROUS
  - ANGER
  - ANIMALS
  - ANXIOUS
  - BUSINESS
  - DANGER
  - DEAD BODIES
  - DEATH
  - EVENTS – previous – day; of the previous
  - FALLING
  - FIRE
  - FRIGHTFUL
  - GHOSTS
  - LIONS
  - MANY
  - MEN
  - MURDER
  - NIGHTMARES
  - PURSUED; BEING

- SNAKES – biting him
- TEETH
- VIVID
- WAR
- **GENERALS**
  - ANEMIA – haemorrhage; after
  - APOPLEXY
  - BLACKNESS OF EXTERNAL PARTS
  - BONES; COMPLAINTS OF
  - CATALEPSY
  - CIRCULATION; COMPLAINTS OF THE BLOOD
  - CLOTHES – tight; too
  - CLOTHING
    § intolerance of
    § pressure of clothing
  - CONGESTION
  - CONSTRICTION
    § External
    § Internally
    § tetanic rigidity
  - CYANOSIS
  - DISCHARGES – amel.
  - DROPSY – internal dropsy
  - FISTULAE
  - FOOD AND DRINKS – cold food – desire
  - FULLNESS; FEELING OF – Internally
  - HEMORRHAGE
    § blood
    § black
    § clots
    § dark
    § decomposed
  - HYPERTENSION
  - HYPOTENSION
  - INFLAMMATION – gangrenous
  - JERKING
  - MENOPAUSE
  - MENSES
    § after – amel.
    § before – agg.
  - NECROSIS
  - PAIN – choking pain
  - PARALYSIS – one side

- PERIODICITY
  - § year – every
- PRESSURE – agg.
- PULSATION – Internally
- PULSE
  - § fluttering
  - § hard
  - § soft
- SEPTICEMIA, BLOOD POISONING
- SLEEP – after sleep – agg.
- SWELLING – general; in
- WEATHER – rainy – agg.
- WOUNDS
  - § bites
  - § bites – snakes; of
  - § bleeding freely
  - § gangrene of
  - § heal; tendency to – slowly

References

1 Lilley D. *Lachesis*. Cape Town. (Accessed in RadarOpus 23rd October 2020.)

2 Fraser P. *Snakes Drawing Power from the Underworld*. Bristol: Winter Press; 2009.

3 Rowe T. *A Proving of Geochelone sulcata (African spurred tortoise)*. Phoenix AZ: AMCH Publishing; 2010.

4 Sankaran R. *Provings – Similia similibus curentur – Crotalus cascavella*. Mumbai: Homeopathic Educational Services; 1998.

5 Master F. *Bitis arietans*. Mumbai, 2003. (Accessed in RadarOpus.)

6 Master F. *Oxyuranus scutellatus – Taipan – A Homoeopathic Proving*. Mumbai, 1997. Available online at: *https://tinyurl.com/2mazre9w* (Accessed 7th June 2021.) (Accessed in RadarOpus.)

7 Joshi B, Joshi S. *Quick Book of Minerals and Animals*. Mumbai: Serpentina Books; 2013.

8 Vithoulkas G. *Essence of Materia Medica* (rev. 2nd edn). Alonissos: B Jain Publishers; 2008.

9 Allen T. *Encyclopedia of Pure Materia Medica – Crotalus cascavella*. New York: NY. (Originally published in 1874.) (Accessed in RadarOpus.)

10 Master F. *A Proving of Moccasin Snake*. Mumbai, 1996–1998. (Accessed in RadarOpus.)

11 Schroyens F. *Synthesis 9.1* (Treasure edn). Ghent: Homeopathic Book Publishers; 2010 (plus author's own additions).

12 Rowe T. *A Proving of Alligator mississippiensis*. Phoenix AZ: AMCH Publishing; 2010.

13 Allen T. *Encyclopedia of Pure Materia Medica – Naja tripudians*. New York: NY. (Originally published in 1874.) (Accessed in RadarOpus.)

14 Klotzsch B. *Proving of Python regia*. Bergisch Gladbach: Self-published; 2001.

15 Gutman W. *Homoeopathy – The fundamentals of its philosophy the essence of its remedies*. New York NY: The Homoeopathic Medical Publishers; 1978.

16 Sankaran R. *The Substance of Homeopathy – Naja tripudians*. Mumbai: Homeopathic Medical Publishers; 2005.

17 Sankaran R. *The Soul of Remedies – Naja tripudians*. Mumbai: Homeopathic Medical Publishers; 1997.

18 Master F. *Naja naja naja*. Mumbai: (Accessed in RadarOpus.)

19 Sankaran R. *Sankaran's Schema* (2nd edn). Mumbai: Homoeopathic Medical Publishers.

20 Hardy J. Two cases of Cenchris contortrix. *Homeopathic Links*, Spring 2000.

21 Neesgard P. *Hypothesis collection – Primary Psora and Miasmatic Dynamic.* Denmark, 2019. (Accessed in RadarOpus.)

22 Clarke JH. *Dictionary of Practical Materia Medica* (Vols 1–3). Mumbai: B Jain; 2005. (Work originally published in 1900.) (Accessed in RadarOpus.)

23 Sankaran R. *Provings – Similia similibus curentur – Denroaspis polylepsis.* Mumbai: Homeopathic Educational Services; 1998.

24 Vermeulen F. *Synoptic Reference – Dendroaspis polylepsis* (rev. 2nd edn). Glasgow: Saltire Books; 2016.

25 Ward J. *Unabridged Dictionary of the Sensations "as If".* Noida Uttar Pradesh: B Jain Publishers; 1995.

26 Serban G. The up and down snake – Elaps corallinus. *Homeopathic Links,* Summer 1998.

27 Marim M. *Simplified Materia Medica of Bothrops jararacussu (lanceolatus).* Buenos Aires, 1996–1998. (Accessed in RadarOpus.)

28 Greenberg A. A bothrops case – Complaints after apoplexy, cystitis. *New England Journal of Homeopathy.* 1999; 8 (2).

29 Wright C. *Bitis arietans arietans and its veno*m. 1997. (Accessed in RadarOpus.)

30 Rowe T. *Heloderma suspectum proving.* Phoenix AZ: AMCH Publishing; 2010.

31 Vermeulen F, Johnston L. *Vista Vintage.* California, 2019. (Accessed in RadarOpus.)

32 Bocok R, Vermeulen F. *Vista Vintage (Transactions of the 51st Session of the American Institute of Homeopathy, 1895).* California, 2019. (Accessed in RadarOpus.)

33 Herrick N. *Animal Mind Human Voices – Maiasaura lapidea – Good mother lizard.* (unabridged edn). Grass Valley CA: Hahnemann Clinic Publishing; 1998.

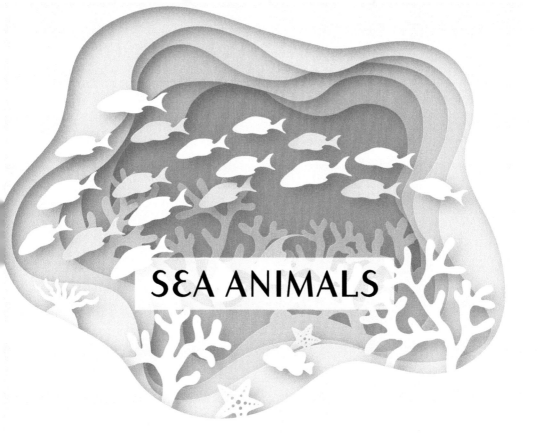

SEA ANIMALS

MYTHOLOGY

- Neptunian forces impel the individual to seek **escapism** from the world of form (materialism) through addiction, fantasy and dreams. There can be also be a profoundly idealistic nature with an urge towards selflessness, dissolving back into the oceanic feeling of the womb. *cf. Series 2, Periodic table – the journey from symbiosis to separateness.*
- Urge to explore spirituality through a sense of unity, merging and oneness with the world.
- Rather than being an individual you become part of the shoal. Lack of boundaries, open to attack.
- The instinctive and intuitive senses are amplified whereas the rational and logical processes are deficient. This can lead to gullibility, naivety and an overly-idealistic view that when shattered leads to disillusionment, disconnection and isolation.

Neptune | Poseidon

Dissolving of form, Sacrifice, Addiction.
Escapism, Oblivion, Dreams, Turbulence.
Oceanic feeling, Idealism, Disillusionment.
Collective unconscious, Evasion of responsibilities.
Victim or victimised, Rescuing or needing to be rescued.
Selflessness, Devotion, Martyrdom.

Astrological Water

The realm of feelings, intuition, deep emotion, overwhelming fears, passions.
Compulsive, irrational, lacking solidity and structure. Desires protection.
Connection, oneness, acceptance, love.
Sensitivity, fluidity, empathy, responsiveness.
Secretive, hidden undercurrents, turmoil beneath a calm exterior.
Needs to be channelled otherwise it is formless.

Mars – Neptune

Escaping from violence. Victims of aggression. Supporting the underdog. Passive aggressive. Strength is only an illusion.

Affinities

- The pineal gland, dreaming, sleep / wake cycles.
- Immune vulnerabilities, lymphatic toxicity.
- Psychic sensitivity, vulnerability, possession, confusion of identity.
- Mental fogginess, confusion, poor boundaries, addiction.
- Victim / Rescuer relationships.

SEA ANIMALS IN HOMEOPATHY

Early life-forms evolved in the sea; the realm of the collective unconscious. The unconscious mind is not shaped by ego experience, but by the collective. Therefore, the ego may be lacking differentiation to the point that one's sense of identity is easily lost and boundaries easily breached. More positively, a strong connection to the Water element can lead to a sensation of merging and of unification with others and one's surroundings. These themes are shared with the Drug group of remedies, which are also affiliated with Neptune.

In Sea cases, there can be heightened sensitivity in common with the early flowering plants such as the Magnoliidae, to which Michal Yakir has assigned predominantly 'watery' characteristics where the ego is in an early stage of development.[5] Water is formless without a container.

Whilst the Water element may be commonly expressed through tendencies such as dependency, weakness and lack of direction, it is also experienced as merging into symbiotic relationships, caring for and nurturing others, victim / rescuer dynamics, seeking the ideal partner, keen intuitive faculties and deeply felt emotions often hidden under a calm exterior.

The themes of sexual abuse and of being abandoned by one's parents also feature in Sea remedies. Sexual liaisons have an impersonal quality and eggs are left unattended to be fertilised later, whilst the young are expected to fend for themselves. These themes often call for a direct comparison with the *Milks* and *Birds*. Of course, some sea animals are indeed mammals or birds themselves. . . .

Whilst Sepia can be considered the 'type-remedy' for sea animals as a family, offering a homeopathic blueprint for the other less well-known remedies, it should be kept in mind that this is a very broad and varied group combining diverse creatures, lifestyles and survival patterns. Water can take many forms; vast oceans, flowing rivers, crashing waves and still lakes. The creatures who make it their home are the originators of animal life on this planet, and like all animals they each need to find their own niche in order to survive.

In the marine invertebrates there is an innate passivity; clinging to rock, filter-feeding and shutting out the dangerous world with a hard-exterior shell. This is necessary to protect their inner softness. Cephalopods have evolved to swap this static world of protection for freedom of movement, internalising their calcareous structure. With this greater sense of freedom comes more danger as they are no longer protected. Instead they need to be on the alert and supreme escape artists; some are also able to leave a decoy so they can flee from danger unseen.

Many fish live together in shoals, gaining anonymity and strength in numbers as protection from predators. Mammals such as Dolphins, Orcas, Whales and Seals are incredibly successful predators of the oceanic realm, utilising a variety of mammalian qualities such as intelligence, teamwork and speed to give themselves a competitive advantage.

Molluscs: Combine mineral and animal themes

Structure *vs.* Fluidity (Earth *vs.* Water); many sea creatures don't move, but they are animals. For example: Oysters. They shut themselves in and keep the world out, remaining static, clinging to rock for safety, filter feeding, eventually creating a pearl of wisdom. This pearl of wisdom reflects the spiritual theme that runs through the oceanic remedies; the ego is relatively undifferentiated when compared to more recently evolved animals. Whilst this may be expressed as dependency or weakness; on the other hand, it can be channelled into spirituality and selflessness.

From *A Proving of Mussel Pearl* by John Morgan,

"*Initially there was this wonderful sense of **connection** with and **empowerment** from a **spiritual** source through my own meditation and channellings. . . . An awareness of and **deep connection** with the Christ energy and an understanding that I was being **cleansed**; spiritually, emotionally and physically. . . .* "[1]

Our homes are made from the calcareous deposits left by the shells of these primitive invertebrates. Home and house and fundamental security are often the issues presented by these patients – *cf. Calc-carb Stage 2, Series 4.*

Like the Milks, Molluscs also have an affinity with the astrological Moon. Here is a reminder of some Lunar keywords: *Family, Nurture, Creature comforts, Habitual, Instinctive, Caring, Sensitive, Touchy, Moody, Waxing and Waning, Yin, Emotional, Sense of self, Place at home, Cyclical, Reflective, Soulful, Fertile, Inward, Mother, Union, Subconscious, Uncompensated, Feelings, Responsive, Receptive, Reactive, Flowing, Oversensitivity.*

Gastropods: Snails. Cypraea eglantina (Cowrie snail); there is a venturing out and retreating back into the shell rather than being shut-in all the time. Murex, Helix tosta (hermaphrodite). Between earth and water; living in rocky terrain. Proboscis, mantle, tentacles, secretions. Polished, smooth shell. Hiding, retracting, camouflaged.

Marine arthropods: Outgrow the shell, begin to feel restricted (*cf. Stage 15 / Nitricums*) and must move house – a very dangerous transition to make. Vulnerability to attack. For example, Limulus, Horshoe crab, Astacus (river crab), Hermit crab, Homarus (lobster). These creatures mark the evolutionary transition from Water to Earth. Homarus is closer in form to Androctonus.

Echinoderms: Asterias rubens (starfish). Extruding stomach to ingest prey. Solitary. Sensations; crushed, beaten, crawling. Theme; regeneration – delusions, limbs longer (the starfish can regrow limbs). Sea urchins; spines, vivid colours, venom, teeth, jaws.

Cephalopods: The soft tissues are formed around the skeletal structure so they are no longer fixed to one place – they can move and enjoy the freedom of the ocean. But this means they lack protection, having sacrificed this for freedom of movement. To survive they must be cunning, quick and a good escape-artist. Or become camouflaged, changing colours, leaving a decoy – for example, ink in the case of Sepia. A shared trait of the group are sucker-bearing tentacles used to seize and hold prey. *Cephalopods reproduce only once in their lifetime.* When females reach sexual maturity they will mate and lay their eggs. In some cases the adults die right away and the eggs are left to the mercy of the ocean. For example, Nautilus, Octopus, Sepia, Squid.

Cnidaria: Hard and soft corals, jellyfish, anemones. For example, Stoichactis kenti (giant sea anemone) has nematocysts to sting their prey. Sensations: stunned, electricity, feeling like jelly. Coralium rubrum (calc-carb and iron oxide). *Look inanimate but are alive and predatory.* Symbiotic relationships; for example, between Stoichactis kenti and the clownfish (which has a mucus layer to protect it from the nematocysts). They can form specific partnerships with the anemone who provides them with shelter. In the Coral Reef, life is experienced as vivid and colourful in health; becoming grey and monochrome when ill. Symbiotic relationships are highly complex and crucial for survival. They provide a nursery and offer protection for young sea creatures to develop.

Sponges: Spongia tosta. Filtering, breathing – respiratory disorders (*tubercular*).

Fish: living as one organism within the shoal offers protection and anonymity. There is a sense of oneness within the shoal that goes beyond that of insect communities (who may work together in a super-society). The way a shoal operates as one is an analogue for Jung's collective unconscious; the shared mythological symbols we inherit as a collective.

The polarity is the theme of evading parental responsibility; eggs are abandoned and the young left to fend for themselves. The popular phrase after a romantic break-up; 'there are plenty more fish in the sea', alludes to matters of grief, loss and disappointed-love that are brought out in provings and cases requiring sea remedies.

Powerful predators: Sharks (ancient, primitive), Orcas (imprisoned to perform clever tricks).

Aquatic mammals: Whales, seals, dolphins, otters. Playful, sports, organised, sociable, inventive, communicative. Taking huge breaths to dive deep into the ocean.

Birds: Penguins, and many more.

Affinities

Menses / Climaxis / Menopause / Hormonal Imbalances / Infertility / PMT / Miscarriage / Hot Flushes / Sexual Excesses / Ailments from celibacy / Menstruation / Femininity / Circulation / Allergic reactions (*Astacus*)

Summary

The sea animals are a challenging group to write about in terms of themes, given that the classification is so broad and encompasses such diverse groups as marine invertebrates, fish, cephalopods, gastropods, cnidaria, mammals and more!

MAPPA MUNDI

Air

Difficulty in communication leading to isolation, solitude, indifference to sex. Indifference to nurture; handing over parental role to the male (*Hippocampus kuda*).
Deceptively calm ocean is another world of danger and darkness. Feeling suddenly threatened.
Rape, abuse, abandonment of young.

Phlegmatic (*Molluscs*)

Dependence on partner for security.
Desire to hide and camouflage oneself (cephalopods).
Shell = Conflict of Protection (*Molluscs*) vs. Claustrophobia (*Crustacea*).
Feeling lost, stupid and weak, they are dependent on another for protection,
especially financial.
Mental dullness.

Sanguine (*Fish*)

Yearn for fun and lightness, freedom and open spaces.
Desire freedom from responsibility.

Choleric

Power and dominance (*predatory sea animals*). Pressure agg.
Self-sufficiency in young, ability to fend for themselves and take on responsibility from a young age (*Aurum, Carcinosin*).

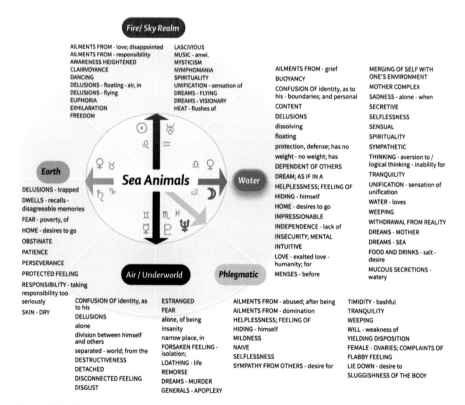

Figure 7.1 Mappa Mundi dynamics for the Sea Animals

Water

Grief, sadness and mood swings.
The gender roles are reversed or questioned. Gender fluidity.
Men take on a mothering role whilst women are independent, focusing on career.
Sea is mother (*la mere*); the watery world of the womb.
Dreams: children in danger – especially drowning; floods, waves, storms, tsunami.
Water expressions: *"Coming over my head . . . Keeping my head above water".*

Earth

Extreme protectiveness. Lack of structure and routine <
Heavy, weighed down, and tied up by responsibility and guilt (*Gold Series*)

Sea Animal source language, according to the Mappa Mundi

Air	Water	Phlegmatic	Melancholic
Abyss	Flow, Balance,	Retreat	Stagnant
I am not myself	Water	Hide	Closed
Rape	Moon	My space	Suffocated
Cheat and	Tide	Sink	Solitary
Deception	Float	Tired	Claustrophobia
Cold	Filter	Sexual desire	Criticise
Disconnect	Drown	reduced	
Undercurrent	Clear/Muddy	Dependence	
	Waves		
	Camouflage		
Fire	**Earth**	**Choleric**	**Sanguine**
Light	Mud, Hard,	Energetic	Open
Power	Heavy	Pressure	Bubbles
Dominance	Cave		Open space
Sexuality	Calm		Freedom
Colours	Grit		Fun
Different world	Protection		
	Detached		
	Sand		

THEMES

Lost, confused and aimless *vs.* Connected, at-one, content

Problems arise for patients suffering from a lack of direction; floating aimlessly, loss of purpose, lacking routines; wanting to go with the flow as opposed to being disciplined or following a structure (*Earth*).

I feel I am in the middle of an ocean, not knowing what direction to swim in. It is the same distance to any shore. And they all seem far away. It makes most sense to flow and see what direction I go naturally. But there are some doubts, that I should exert some effort in some direction. I just want to lie still and let the sun fill me with warmth and light. But then the night comes; it is cold and lonely. I want to be somewhere other than where I am. _{galeoc-c-h.}[2] *Feel in a daze all day, as if not really awake . . . I feel unclear in my thinking; I feel a bit dopey . . . I can't make my mind up about anything. Where shall I park? What shall I buy? What shall I do first?* _{clup-hr.}[3]

There may be a distinct lack of ego, expressed through qualities such as a yielding disposition, phlegmatic temperament, mildness, submissiveness, selflessness etc. These qualities can manifest both positively; in the form of meditation, selfless service to others and humility; or negatively, as being used, abused and becoming a doormat. Sensations or feelings such as being "helpless, frozen in a vacuum, unapproachable, disconnected, distant" may be expressed. _{Cypra-eg.}[4]

The evolutionary imperative for sea animal patients may be to allow the ego to dissolve and experience the oneness of connection (as if back in the womb). This is perhaps most true for fish whose individual identity is bound up with the collective of the shoal. The Oyster also produces pearls of wisdom to highlight the importance of spiritual themes throughout the watery realm. "Strong desire for spiritual connection, strong empathetic feelings, increased sensitivities" _{hippoc-k.}[5] For someone over-identifying with their own ego, the vast ocean can be lonely and unforgiving. There are feelings of isolation, abandonment and of being forsaken:

Felt very remote. . . . Woke feeling out of it, as if I am not all there. . . . Feelings of detachment . . . remote and detached. . . . Completely cut off and alienated from everybody. . . . Feeling exposed, vulnerable. _{oncor-t.}[6]

Rubrics
Absentminded – dreamy | Blissful feeling | Confusion of mind – identity, as to his – boundaries; and personal | Connection; sense of | Content | Delusions – dissolving, she is | Delusions – floating | Delusions – lost; she is | Disconnected feeling | Dream; as if in a | Floating sensation | Grounded – not grounded | Idealistic | Impressionable | Merging of self with one's environment | Mysticism | Naive | Spirituality | Unification – sensation of unification | Withdrawal from reality

Escape artists; hiding, deception, decoy and camouflage

Many sea creatures (as exemplified by Sepia) rely on camouflage as a survival strategy; changing colours to dazzle predators or hiding behind a cloud of ink. In human terms, this equates to an urge to escape or hide away from difficult situations rather than confront them head-on (*as might Lac Leoninum*). The ability to go unseen and escape quickly when necessary is reminiscent of those who always seem to flee from problems, looking for a 'get-out-clause' at the first hint of trouble. This tendency may also be expressed as secrecy, a yielding and introverted nature, preferring to remain private or withdrawn from the outside world.

Sea animal cases can have themes of vulnerability and helplessness, of being surrounded by undercurrents of danger that threaten to overwhelm the individual. There is nowhere to hide in the deceptively calm ocean where violence lurks hidden in murky depths. In this way, these patients may seem less overtly 'animal' as Snakes, Spiders and Insects, associating more as the victim than the aggressor. *"Feeling of being a helpless victim. Helpless, hopeless; given up completely. I don't care. No resistance at all."* oncor-t.[6]

Another survival strategy, exemplified by the Molluscs, is to cling to another for support, protection and safety. With the support of 'their rock', they can feel at-home as long as they are not asked to go outside of their comfort-zone.

Rubrics
Delusions – protection, defence; has no | Delusions – safe; she is not | Delusions – victim; she is a | Escape, attempts to – run away, to | Helplessness; feeling of | Hiding – himself | Impressionable | Insecurity; mental | Introspection | Secretive | Will – weakness of | Yielding disposition

Idealism and selflessness *vs*. Escapism, disillusionment and gullible naivety

Desire for meditation, stillness and dissolving of the ego *vs*. turbulence, stormy emotions, feeling suddenly under threat; *"Fear of being attacked and fear to die. . . . There is a feeling of threat."* stych-gig.[7]

Seeking to escape reality; indulging in the imagination, evading responsibility, day-dreaming, addictive behaviour; dependency on drugs, alcohol, sex or food.

Escapism may also be creatively expressed through indulging in music, novels and fantasy; anything which transports you out of the humdrum and into a more idealised or imaginal world. *Row 2 of the periodic table also has a strong water-element to it, being an analogue for the journey from symbiosis to separation; the process of arriving into the world from the womb.*

Rubrics
Absentminded – dreamy | Blissful feeling | Depersonalisation | Dream; as if in a | Meditating | Withdrawal from reality

Weightless, floating, directionless *vs*. Pressure, heaviness, weight

Light, bubbles, buoyant, floating vs. Heaviness, depth, pressure.

"I just let things float. I am trapped. I can't do anything about it. . . . I feel weightless and free." oncor-t.[6]

There may be hand gestures that show a wave-like or undulating pattern and characteristic language such as 'being pulled under, submerged, drowning, finding my flow, going with the flow, riding the wave.' Floating, weightless sensation. *cf. Birds*; where it may be described as soaring high up in the rarefied mountain air. In Sea animals the floating is described like a flowing, bobbing or a suspended feeling. *(cf. Hormones, Drugs and Gases – Deep sea divers can get nitrogen narcosis when under the heavy pressure of deep water.)*

Sea Animals 411

The journey of Row 2 goes from the floating, drug-like sensations of Lithium through to the fear of downward movement in Borax and pressurised feeling of Nitrogen. The provings of several Sea animal remedies feature **sensations of pressure**, as detailed in Hering's Guiding Symptoms:[8]

- Violent pressure upon anterior lobes of brain, extending beneath eyes Aster.[8]
- Violent palpitation, with pressure in chest, as if a lump lay there Ambr.[8]
- Pressure in stomach: as from a stone; as if it were sore internally; after a meal and from touch Sep.[8]

As if crushed. There can also be a fear of being crushed, trapped, suffocated. (*Earth element*)

- Asterias rubens: "pain as of cranium being crushed" Hughes[9]
- Sepia: "As if brain were crushed." Hering[8]
- Calcarea: "Deep-seated pain in right orbit, as if the eyeball would be crushed;" Buck[10]

Carrying a heavy burden

"Heaviness. Every pain is dragging, heavy, like a stone, like a burden. Something that drags them down. The whole system is very slow. Trying to save their energy as much as possible." Ven-m.[11]

The clinical picture of Sepia can be brought to mind with the phrase *'Sag, Nag, Drag'*. In such cases, there is a feeling of being over-burdened and weighed down, with a feeling of dragging in the abdominal / womb area.

Rubrics

Buoyancy | Delusions – floating – air, in | Delusions – weight – pressing down from above | Delusions – pressed down by a great force | Floating sensation | Pressure; external

Boundaries dissolved: Letting life flow in *vs.* Withdrawing to the shell and closing off

Dreamy, spaced-out, drifting, intuitive; tuned-in to an oceanic reality; a world of dreams, feelings, imagination and spirituality. This Neptunian realm comes through in the proving of Atlantic herring;

> *Feeling very far away and dreamy. . . . It is like you're looking at the world and then you realise it is just a picture, like you are separate, not a part of it, like a movie, like a 3D picture. Just for a split moment just a glimpse of something, of other consciousness.* clup-hr.[3]
> And in Stingray; *Increased intuitive awareness – saw what took place where my friend died. . . . When people look at me, I feel they are looking at my energy – not a good feeling. . . . Intuition improved – saw a patient and diagnosed throat cancer intuitively.* urol-h.[12]

As with the Aids miasm, in the ocean there are no boundaries; the ego must be dissolved. There can be free flow from without to within and there are no defences anymore. Like the filter-feeding Oyster who lets the nutrients flow-in whilst keeping the dangerous world at bay. Adopting this strategy means a static existence, staying within one's comfort zone and a lack of freedom. To be free-flowing in the ocean means opening yourself up to the inherent danger of predators.

> *No boundaries in water . . . Caressing body, water, bliss. Deep, unexplainable memories of pain in the hands of men; innocent trust. Seas have no borders but there are barriers.* oncor-t.[6]

Neptune rules the immune and endocrine systems; when these are compromised the body's boundary is too easily breached. *"I feel completely and utterly vulnerable and open, everything comes into me, I have no defences."* clup-hr.[3]

The oceanic sense of reality, as Freud termed it, is a world of blurred boundaries, merging and unity; as if still connected to mother in the amniotic fluid of the womb. The ocean, whilst offering an environment of merged boundaries and unity, is also the most impersonal environment in which to live. Unless you let go of attachment to form and ego (*Earth element*), there can be extreme feelings of loneliness and abandonment (*Air element*). Isolation is ameliorated by connection with others, meditation, mindfulness or some form of spiritual practice (*Fire element*).

> Dream: *My first love comes to see me and immediately all the love I felt for him and the passion develops all over again – I tell him that and try to kiss him and he puts me off – I get very upset and tell him I don't want to lose him again – I plead with him not to go –* **I felt totally closed out and abandoned** *– he is very cold and this makes me even more desperate – I am churning inside, begging him to stay – I feel as if every atom of me will fly away and shatter me into pieces.* urol-h.[12]

Rubrics
Confusion of mind – identity, as to his – boundaries; and personal | Forsaken feeling – isolation; sensation of

Yearning for fun and lightness, freedom and open spaces
(*cf.* Birds, Sanguine temperament)

- Idealistic / naive attitudes towards care, nurture and love relationships (*cf. Lepidoptera*).
- Blissfully unaware of their own separateness until this dream is shattered as an illusion by painful life events (*cf. Row 2*).
- "Desire to touch people, be near them, feel their presence, feel connection, to have fun with them, to laugh with them. Normally I want time to myself." lac-del.[13]
- "Desire to be free and wild / run to the mountains." oncor-t.[6]
- "Flightiness has gone, I feel relaxed, in flow, playful and fun. . . healthy devilment, attitude and fun, sensuality. A kind of, this is me, and that's the way it is." clup-hr.[3]

- This is contrasted with feeling flat, lifeless and colourless when decompensated. The Coral reef is vividly colourful with luminescence when healthy *vs.* grey, flat and monochrome when dying.

Rubrics

Blissful | Connection; sense of | Elated | Euphoria | Exhilaration | Freedom | Love – exalted love – humanity; for | Mirth | Pleasure | Vivacious

Abandonment, evasion of parental responsibilities *vs.* Selflessness, devotion and martyrdom

Lack of mother, abandoned, isolated, forsaken feeling. *cf. Halogens; chlorine, bromine and iodine are all present in the sea.* In the oceans, reproduction has an impersonal quality; abandonment of children with no parental supervision. Eggs are abandoned, children left to fend for themselves and must grow up early, becoming self-sufficient and taking early responsibility (*cf. Carcinosin*).

> *Feeling intensely preoccupied and feel like pondering and re-assessing my personal situation. Also feeling extremely lonely.* chir-fl.[14] *Disassociated feeling. Heard people talking, sounded like the hum of bees. Felt separate from this, not a part of it. Felt really like I wanted to isolate. Feeling like a loner. Spacey floating feeling, and again next day. Just stay on the beach and relax and not participate.* lac-del.[13]

There is a danger of overcompensating for having felt abandoned by associating oneself too readily with other victims; always coming to the rescue of those less fortunate. This can result in being taken advantage of through one's desire to rescue and nurture others.

Tuna fish – produce millions of eggs which are abandoned in the sea to fend for themselves. This is contrasted by Salmon, who dutifully swim back to the source of the river where they were spawned, risking their lives against the elements (including ravenous bears) to give birth to their young. They undertake this perilous journey only to die immediately after spawning. Hence the urge to become a mother and beget children is very strong indeed, despite the journey being fraught with danger and ultimately resulting in the loss of their own identity. Like the journey of the salmon to its place of spawning, patients undergoing IVF may experience a sense of desperation to conceive. The process of IVF involves repeated *cycles* (a keyword in Water-element cases) of ovarian stimulation, egg retrieval and implantation.

In sea-animal cases, the whole process of reproduction may be equated with death or loss of identity. This is expressed in cases of post-natal depression where Sepia is often a sterling remedy.

Rubrics

Abandoned | Delusions – division between himself and others | Delusions – separated – world; from the – he is separated | Delusions – victim; she is a | Dependent of others | Detached | Disconnected feeling | Estranged – friends and relatives | Fear – alone, of being | Forsaken feeling

Ailments from abuse (*cf.* Birds, Milks)

- Urolophus helleri – *There was a strong theme of rape. Provers saw sexuality as torture in several dreams. The female stingray is often abused with many scars by the male stingray. The reverse side of this came out in one male prover who saw women as very powerful and in control of everything. . . . Dream in which two men tried to rape me and I killed them with a broom – there was no feeling.* urol-h.[12]
- Stoichactis kenti – *Dreams – Abused sexually; being*
- Asterias rubens – *Ailments from – abused; after being – sexually – rape*

Grief and loss *vs.* Letting go of attachments

Ailments from grief, bereavement, emotional trauma, unrequited love.

> *Woke up crying, remembering mother's death. My boyfriend held me as I sobbed through the pain and story of those days. I cried for nearly an hour. I thought most of that grief had been cleared so was very surprised at the intensity of it. We made love, I needed that connection.* hippoc-k.[5]

The highest ideal of romantic partnership is sought after for the feeling of merging into unity. When this separates or breaks apart, the ensuing feelings are of profound grief, deep depression, forsaken feeling, loss, being lost at sea, total isolation (*cf.* Nat-m, Sepia, Cygnus cygnus, Ignatia).

> *It is a feeling of isolation – I want to talk to somebody. I feel like a big wall has come down in front of me. . . . During the proving, I had been plagued by a sense of isolation, as if I were trapped behind glass, looking at the world but completely separate from it.* hippoc-k.[5]

Feeling detached from or unable to establish one's true identity; too easily influenced by other people's currents of emotion. Where there was once a feeling of unity and blissful connection, there is now separation. This may also be expressed as a loss of purpose, particularly after trauma, grief, or becoming a parent; '*I am not myself anymore*'.

The feeling may arise that one's true self becomes obscured / dissolved / diluted / murky / washed-away under the heavy burden of responsibilities to the family. Or following the pain of separation.

Emotions that 'come in waves' or 'tides' overwhelm the individual, leading to a variety of compensations; walling oneself off (in the oft-observed Nat-m. way), wallowing, weeping, floating aimlessly etc. Healing may lead to a balance between over-identification with the intuitive, unconscious 'selfless' person and the conscious 'selfish' drives of the ego. In the case of sea remedies, balance may be achieved by claiming back something for themselves rather than by continuing to over-give in their responsibility to others.

Rubrics
Ailments from – grief | Ailments from – love; disappointed | Grief | Weeping

Static, immovable hard shell for protection *vs.* Moving house, suffocated by home life

(Molluscs, gastropods, marine arthropods)

- Conflict of protection (hard outer shell) and claustrophobia (restricted by the shell). *cf. Coleoptera* (*beetles*)
- In Crustacea, moving home is an important theme. The crab gets more and more tight; leading to a feeling of 'not enough room' in the home. Eventually they outgrow their shell and must leave home to find a bigger one.
- The crab carries its home wherever it goes; these are people who like to bring a bag full of homely creature-comforts around with them.
- Often, problems with close family and relationships will come through in the case-taking.
  (*cf. Row 3 and 4*).
- In terms of Mappa Mundi dynamics, the Molluscs, Gastropods and Marine arthropods are positioned between the realms of Water and Earth.

Rubrics
Protected feeling | Fear – narrow place, in

Gender reversal, imbalance of Yin and Yang energy

The loss of identity after motherhood means that gender roles can become reversed – an absent mother who would like to return to work and a nurturing father who stays at home. Sea remedies will often involve an imbalance between, or reversal of, the fundamental Yin and Yang principles, typified in "the [Sepia] woman [who] seeks to emancipate herself from the passive, receptive female role, the world of home and emotions, into a life of action. [Or by] the male who wants to disengage from the active world of politics and business and lead a quieter, more contemplative life." Coulter[15]

- Some fish will change gender in later life, morphing from female to male.
- In Sea horses the father takes on the role of mother.
- In Sepia, the more successful males 'cross-dress' in order to sneak past the larger males who are fighting over breeding rights.

Rubrics
Confusion of mind – identity, as to his – sexual identity

Symbiotic relationships, dependency

- Yielding and soft; these patients can become dependent on another for protection and consolation (the fleshy oyster requires a hard shell). Or they rely on another to provide financial security, structure and routine (*lacking Earth element*). This dependency can eventually result in feelings of lowered self-worth.

- Clownfish and Anemone rely on an intimate, long-lasting relationship that mutually benefits their chances of survival.
- It can be very hard to find a partner in the deepest depths of the ocean, although paradoxically we use the saying 'plenty more fish in the sea' following break-ups! Certain fish will attach themselves to their mate so they can never come apart again.

Clean, cleansing, clarity *vs*. Dirty, murky, absent, dull

Rational processes can become very dull (*cf. Alumina*) with absentmindedness and slow thinking. The intuitive faculties might be intensified with heightened sensual awareness, expressing an imbalance between the earth and water elements.

Rubrics
Dullness | Confusion of mind | Intuitive | Sensual | Thinking – logical thinking – inability for

Dirtiness, disgust, leprosy miasm

Sepia, Ambra grisea and Stoichaktis kenti have all been assigned the leprosy miasm by various homeopaths.

- "I wanted to go to the temple but didn't go, 1000 people, infection, dirty place. . . . Intense reaction to being moved into a dirty house, not OK, cried all night." stych-gig.[7]
- Ambra grisea – *Disgust – body; of the – own body; of one's – odour; of the.*
- Sepia – *Disgust – oneself.*
- Asterias rubens – *Dirty – he is – inside and smells badly.*

Dancing, movement and flowing with the senses

This group of remedies gain more enjoyment from life when they can be led by their intuitive, rather than their logical faculties. They may seek involvement in the arts, music and poetry over a typical career. Indeed, many sea remedies have a desire for motion in general and dancing in particular. The following remedies are all listed under the rubric 'Mind – Dancing':

chir-fl.	clup-hr.	hippoc-k.	lac-del.	lim.	medus.	oncor-t.	sea-an*	sep.	spong.

Sepia is especially well known for this symptom as is Tarentula. However, the type of dancing may be quite different. Somebody with a strong Water dynamic will prefer flowing movements, whereas the Insects and Spiders may prefer a faster and more rhythmical style of dance.

Sea Animals 417

Financial worries, fear of poverty; lack of earth element

These patients might develop a fixation about money due to a lack of structure in their lives; where is the next reliable paycheck going to come from? Will they be stuck in an impoverished state by staying true to their intuition and creativity?

> *Money problems still make me feel worried. The finances are not working out. Rent late again . . . feel anxious – my mind runs through a very long list of worries – money, future, children's education, college work. Feels better by keeping busy putting everything back in order.* chir-fl.[14] *She tells me that I can make two million dollars but I don't see how and I am appalled at the idea of it. . . . Inherited a great deal of money and gave it all away – felt exhilaration.* urol-h.[12]

The following Sea remedies are present in Sherr's 'Money' rubric in Q Repertory[16]

ambr.	calc.	caras-aur.	chir-fl.	cypra-eg.	oncor-t.	sep.	spong.	stych-gig.	urol-h.

Calcarea has the following rubrics relating to money:

- Anxiety – business; about
- Anxiety – money matters; about
- Avarice
- Delusions – ruined – is ruined; he
- Fear – business failure; of
- Fear – poverty; of
- Fear – starving; of

Differential Diagnosis

Aids Miasm (no boundaries)
Halogens
Noble Gases
Stage 13 (confusion, liquid metals)

Cruciferae (flowing, blocked)
Magnolianae (confusion, floating)
Papaveraceae (numb, anaesthetic)
Ignatia; the acute of Nat-m.

Source words

Drained, Flowing, Detached, Floaty, Absent, Estranged, Suffocated, Dependency, Cyclical, House, Shell, Salty, Fluidity, Power, Turmoil, Shoals, Floating, Flying, Undulating, Phosphorescence, Colours, Luminescence, Dissolve, Flow, Wet, Wave-like, Swimming, Diving, Bubble, Salt, Beach, Sand, Holding your breath, Syphons – filter feeding.

Sea Animal Dreams

Carousing / Children; about / Danger / Dead; of the – Relatives / Embarrassment / Family, Own / Fantastic / Fish / Flood / Flying / House / Journeys / Lost; being / Pursued; being / Running / Sea

REMEDIES

Sea Animals

acip-st-ov, **AMBR**, anthop-xa, arde-he, **aster**, aurel-a, bad, barb, <u>CALC</u>, caras-aur, caruk-b, **chir-fl**, cigua, clup-hr, conch, **cor-r**, **cypra-eg**, diplor-cl, eryth, gad, galeoc-c-h, guan, **hippoc-k**, hom-am, hydroph, ichth, **lac-del**, lac-ph-v, lim, medus, **murx**, oct-mac, ol-j, **oncor-t**, pect, pelec-o, pern-c, physala-p, pleur-pt, prop, pyrar, saxitox, <u>SEP</u>, ser-ang, silur-gn, sphen-h, spong, **stych-gig**, synan-hr, synan-vr, trach, trach-v, **urol-h**, **ven-m**.

Ambra grisea (Excretion of the sperm whale)

Phylum: Chordata
Class: Mammalia
Order: Artiodactyla
Family: Cetacea

Ambergris; waxy substance formed in the lower intestine of the sperm whale. Freshly produced ambergris has a marine, faecal odor. It acquires a sweet, earthy scent as it ages, commonly likened to the fragrance of rubbing alcohol without the vaporous chemical astringency.

Provings by: **S. Hahnemann, Germany (1827); Krassning, Austria (1985).**

Fundamental delusions
- Faeces, sees – diabolical faces crowd upon him – get away from them cannot
- Influence; one is under a powerful
- **Mind – out of his mind; he would go**
- Assembled things, swarms, crowds etc.
- Enemy – surrounded by enemies
- Hearing – wrist-watch; winding up of
- Images, phantoms; sees – sleep – preventing
- Light [= brightness] – too much light in room on falling

Important symptoms
- Ailments from – business failure
- Anxiety
  - Conscience; anxiety of – masturbation; after
  - Crowd; in a
  - Speaking, when
- Company – aversion to – strangers, aversion to the presence of – stool; during
- Disgust – laughing of others; at
- Flattering – seducing behaviour in children

Essence

Extreme bashfulness cannot pass stool in presence of others. Big problem with sleep – can see diabolical faces crowding him. Phatak[24] says it is indicated for society girls – people who used to go out partying and used alcohol to dampen their anxiety around strangers, which is very strong. Embarrassment is a big keynote of the Rx. There are Sycotic growths around the genitals. Hints of the Leprosy miasm picture with the disgust element of the Rx. Disgust at stool, or of one's own body odours. Imagines others are laughing at him – which goes further than Calc – who does not want others to observe his confusion. It is more like Baryta who assumes everyone is laughing and mocking him for his idiocy. Patient is very bashful, cannot get much out of them – don't like answering questions.

Source words

DEEP: depth, 'out of my depth', 'hidden depths', dark, sinking, submerged, underwater, unseen things, drowning, gasping for breath, suffocated, diving, timeless, vast space, immense.

Affinities – (Boger)

- Nerves
- Pneumogastric
- Solar Plexus
- Spinal
- Mind
- Female Organs
- One Side
- Chest, Left

Modalities

- agg. Before Sleep
- agg. Lying in Bed
- agg. Mental Exertion
- agg. Warm, becoming, in bed
- amel. Eating, while
- amel. Open air, walking in
- amel. Walking
- amel. Cold, in

Provers speaking as one [Hering][8]

§ "Comprehension slow, has to read everything three or four times, and then does not understand it. Is not able to reflect upon anything properly, feels stupid. . . .

§ Confusion of head; of occiput. . . . Difficult thinking in morning. . . .

§ **Distorted images, grimaces; diabolical faces crowd upon his fancy**. . . .

§ She is excited, loquacious; talking fatigues her; was unable to sleep at night, or averse to talking and laughing. . . . Melancholy, sits for days weeping; with great weakness, loss of muscular power and pain in small of back with constipation. . . .

§ Fear of becoming crazy. . . . Despair; loathing of life. . . . Anguish and sweat all over at night. . . . Anxiety, oppression, nervous weakness, with irritability and impatience. . . .

§ After business embarrassment cannot sleep, must get up. . . . Hurries too much while engaged in mental labor. . . . Embarrassed manner in company. . . .

§ Cough agg when many persons are present. . . . The presence of other people aggravates the symptom. . . ."

Asterias rubens (Starfish)

Phylum: Echinodermata.
Class: Asteroidea.
Order: Forcipulatida.
Family: Asteriidae.

The common starfish is an echinoderm – the body consists of five equal segments with radial symmetry, each arm radiating outwards from a central body. They have no heart, brain, nor eyes, but some brittle stars seem to have light sensitive parts on their arms. When feeding on molluscs, they attach their tube feet to each shell valve to exert a force strong enough to prise them apart. They then extrude a fold of their stomach, secrete enzymes and start digesting the mollusc body. In the spring, the females release up to 2.5 million eggs into the sea to await the males' sperm so that fertilisation can takes place in the water. The larvae are planktonic and drift for about 87 days before settling on the seabed to undergo metamorphosis into juveniles. The common starfish produces a saponin-like substance designed to repel predators. Famously, they are capable of re-growing severed limbs.

Provings by: **Petroz, France (1850); Günther, USA (1853); Berridge, UK.**
Seminar trituration proving by: **E. Schulz (2000).**

- **Fundamental delusions**
  - Answers to any delusion
  - Betrayed; that she is
  - *Dirty – he is – inside and smells badly (Aids/ Leprosy miasm)*
  - Enlarged – body is – parts of body – growing too long; as if
  - Invaded; one's space is being
  - Sinking; to be
  - Strangers
    - § Control of; under (*Snakes*)
    - § Surrounded by (*estranged from family*)
  - Sucked up; she is being
  - *Suffering – women through the ages; conscious of (Lac-lup)*
- **Fears**
  - Alone; of being
  - Apoplexy; of
  - Cancer; of
  - Evil; fear of
  - Fainting; of
  - New enterprise; of undertaking a
  - Waking; on
  - Weeping amel.

Mind

- Ailments from – abused; after being – sexually
- Ailments from – mortification
- Anxiety – conscience; anxiety of
- *Aversion – children, to her own – guilty feeling; with*
- *Benevolence*
- Confusion of mind – identity, as to his – boundaries; and personal
- Confusion of mind – muscles refuse to obey the will when attention is turned away
- *Disgust – sex, kissing etc.*
- Egotism

- Estranged
  - Family; from his
  - Menopause; during
- *Euphoria – alternating with – sadness*
- *Housekeeping – aversion to*
- **Independent**
- Indignation – alternating with – mirth
- Irritability – coition – after
- **Lascivious**
- *Neglecting – children; her*
- **Nymphomania**
- Order – desire for
- Sensitive
  - Criticism; to
  - Moral impressions; to
- Superstitious
- Sympathetic
- Thoughts – sexual
- Unification – desire for
- Weeping
  - Emotions – slight; after
  - Sexual excitement; with
  - Telling – sickness; when telling of her

Compared to Sepia, who gets dragged down by domestic duty; in the case of Asteria rubens, it seems that there develops a complete aversion to domestic life in an attempt to maintain independence. This may be contrasted with a more sympathetic and benevolent side; nurturing and caring for others spontaneously and freely.

Clinical _{Clarke}[22]

Acne / **Apoplexy** / **Cancer** / Constipation / Convulsions / Epilepsy / Headache / **Heart** – affections of / Hysteria / Salivation / **Sycosis** / Tongue – paralysis of / Tongue – swelling of / Ulcers / Uterus – affections of

Clinical _{Ward}[23]

Ants limbs / Anxiety afternoon / Arm wind / Awake illusion / **Beaten arm** / **Beaten limbs** / Brain shaken / Brain tired / Break skull / Bursting head / Ceased heart / Constriction epigastrium / **Discharge womb** / Distress epigastrium / Distress womb / Eyes drawn / Fullness brain / Fullness chest / Hallucinations home / **Head hot** / Home away / Leg drawn / Limbs crawling / Locomotion impeded / Long leg / Misfortune impending / Needle jaw / News bad / Pressure abdomen / **Protruding womb** / Pushing womb / Restless mind / Roughness larynx / **Shocks electric** / Sunken eyes / Teeth piercing

Pathogenetic _{Ward}[23]

Air head / Bruised skull / Bursting head / Ceased heart / Consciousness extinct / Crushed skull / Distension breasts / Electricity head / Expulsion womb / Home hallucinations / Hot-air head / Long leg / Misfortune impending / News bad / Protruded womb / Pulled breast / Shocks brain / Shocks head / **Surrounded hot-air** / Waves ears / Wind arm

Calcarea carbonica (Oyster)

Phylum: Mollusca.
Class: Bivalvia.
Subclass: Pteriomorphia.

As a keystone species, oysters provide habitat for many other marine species. The hard surfaces of their shells and the nooks between them provide places where a host of small animals can live. They usually reach maturity in one year and are protandric; during their first year, they spawn as males by releasing sperm into the water. As they grow over the next two or three years and develop greater energy reserves, they spawn as females by releasing eggs. A single female oyster can produce up to 100 million eggs annually which become fertilised in the water and develop into larvae. Oysters filter large amounts of water to feed and breathe (exchanging O_2 and CO_2 with water) but they are not permanently open – they regularly shut their valves to enter a resting state. In the early 19th century, oysters were cheap and mainly eaten by the working class. Oysters are an excellent source of zinc, iron, calcium, and selenium, as well as vitamin A and vitamin B12.

Proving by: **S. Hahnemann, Germany (Date unknown).**

Fundamental delusions
- **Confusion; others will observe her**
- Body – dashed to pieces, being
- Disease – incurable disease; he has an
- Annihilation; about to sink into
- Brain – dissolving and she were going crazy; brain were
- Friend – fantasy world of imaginary friends; lives in a
- Home – away from home; he is – must get there

Important delusions
- Animals – persons are animals – rats, mice, insects etc.
- Inanimate objects are persons
- Money – talks of
- People – beside him; people are – walking beside her
- Room – house; room is a
- Ruined – is ruined; he
- Tumble – he would tumble
- Vermin – seeing vermin crawl about
- Walking – cotton; he walks on
- Watched; she is being
- Wealth; of
- Wrong – everything goes wrong

Oyster is a primitive life form whose existence is defined by having an external skeleton, which necessitates stasis and immovability (two key themes in the remedy picture of Calc Carb, whose hesitancy, indecision and timidity are renowned across the materia medica). The inherent fragility of the Mollusc's survival, dependant on clinging to a rock surface its whole life, is an apt metaphor for the individual who is 'slow to resolve or decide as well as to act or achieve . . . [who is] full of anxieties which give him a mild exterior.'[20]

In Oyster, there is only one natural defence mechanism – to snap the jaws tightly shut when stimulated by the presence of an irritant. This muscular spasm keeps out invaders and facilitates the painstaking creation, over lengthy duration, of a pearl of prized value and beauty. The response of Oyster to invader is to repeatedly cover the parasite with Nacre, a strong, resilient type of lacquer that encases the offender, nullifying their toxicity. Taken as a metaphor for human behaviour, this provides a nice signature for Calc Carb in potency; people who are slow in their development, and develop fixed ideas in the defence of unwanted intrusion (such as the plethora of fears, anxieties and monomania that plague these people when the boundaries they set up are breached).

The Calc carb child is plodding along quite happily in life, enjoying creature comforts and the nurturing bosom of familial life, until the first major physiological shock; vaccination, humiliation, vexation, or other such set back could all be candidates. This stimulates the active Psoric root in such a child to erect a protective barrier to compensate for feelings of inner weakness (the Oyster snapping shut its jaws to create an impenetrable barrier to further invasion). As the Oyster is a filter feeder (so this child is a passive observer), and relies on passing sea minerals for nourishment; if this appropriate action of defence in order to keep out hostile parasites is prolonged beyond the actual need, then there is going to be a problem – that of under-nourishment. Here we can see the principal aspect of the Calc Carb state – a problem of ineffectual assimilation (for example, < mother's milk) resulting from the prolonged action of clamping shut to keep unwanted things out.

Untreated, we can witness pathology progress along the theme of improper assimilation, with affiliation in particular to the glands, skin, bones and blood. In fact, Calcium is such an important mineral in metabolic processes that an inability to assimilate it can have disastrous effects globally and helps explain the long list of rubrics for this remedy. To paraphrase Gibson[36] Calcium acts as part of a metabolic quartet with Sodium, Potassium and Magnesium. It is the most important inorganic element in the body and is contained in the highest proportion. Without enough Calcium, 'the unrestrained influence of Potassium and Magnesium keep the muscles in a state of constant hypertonus resulting in tetany and finally paralysis through exhaustion'. Hence, Calc Carb's aggravation mental / physical over exertion.

On the other hand, too much Calcium can lead to oedema and the guiding symptom – generalities: feeling flabby, 'tissues plus quantity and minus quality.' [Tyler][37] This is because excretion of water and other solutes is cut down as all membranes turn from 'filter paper into parchment'[36] as Gibson puts it. Disorders in Calc Carb are disorders of equilibrium as Calcium swings like the tide from repletion to depletion.

Calcium is the main constituent in bone (indeed the word Oyster derives from the Greek word for bone) and forms a crystal lattice of calcium carbonate and phosphate, indicating the possible skeletal derangements that this great polychrest can act upon when Calcium is in deficiency, such as tardy dentition, late closing of fontanelles, rickets or curvature of the spine. Calcium is essential for proper clotting of the blood (hence we see anaemia when it is in deficiency) and is vital in many physiological activities because of its ability to form compounds by combining with proteins, accounting for the extraordinarily wide-ranging sphere of influence this remedy has.

Progression to the mental level, when left unchecked, can lead to expressions of the Psoric constitution defined by deficiency, immobility, insufficiency, debility. Ortega, speaks of the Calc Carb nature as being:

> *reserved, lax or indifferent; any possible irritation or transient excitement will . . . leave him feeling drained . . . [he is] cold and sensitive, delicate because of his scanty natural resistance . . . extremely reserved and tends to feel disappointed which makes him taciturn, obstinately engaged in depressing thoughts.*[20]

A look at the meaning of the word timidity, yields some interesting synonyms for the Calc Carb state: An awkwardness / lack of self confidence in presence of others (which leads us directly to the rubric – Fear: of his condition being observed); backwardness, bashfulness, coyness, retiring, shy, hesitant, restraint, indecision, vacillation, tentativeness. The end-stage of the mental level of Calc Carb is written in the books as depression, melancholia, thoughts of suicide, and fear of insanity. All of which can be linked via the signature of this remedy to the situation of the Oyster and to the theme of improper assimilation and subsequent feeling that, *'I must cover up for the fact that I have insufficient energy to accomplish my tasks'*.

On the mental level, this inability to assimilate leads to confusion of mind and incompetence at basic mental tasks. This is covered up (with the visage of a competent outer shell) and compensated for, whilst underneath there is turmoil of anxieties about their confusion and being noticed in public, which underpins the nucleus of potentised calcium carbonate.

Chironex fleckeri (Box jellyfish)

Phylum: Cnidaria.
Class: Cubozoa.
Order: Chirodropida.
Family: Chirodropidae.

Chironex fleckeri, commonly known as the sea wasp, is a species of extremely venomous box jellyfish in the Cubozoa class – found in coastal waters surrounding Australasia. Cubozoans have cube-shaped, transparent medusae and are heavily-armed with venomous nematocysts. The box jellyfish actively hunts its prey (small fish), rather than drifting as do true jellyfish. When they are swimming the tentacles contract, but whilst hunting, they become thinner – extending to about 3 m long. Their tentacles are covered with a concentration of stinging cells called cnidocytes, which are activated by pressure and a chemical trigger; reacting to proteinous chemicals. The sting produces an excruciating pain accompanied by an intense burning sensation, like being branded with a red-hot iron. They have planula larvae, which settle and develop into sessile polyps, which subsequently metamorphose into sexual medusae, the oral end of each polyp changing into a medusa which separates and swims away.

Proving by: **Alastair Gray, Australia (2001).**[14]

Mind

- **Abrupt – harsh**
- Absentminded – conversing, when
- Anger – vexations; about former
- Awkward – strikes against things
- Blissful feeling
- *Censorious – friends; with dearest*
- **Clairvoyance**
- **Coma**
- Concentration – **vacant** – attempting to concentrate; on
- Confidence – want of self-confidence – **failure**, feels himself a
- Confusion of mind – concentrate the mind, on attempting to
- **Contemptuous**
- *Content – forgets all his ailments and pains*
- **Cruelty**
- Dancing
- **Defiant**
- Delusions
  - alone, being – always alone; she is
  - butterflies, of
  - floating – air, in
  - head – pulled backward
  - whispering to him; someone is
- **Dictatorial**
- Elated
- Exhilaration – blissful
- Fear
  - alone, of being
  - dark; of
- **Fight**, wants to
- Indifference
  - duties; to – domestic, to
  - suffering; to
- Irritability – alternating with – indifference
- Jealousy
- Joy
- *Obstinate – plans; in the execution of*
- *Order – desire for – life; in one's*
- *Perseverance – duties; in performing irksome (**cf.** limulus)*
- **Prophesying**
- Thoughts – vagueness of
- Unconsciousness – semi-consciousness
- Unsympathetic – friends; towards

From these rubrics, one can find some interesting characteristics of the remedy. There are Sea themes of bliss, vacant thoughts, clairvoyance, prophesying *vs.* predatory, themes of cruelty, defiance, harshness, desire to fight. There is an interesting parallel with Limulus cyclops in the rubric *persevering in irksome duties*. This couples with being *obstinate in the execution of one's plans*. These rubrics are fitting for this species whose habits and mode of survival have remained unchanged since the Cambrian period; 430–590 million years ago.

Dreams

Children; about / Coition / Coloured – orange & yellow / Competition / ***Continuation – dreams, of – sleep; former dream is continued on going to*** / Embarrassment / Flashes, like still pictures in a movie format / Flying – people / Friends – seeing friends / Gardens – overgrown / House / Humiliation / Insults / Long / Lost; being / Moths / Provoked; being / River – banks crumbling; river / School – old; goes back to / Sea / Sexual / Shoes – dancing shoes; cannot get on / Teacher – yelling at me; old teacher / Tongue – large; too / Trees – removing and replanting / Visits – making visits / Wandering / Waves

Characteristic physicals

- **Vertigo**
  - Fall, tendency to – backward
  - Rising – sitting; from – after
  - Waves; in
- **Head**
  - Lightness; sensation of – contents had greatly diminished in weight; as if the whole
  - Pulled backward – sensation as if
- **Eye**
  - Heaviness – Lids – pressed down; as if
- **Vision**
  - Colours before the eyes – black – outlines; and white
  - Loss of vision – head – turning agg.
- **Face**
  - Eruptions – acne – Chin & Forehead
  - Pain – burning – chemical; like
- **Mouth**
  - Froth, foam from mouth – convulsions – during
  - Pain
    - § Tongue – eating – after – agg. – burning
    - § Tongue – Tip – burnt; as if
    - § Tongue – Tip – excoriated; as if
    - § Prickling – Tongue – scalded; as if
  - Taste
    - § clammy
    - § nauseous
- Lump; sensation of a – swallowing – agg.
- Mucus – sensation of
- Swallow, constant disposition to
  - § lump in throat, from
  - § mucus, from thick
- **External Throat**
  - Induration of glands
- **Abdomen**
  - Pain – cutting pain – knife; as with a
  - Pain – Solar plexus – blow; pain as from a
- **Male**
  - Sexual desire
    - § excessive – ailments from
    - § increased – erections – without
    - § increased – women – company of women; in
- **Female**
  - Sexual desire – increased – menses – during – agg.
- **Larynx and Trachea**
  - voice – husky
- **Respiration**
  - Gasping
  - Irregular
  - Superficial
- **Expectoration**
  - Frothy
- **Chest**
  - Oedema; Pulmonary
  - Lightness; sensation of – expansive

- Oppression – expiration – deep – amel.
- Oppression – inspiration – agg.
- Pain – Mammae – menses – before – agg.
- Palpitation of heart – irregular
- **Sleep**
  - Sleepiness – sudden
  - Tiredness; without
- **Chill**
  - Heat – overheated; when
  - Perspiration – with perspiration; chill
- **Skin**
  - Cicatrices
  - Discoloration – spots – burnt; as if
  - Eruptions
    - blisters
    - erythema
    - red
  - Inflammation
  - Prickling
  - Swelling – Affected parts; on
- **Generals**
  - Bathing – sea; bathing in the – amel.
  - Breathing – deep – desire to breath deeply
  - Collapse – sudden
  - Comfortable feeling
  - Convulsions – pain – during
  - Hypotension
  - Infectious disease – streptococcus
  - Necrosis
  - Pain
    - burning – hot coals; as from
    - intolerable
    - intractable
    - radiating
    - screaming; from
    - shooting pain
    - waking – on – sore
  - Wounds
    - granulations, proud flesh
    - heal; tendency to – slowly
    - painful

Clupea herangus (Atlantic herring)

Phylum: Chordata.
Class: Actinopterygii.
Order: Clupeiformes.
Family: Clupeidae.

The earliest vertebrates were primitive fish that had evolved during the Cambrian period from yet more primitive creatures with notochords. Fish are generally cold-blooded, breathe underwater through gills, are covered with scales and have fins to help them move easily through water. Most species live either in fresh water or the sea, while some species are able to live in both, moving from one environment to another at various stages of their life cycle. This group contains the largest number of vertebrates on the planet. Fish generally take no responsibility of their young other than releasing eggs or sperm.

The Herring is the most numerous of all the fish in the ocean. It is an obligate schooler, which means it can only survive as part of a large school. These schools can be enormous, there are records of schools being 4 cubic kilometres in size and containing several billion individuals. They move at considerable speed, up to 4 km/hour. They feed by capturing plankton in their gill rakers as they swim through the water with their mouth open. They form a major part of the diet of many ocean fish and cetaceans.

Proving by: **Misha Norland and Peter Fraser, UK (2008).**[3]

Themes in rubrics

- Inclination to sit and meditate
- Affectionate – Sympathetic
- *Amorous – Lascivious*
- *Carefree – Playful*
- Change – desire for
- Undertaking – many things, persevering in nothing
- Disorder; sensitive to
- Rest – cannot rest when things are not in the proper place
- Confusion of mind – identity, as to his – *boundaries*; and personal
- *Connection*; sense of
- *Content*
- Dissolving, she is
- Depersonalisation
- Ease, feeling of
- *Merging of self with one's environment*
- *Tranquillity*
- Danger, impression of
- Escaping – danger; from
- Hiding – danger; from
- Alone
- Detached
- Division between himself and others
- Disconnected feeling
- Estranged
- Isolation; sensation of
- Dream; as if in a
- Unreal – Everything seems
- Confusion of identity
- Dreams – *escaping*
- *Floating* – sensation of
- Out of body experiences
- Helplessness; feeling of
- Impressionable
- Insecurity; mental
- Overwhelmed
- Dreams – hiding
- Activity – desires
- Busy
- Occupation – amel.
- Energy – excess of energy
- Clairvoyant dreams
- High-Spirited
- Mirth
- Vivacious
- Low self-confidence
- Reproaching oneself
- Rejected – unappreciated
- Dreams – pursued, being
- Dreams – prisoner – being taken a
- Trapped

Proving extracts[3]

ᚦ The remedy has **distortions of space and time**. . . . Being able to go with the flow of time and circumstance and everything will work out. This results in a feeling of **calmness and contentment**. There were also feelings of being lucky and happy with gratitude and benevolence. These feeling become more pathological in a feeling of lethargy and a sense of 'I can't be bothered'.

ᚦ Physically there is great heaviness, exhaustion and sleepiness. Provers just wanted to curl up and go to sleep. They felt they couldn't move. There was a polarity of being energised and able to do many things at the same time.

ᚦ There was also considerable **confusion**. This could be of **space and time and of identity and personal boundaries** but was most often expressed as **confusion in communication**. They were unable to connect brain and mouth

Sea Animals

to speak effectively, but could also not follow conversations and were easily distracted.

§ Provers got colds that affected the nose, the ears and the eyes with, often severe headaches and an irritating cough. These were the symptoms of a cold rather than a flu. . . . There were many symptoms of the limbs including heaviness, numbness and pain, which were sometimes severe and prevented walking.

Conchiolinum (Mother of pearl / nacre)

Phylum: Mollusca.
Class: Bivalvia.
Subclass: Pteriomorphia.
Substance: Inner shell layer of bivalve molluscs.

Gordon Adam writes:
*Conchiolinum is the innermost layer of the oyster shell, a beautiful form of calcium carbonate, and many times stronger than the middle layer, from which calc-c is derived. If calc-c is concerned that others might observe their confusion, **conchiolinum has the feeling 'How am I seen?'** Conchiolinum has had a limited proving but is better known for its propensity towards bone and joint inflammation, as well as benign bone tumors. Conchiolinum is the "secretion" which ultimately creates the oyster pearl.*[29]

Proving by: **Claudia Klun and Reinhard Flick, Austria (1992).**

Delusions
• **Crime** – committed a crime; he had
• **Fail**, everything will

Rubrics based on my repertorisation of a case by Anne Vervarcke.[30]

• **Delusions**
  ○ Alone; being
  ○ *Bubble*; as if in a
  ○ *Danger*; impression of
  ○ Fail; everything will
  ○ Floating
  ○ Hard; everything is
  ○ Safe; she is not
  ○ Separated – world; from the – he is separated
  ○ Wrong – something were wrong
• **Fear**
  ○ Night
  ○ *Alone; of being*
  ○ *Betrayed*; of being
  ○ Cancer; of
  ○ Control; losing
  ○ *Death; of*
  ○ *Disease; of impending*
  ○ *Everything; constant of*
  ○ Happen; something will
  ○ *Heart – disease of the heart*
  ○ Poverty; of
  ○ *Rejection; of*
  ○ *Solitude; of*
• **Alert**
• Confidence – want of self-confidence – *support*; desires
• Escape; attempts to – run away; to
• *Estranged*

- Forsaken feeling – *isolation*; sensation
- *Freedom* – desire for
- Hiding – himself
- Inhibition
- Insecurity; mental / Vulnerability
- Intuitive
- Quiet; wants to be
- Reserved
- Sadness
- Sensitive
- Space – desire for
- *Stability – desire for stability*
- Swimming – desires
- Timidity
- Unification – desire for
- Yielding disposition

Mind

- Content
- Forgetful – words while speaking; of
- Forsaken feeling
- Hurry – eating; while
- Indifference – adverse circumstances; to
- Indifference – appearance; to his personal
- Jesting
- Laughing – paroxysmal
- Memory – weakness of memory – say; for what he is about to
- Mood – alternating – wavelike
- Morose
- Quarrelsome
- Quiet; wants to be
- Taciturn
- Tranquillity – cheerful

Dreams

Attacked, of being / Divided – two parts; into / Frightful

Physicals

- Head – Pain
  - Forehead
  - Constant
  - Nose; above – pressing pain
- Teeth – Pain – Roots – sore
- Female
  - **Coition – aversion to**
  - Itching – Vagina – menses – before – agg.
- Larynx and trachea – Voice – deep
- Back – Pain – Spine – rubber; as if made out of
- Pain
  - Joints – boring pain
  - Joints – stitching pain
  - Knees – walking – agg. – stitching pain
  - Shoulders – left – sprained; as if
  - Shoulders – dislocated; as if
  - Wrists – boring pain

Generals

- **Inflammation – Bones; of**
  - *Bone marrow; of*
  - *Periosteum*
- **Pain**
  - *Growing pains*
  - Bones – sore
- Swelling – Bones; of – Condyles – Epiphyses; and
- Tumors – enchondroma

Extremities

- Awkwardness – Lower limbs – stumbling when walking
- **Exostosis**

Sea Animals   **431**

Corallium rubrum (Red coral)

Phylum: Cnidaria.
Class: Anthozoa.
Order: Gorgonacea.
Family: Coralliidae.

Corals, sea anemones, jellyfish and hydras are among the 9400 species in the phylum Cnidaria. *Corallium rubrum* is a soft coral with a rock-hard but brittle internal skeleton. The distinguishing characteristic of precious corals is their durable and intensely coloured red or pink-orange skeleton, which is used for making jewellery. They grow on the rocky sea bottom with low sedimentation, typically in dark environments – in the depths, dark caverns or crevices. Their valuable skeleton is composed of intermeshed spicules of hard calcium carbonate, coloured in shades of red by carotenoid pigments. The skeletal branches are overlaid with soft bright red integument, from which numerous retractable white polyps protrude, exhibiting octameric radial symmetry.

Proving by: **Attomyr, Germany (1830).**

- **Delusions**
  - *Intoxicated* – is; he
  - *Outcast*; she were an
  - *Poisoned* – he – has been
- **Fear**
  - Pain – of the pain
  - Rain, of
  - *Suffering, of*
- *Abusive* – pains; with the

- Confusion of mind – intoxicated – as after being
- *Cursing* – amel.
- Cursing – pains, at
- Late – too late; always
- Quarrelsome – pains – during
- *Slander*, disposition to
- Starting – dreams, in – from a dream
- Starting – sleep – going to sleep; on
- Unconsciousness – cough – during

Bold type respiratory symptoms
- **Larynx and trachea**
  - Catarrh
  - Constriction – Larynx – cough – during – agg.
  - Irritation – Larynx
  - Irritation – Trachea
  - Laryngismus *stridulus*
- **Respiration**
  - Arrested – cough – during – agg.
  - Gasping – cough – during – agg.
  - Loud
  - *Paroxysmal*
  - *Suffocation*; attacks of

- **Chest**
  - Coldness – cold air – breathing
  - Pain – Sides – pressing pain
  - Sensitive – cold air; to –
- **Bronchial tubes**
- **Cough**
  - Cough in general
  - Breathing – deep – agg.
  - Cold – air – *sensation of icy cold air in air passages; from*
  - Constriction; from – Larynx; in
  - *Inspiration agg. – crowing, violent, spasmodic cough – beginning with gasping for breath – followed by*

repeated crowing inspirations – face becomes black or purple and patient exhausted; till – Night and after a meal agg.
- ○ Paroxysmal
  - § Attacks follow one another quickly
  - § Consisting of – short coughs
- ○ **_Rapid, until patient falls back as limp as a rag_**
- ○ Spasmodic
- ○ Tuberculous persons, in
- ○ Whooping
  - § Spasmodic phase
  - § Violent
- ○ Expectoration
  - § Bloody
  - § Cool

Therapeutics Lilienthal[32]

"Nervous, hysterical, spasmodic cough; firing **minute guns of short barking cough**, all day and for half an hour, about evening increasing to a violent spasmodic paroxysm; during deep inspiration sensation as if the air passing through the air-passages was icy cold, with inclination to cough and difficult hawking up of bronchial mucus; cold expectoration; **every atmospheric change causes coughing**. Tuberculosis."

Cypraea eglantina (Cowrie snail)

Phylum: Mollusca.
Class: Gastropoda.
Clade: Hypsogastropoda.
Family: Cypraeidae.

The 'Dog-Rose Cowry' is a species of sea snail. The cowrie was the shell most widely used as money and are also commonly worn as jewellery or used as ornaments or charms. In Mende culture, cowrie shells are viewed as symbols of womanhood, fertility, birth and wealth. They exude a prodigious amount of slime and have a wide, strong, extendable foot that enables them to move at a surprising speed for a snail. Their shells are extremely smooth and shiny because they are nearly always fully covered by the mantle. The mantle itself can be ornamented with papillae of various shapes and colouration which serve to camouflage the animal in its habitat. They have a long sensory tentacle on each side of the head. The prehensile proboscis is located between the two tentacles and there is a well-developed radula that is used to scrape off morsels of algae and other prey.

Proving by: **Anne Schadde, Germany (1996).**[4]

Delusions
- Alone, being – castaway; being a
- Fantasies are forced upon him; a multitude of
- Ground – gave way beneath his feet
- Jelly; the body is made of

- Net; as if in a
- Poisoned – medicine; being poisoned by
- Space – decomposition of space and shape
- Space – expansion of
- World – she has her own little world – clear, but outside is uncertain; in which things are

Characteristic mind rubrics
- Confusion of mind – identity, as to his – *own, as if not his*
- Exhilaration – intoxicated; as if
- *Finances – inability to manage*
- Love – exalted love – humanity; for
- Magnetised – easily magnetised
- Moonlight AGG.
- Sensitive – certain persons, to
- Susceptible (impressionable)

Dreams
Confused / Devils / Historic / Money – gold, of (*Cowrie shells used to be exchanged for financial transactions*) / Teeth – falling out

Characteristic physicals
- **Vision**
  - Darkening of
- **Ear**
  - Water; sensation of – out of ears; running
- **Nose**
  - Odours; imaginary and real – fish-brine, of
- **Throat**
  - Pain – right – extending to – left
- **External Throat**
  - Swelling – cervical glands – lymphatic tissue
- **Bladder**
  - Urination paroxysmal

- **Female**
  - Condylomata – vagina
  - Formication
  - Menses – painful – flow – amel.
- **Extremities**
  - *Eruptions – Legs – urticaria*
- **Generals**
  - Electricity; sensation of static
  - Flabby feeling – internally
  - Food and drinks
    - § Rich food – desire
    - § Yoghurt – aversion
  - Moon – full moon – amel.
  - Twitching – electricity, as from

Extracts; paraphrased from the proving diaries and supervisor's comments.[4]
- ∮ Main polarity of "over-sensitivity, sensibility, tenderness, emotion, romance, love and on the other side hardness, emotional coldness, dullness, cruelty, desire to kill, persecute, rape, guilt".
- ∮ [They] **demand a great deal of attention / affection**. . . they don't have a sense of time, they take everything, they basically consume others due to their complete self-centredness. . . . Every possible demand is harshly expressed . . . at the same time she has a great want for closeness and affection. . . .

$ She is only physically present; **her spirit and her soul are distant**. . . . She wants me to love her but **expects that I notice her needs** – without her having to express them. . . . They are very **attached** and want physical contact, but they send the message **'don't touch me'**. That is why they feel misunderstood by everyone. . . . It is the picture of hysteria; "female narcissism". . . .

$ [However] One prover felt herself *becoming 'more feminine, lively and mature . . . moving towards greater personal freedom'*. . . . *Blockage of communication with the feeling of being paralyzed, unable to act or make decisions. . . .*

$ The outside world cannot understand their state of being. . . . Becoming *isolated, helpless, cornered and powerless; at the mercy of something terrible. . . . Helpless, frozen in a vacuum, unapproachable, disconnected, distant. . . .* Depth, the unconscious, cosmic, deepest emotional levels, into worlds that cannot be described in words. . . .

$ **Something childlike is destroyed, very violent**. . . . Sexuality turned into cosmic union. Tragedy like Romeo and Juliet. Guilt and atonement. **Escapes into dreams of longing – reality is too harsh**. . . . **Defenceless and sensitive**, no sense of time. Confusion . . . Chills alternating with redness of the face; headache with redness of eyes and lack of appetite.

Erythrinus (Red mullet fish)

Phylum: *Chordata*.
Class: *Actinopterygii*.
Order: *Perciformes*.
Family: *Mullidae*.
Genus: *Mullus*. For species see text.

The **red mullets** or **surmullets** are two species of goatfish, *Mullus barbatus* and *Mullus surmuletus*, found in the Mediterranean Sea, east North Atlantic Ocean, and the Black Sea. Both "red mullet" and "surmullet" can also refer to the Mullidae in general.

Erythrinus is an unidentified fish introduced by Compton Burnett on the basis of 'pityriasis rubra' case which was difficult to cure. According to Howard, Erythrinus (which simply means "red" or "reddish") is used as both a generic and specific name for various species of fish, and although the remedy is consistently given as belonging to the Erythrinidae of South America, it is also referred to by the common name of "red mullet" in the 19th century homeopathic literature, introducing confusion, if not a total red herring, into the picture.[27]

Proving by: **Joy Lucas, UK (2007)**.[27]

Themes of the proving. Edited and paraphrased.
Negativity / Anxious nervousness / Dissatisfied and unsettled / Indifferent / **Vulnerable** / **Helpless** / Confused / Inability to concentrate / **Weeping** / **Grief** / Irritability / Separated / **Disconnected** / Identity / Negative feelings / Separated

from friends / Wanting to be separated / Not communicating / Arguing / **Unity** / **Elation** / **Calmness** / Sense of well-being / Excited and happy / Feeling especially fresh and happy in the morning / *Laughing* / *Amusement* / *Desiring company* / Caught between negative and positive / Wrong, everything seems / Change is about to happen / Time distortion / Sensation as if ahead of time / Sensation as if losing track of time / Making plans for the future / Separation / Dwelling on sexual matters / **Feeling of having no will in male presence** / Aversion to men / Being **massively pregnant with the whole earth** / **Hears a man calling her but no-one there**

Delusions
- *Alone, being – world; alone in the*
- *Betrayed – being*
- *Calls – someone calls her*
- *Friend, beloved one – affection of; has lost the*
- *Pregnant; is*
- *Separated – world, from, one is*
- Wrong – everything is
- Wrong – he has done

Mind
- Brooding
- *Censorious, critical – friends, with dearest*
- Company – aversion to – avoids the sight of people
- Compulsive disorders
- Disappointment, deception agg., ailments from
- *Duty – aversion to*
- Dwells – events, on past disagreeable – sexual matters
- Egotism, self-esteem
- *Emotions – controlled by the intellect, need to be*
- Ennui, boredom
- Estranged
- Euphoria, elation
- Fear
  - Eating, of – too much
  - *Observed, of her condition being*
- Forgotten – something, feels constantly as if he had
- Grief – events, about past – long past offenses
- *Grief – silent, pent up*
- Indifference, apathy – ennui, boredom, with
- *Introverted*
- *Men – aversion to*
- Mortification – ailments from, agg.
- Occupation, diversion – desire for
- *Opinion – expects others to pay respect to her*
- Plans – making many plans
- Recognise – does not – people, anyone – relatives, his
- *Respect – desires*
- Sensitive, oversensitive – complaints, to the most trifling
- Unification – desire for
- Vulnerable, emotionally
- Will – loss of

Dreams

Amorous; feeling, without / Arrested, caught, of being / *Attacked*, of being / Birds, of; prey / Castles, of / Danger; brother in / Examinations / *Excrements* / Face; glass, of translucent / Food; refusing / Itching / Killing / Punishment, of / Pursued, of being / Spiders; squashing them / Trapped, he is / Unification, of / Walking, of; unable of, is / Watched, being

Skin eruptions (*cf. Rhus-t., Mez., Sep., Graph., Ars., Led.*)

Extending downward / Elevated / Maculae / Pustules; burning / Pustules; painful / Pustules; stinging, stitching / Rash; scratching; agg. / Rash; itching / Smallpox, variola / Stitching / **Pityriasis rubra** / Uncovering; agg.

Generals – Syphilis

Extracts from the proving (*Wendy Howard*)[27]

- ∮ Strong **aversion to male energy, specifically bullying, aggressive and predatory male energy**. The sort that believes its view of the world is the only one possible. I felt *unusually defensive and vulnerable in its presence*, and **preferred to avoid it**, or, if forced to confront it, to make it plain that there are other ways of seeing the world. . . .
- ∮ Unity consciousness is generally heightened in many provings, it was particularly strong in this one. Sudden eruptions of fury arose in response to separation issues . . . my happiness with my single lifestyle seemed in danger of collapse and frequent dreams in which there was an **overwhelming desire to physically merge with another in a very earthy way**. It was physical contact over the greatest surface area possible that was important, sex being only a natural extension of that. . . .
- ∮ The most dramatic and long-lasting symptoms of the proving, which began post-menses and coincided with the episode of cystitis, were a series of **eruptions which appeared in successive batches**. Initially these were mostly on my inner arms, backs of the hands, and upper legs, then over the course of 3 months they spread and gradually resolved from the top downards and from front to back with the last eruptions on the backs of my legs above the Achillles' tendons . . . eruptions appeared as **papules** with **pseudo-vesicular** centres on raised erythmatous bases with the small "**blisters**" rapidly turning into **flaking skin** or **scabs** surrounded by **dry skin**. The papules were **hyperkeratotic**. . . . The itching felt very deep and was concentrated in the bends of joints – knees, elbows and groin. In my half-waking, half-dreaming state, the itching was associated with website links where the HTML syntax was incorrect and it seemed to me that if I corrected the syntax, the itch would go away. . . . I finally managed to identify the rash as **pityriasis lichenoides**. . . .

Clinical

"Burnett is the authority for the action of this remedy. He based its use from the effects on sailors who ate the fish. They came out with a peculiar red rash which became chronic and which the doctors took for a form of syphilis. Dr. Burnett cured, with it, a case of pityriasis rubra appearing in a large patch on the chest and benefited other cases. He believes this form of skin affection to be a manifestation of syphilis in the second generation, the father of the patient he cured having had syphilis. Aur-m. is the complementary remedy. *Erythrinus might be a remedy highly valuable in forms of chronic skin disease.*" Grimmer[28]

Gadus morhua (Cod)

Phylum: Chordata.
Class: Actinopterygii.
Order: Gadiformes.
Family: Gadidae.

Atlantic cod are a shoaling species and move in large, size-structured aggregations. Larger fish act as scouts and lead the shoal's direction, particularly during post spawning migrations inshore for feeding. Cod actively feed during migration and changes in shoal structure occur when food is encountered. Shoals are generally thought to be relatively leaderless, with all fish having equal status and an equal distribution of resources and benefits. Atlantic cod are apex predators in the Baltic and adults are generally free from the concerns of predation. Juvenile cod, however, may serve as prey for adult cod, which sometimes practice cannibalism. Atlantic cod reproduce during a 1- to 2-month spawning season annually. Adult cod form spawning aggregations from late winter to spring. Females release their eggs in batches and males compete to fertilise them. Fertilised eggs drift with ocean currents and develop into larvae ("fry"). Cod males experience reproductive hierarchies based on size. Larger cod males are ultimately more successful in mating and produce the largest proportion of offspring in a population.

No provings. Self-experiment: **Petroz, France (1830s)**; trituration of cervical vertebrae of the fish.

- **Mind**
  - Death – desires
  - Despair – recovery, of
  - *Express oneself – difficult*
  - Helplessness – sudden, paroxysmal
  - *Pessimist*
  - Thoughts – vanishing of
  - Torpor

- Respiration
  - *Accelerated*, quick – waking, on
  - *Constriction*, contraction – trachea, in
  - *Asthmatic / Painful / Slow*
  - *Chest – Phthisis pulmonalis*
  - *Cough* – whistling, wheezing

Other Physicals

- **Head**
  - Pain, headache – night – agg. – fever, During
- **Hearing**
  - Ticking sound
- **Nose**
  - Motion of wings – fan-like, waving
- **Teeth**
  - Corroded sensation
  - Sensitive, tender
- **Throat**
  - Choking, constricting – night
- **Abdomen**
  - Heat – hypogastrium
  - Heat – burning
  - Pain – stitching – sides – right – pain in Chest, with
- **Rectum**
  - Cholera / Diarrhea – summer
  - Diarrhea – warmth – agg.
- **Larynx and trachea**
- Obstruction, stopped sensation
- **Expectoration**
  - Difficult – lumps seem attached to sides of Chest

- **Back**
  - Pain
    - § Lancinating – dorsal region – spine
    - § Tearing pain
- **Extremities**
  - Pain
    - § Hips – extending to knees – patella
    - § Sore, bruised – hips – extending to – knees
- **Generals**
  - Congestion – blood; of
  - Inflammation – cellular tissue, cellulitis
  - Pain
    - § Sore, bruised – inspiration, deep, agg.
    - § Sore, bruised – bones – long
    - § Stitching – burning
  - Weakness – afternoon – 16 h
- **Clinical**
  - **Diabetes** – insipidus

Galeocerdo cuvier hepar (Tiger shark liver)

Phylum: Chordata.
Class: Chondrichthyes.
Order: Carcharhiniformes [ground sharks].
Family: Carcharhinidae.

The tiger shark is a solitary, mostly nocturnal hunter. It is an apex predator and has a reputation for eating almost anything. Their teeth are unique with very sharp, pronounced serrations and an unmistakable sideways-pointing tip. Such dentition has developed to slice through flesh, bone, and other tough substances such as turtle shells. The skin of a tiger shark can typically range from blue to light green with a white or light-yellow underbelly so that when prey looks at the shark from above, they will be camouflaged, since the water below is darker. Females mate once every three years. They breed by internal fertilisation. The male inserts one of his claspers into the female's genital opening (cloaca), acting as a guide for the sperm. The male uses his teeth to hold the female still during the procedure, often causing the female considerable discomfort.

Proving by: **Melanie Grimes, USA (1997).**[2]

SRP Delusions
- Body – out of the body – someone else saw or spoke outside
- Hearing – tone – world; as from another
- Hollow – organs; being hollow in
- *Injury – about to receive injury; is (snakes)*
- *Ocean – middle of the ocean, not knowing what direction to swim; being in the*
- *Pregnant, she is*
- Strange – voice seemed strange; her own
- *Strangers – control of; under – aliens (snakes)*
- Talking – someone is talking – echo chamber; in an
- Time – hum of time; can hear
- Women – dark-haired – dripping black teeth

Mind
- Anxiety – health; about – own health; one's – *pregnant; wondering if she is*
- Fearless
- Hiding – himself
- Hurry – everybody – must hurry
- Insecurity; mental – hiding it; but is
- Patience
- Pessimist
- Pleasure – wakefulness at night; during
- Secretive – exposure; fear of
- *Thoughts – persistent – sexual desires; about*
- *Threatening – destruction; words of*
- **Fear**
  - Control; losing – ocean; to the
  - Dentist; of going to
  - Destination, of being unable to reach his
  - Ocean – power of the
  - *Separation; of – partner; from*

Dreams
Beaten, being / **Betrayed**, having been / Commune – living in / Flood – floor of house; on / **Homosexuality** – tell her she is homosexual; people / House – other people's; being in / **Identity – search for her** / *People – gatherings – groups, school boards, church commune* / Women – boy; short-haired, thin, blond, no curves, like a / Women – coming to my house – inspecting me and my house / Women – curled up; sitting / **Women – discrimination; against** / Women – underwear; dressed in winter / <u>**Women – widows; we were**</u>

Physicals

- **Vertigo**
  - Driving – curves; on
- **Head**
  - Eruptions – moist – Margin of hair – pustular
- **Eye**
  - Pain – Canthi – Inner – aching
- **Hearing**
  - Strange, her own voice sounds strange in her ears
- **Nose**
  - Discharge – copious
  - Hollow sensation in nose
- **Male**
  - Sexual desire
  - Increased – night – rousing / sleep – disturbing sleep
  - Violent – irresistible
- **Female**
  - Itching – morning
  - Leukorrhea – night / clots; in / cream-like / offensive – putrid – night / scanty
  - Menses – suppressed menses – menopause; during
  - *Sexual desire*
    - § Increased – night – rousing / sleep, disturbing
    - § Insatiable
    - § Violent – irresistible
- **Chest**
  - Fluttering – sensation; of – Heart – excitement agg.
  - Pain – Mammae – right – stitching pain
- **Back**
  - Consciousness – bones; of
  - Pain
    - § Coccyx – lying – agg.
    - § Dorsal region – Spots; in
    - § Spots; in – burning
- **Extremities**
  - Itching – eruptions; without
- **Sleep**
  - Need of sleep – little
  - Waking
  - Easy – senses; acute
  - Periodical – hour – every
- **Generals**
  - Emptiness, sensation of – Whole body is hollow; as if
  - Heaviness – internally – waking; on
  - Pain – motion – amel. / pressure – amel. / tingling pain
  - Touch – agg. – limbs touch each other at night; cannot bear
  - Touch – clothes agg.

Provers speaking as one[2]

ʃ **Hard** feeling toward cat's cry. Usually I would get up quickly to let the cat out, can't stand the cry. Today I would prefer **coldly** throwing the cat against the wall to shut it up . . . felt like throwing her through the window. . . . I lost my temper in front of male visitor and I never lose my temper. I felt like I was trying to bite her head off. I was **attacking**. . . .

ʃ **Embarrassed** about increased **sexual** thoughts. . . . I had sexual desire anytime I was not focused on anything else. Like when I was making dinner, or driving, the desire was high. Constant thoughts of **desiring sex**. I was frustrated because it was often impractical to have sex. . . My mind always comes to rest on sexual thoughts. The desire has reached the point of being uncomfortable and I seriously consider antidoting this remedy. . . .

ʃ *Like my mind is somebody else's. Like being in somebody else's shoes. . . . I feel I am in the middle of an ocean*, not knowing what direction to swim in. It is the same distance to any shore. And they all seem far away. It makes most sense to **flow** and see what direction I go naturally. . . .

§ I just want to lie still and let the sun fill me with **warmth** and **light**. But then the night comes; it is **cold** and **lonely**. I want to be somewhere other than where I am. . . .

§ I fear the **power** of the **ocean** and **fear of being taken over**. . . . It feels **harsh** to me . . . **Depth** of ocean is a **void**. . . . I felt like someone **pulled a plug** on my energy. . . . I felt differently extended, **solid** but **unstable**. This alternated with feeling my **bones**, my **structure** quite firmly. (*Earth – water polarity*). . . .

§ [Thoughts of] Something higher in food chain. What came up for me was that something was *higher in the order of existence*.

Clinical
Sea creatures seem to have a special affinity with the reproductive system. Sepia seems to be for the stage of life of childbearing or just after. Onchorynchus, Salmon is for adolescence. Galeocerdo, Shark, seems to be a menopausal remedy, an old crone.[2]

Hippocampus kuda (Seahorse)

Phylum: Chordata.
Class: Actinopterygii.
Order: Syngnathiformes.
Family: Syngnathidae.

The Seahorse has a carnivorous diet, feeding on small crustaceans and other planktonic organisms. Their body is quite large, elongated and has no spines – all bumps are rounded. The head is relatively large compared to the body. The male broods the eggs in its ventral pouch which contains villi rich in capillaries that surround each fertilised egg – creating a sort of placenta supplying the embryos. Pups exit the pouch once fully grown and go on to live autonomously. Seahorses have no stomach or teeth – they suck in prey through a tubular snout and pass it through an inefficient digestive system. Like other fish, they breathe through gills, extracting oxygen from the water that passes over them. They have one dorsal fin which is rapidly used to propel them through water, and two pectoral fins on either side of the body – used for steering and stability. They are masters of the art of camouflage, changing colour and growing skin filaments to blend in with their surroundings and avoid detection by predators. They are built for manoeuvrability rather than speed as they cannot outrun their hunters.

Provings by: **Chetna Shukla, India (1996); Susan Sonz, USA (2002)**[5]**; Alastair Gray, Australia (2006).**

Mind

- Ailments from
  - Grief
  - Love; disappointed
- Anxiety – conscience; of
- *Aversion – persons – all, to*
- Blissful Feeling
- Company – aversion to – desire for solitude yet fear of being alone
- **Delusions**
  - Breathe
    - § Cannot breathe
    - § Water; can breathe under
  - Control – under his control; nothing is
  - *Division between himself and others*
  - Floating – air; in
  - Heavy; is
  - Light = low weight – is light; he
  - *Lost; she is*
  - *Love is impossible*
  - *Insulted; he is*
  - *Paralyzed*; he is
  - Seasick; he is
  - Separated – world; from the – he is separated
  - *Sounds – muffled*
  - Trapped; he is
  - Water – under water; he is
  - World – cold and dark
- Despair
- Detached
- Elated

- Emotions – unaffected by
- Ennui
- Euphoria – alternating with – sadness – lightness; feeling of
- Exhilaration – alternating with – sadness
- Fate – reconciled to
- Fear – crowd, in a – public place; in a crowded
- Forsaken feeling – isolation; sensation of
- Freedom – doing what he had to do; remarkable freedom in
- Frivolous
- Fun – desire to make
- Giggling
- Grief – loved ones; long lost
- Hair – cut; having hair – desires – bald; desires having hair cut
- Independent
- Joy
- Sensitive – colours, to
- Sensitive – people; to presence of other
- Sensitive – sensual impressions, to
- Spaced-out feeling
- *Spirituality*
- Spoken to; being – aversion – alone; wants to be let
- Suicidal disposition
- Taciturn
- *Tranquillity*

Dreams

Birds / **Breathing under water** / Buildings / Cats / Children; about – **newborns** / Clothes – brightly coloured / Clothes – changing clothes in public / Coloured – black – white; and / Coloured – **exaggerated colours** and proportions / Danger – **escaping** from a danger / Dead; of the – relatives / Destination – reaching – unable / Difficulties – journeys, on / Dogs – buttons instead of eyes / Ducks – mothers and babies / **Excrements** / Fantastic / Fish – **people who are fish** / Gardens / Grass / Guns / **Helpless** feeling / Hiding – danger; from / Hospitals / Ice / Jewellery / Journeys / Killing / Kings – royalty / Light; of – neon / **Locking and unlocking** / **Magic** / **Moon – multiple** / Moon – orange / Mother – dead mother appearing / Music / Mystic / Ocean / Paradise; view of / **Paralyzed** /

Paranormal phenomenon – children / Peaceful / People – old – young; being / **People – transformed** / Pets – dead and beloved / Plants – growing – water; in / Powerful / Rings / Ship – submarine – stone; made of / Snow / Soldier / Spiritual / Stones – floor / **Suffocation** / Threats / Toe – falling off / Treasure / Tunnel / Uniforms / Visionary / Vivid / Water – swimming in

Provers speaking as one[5]

§ **Muffled**, underwater feeling immediately after taking the first dose ... she clearly associates this sensation with the feeling of being **isolated**, sad and **dissociated**. ... Feels like a blanket has covered the day. Muffled sensation, sound, light – **everything far away**. I felt **cut off, inward, trapped, dis-associated**. I felt like I was under water. It was distressing, I was inward focused. The disassociated feeling reminds me of my late teens – It would paralyse me. ... What that "**underwater**" feeling represents is a "cut-offness". ...

§ I was acting **disconnected** ... "Underwater blanket" sensation ... like the feeling in your ears and head when you go under water, **muffled and iso-lating**. The sounds from the outside are muffled, and the sound in your head is amplified. ... I feel **un-grounded**, like I am going to **float** away or lose my mind. I still don't want to see people. I **hide** from them. ...

§ I came away with the feeling that **God has given me a new way of seeing the world**. ... Although Hippocampus does feel isolated, perhaps this is a **desired isolation**, not unlike the natural solitude of the sea horse itself? (It is possible that being alone is conducive to the **spiritual insights** and **mystical realisations** that are mentioned in this proving.) This may indeed be the distinguishing feature of this remedy: a kind of pro-active aloneness, a **positive, colourful relationship with solitude**.

Homarus (American lobster)

Subphylum: Crustacea.
Class: Malacostraca.
Order: Decapoda.
Family: Nephropidae.

The American lobster can reach a body length of 64 cm and a mass of over 20 kg, making it not only the heaviest crustacean in the world, but also the heaviest of all living arthropod species. Mating only takes place shortly after the female has moulted and her exoskeleton is still soft. The female releases a pheromone which causes the males to become less aggressive and to begin courtship, which involves a courtship dance with claws closed. Eventually, the male inserts spermatophores into the female's seminal receptacle using his first pleopods; the female may store the sperm for up to 15 months. The female releases eggs through her oviducts, and they pass the seminal receptacle and are fertilised by the stored sperm. They are then attached to the female's pleopods (swimmerets) using an adhesive, where they are cared for until they are ready to hatch. The larvae go through many moulting phases during their metamorphosis, during which time they are incredibly vulnerable to predation. When threatened, adult lobsters will generally choose to fight unless they have lost their claws.

No provings: **Self-experiments by Cushing, USA (1888).**[34]

Mind
- Anger; violent
- Delusions
  - Move – not move; he could – yet amel. by motion (*Earth-Water*)
  - Shadows, of
  - Superhuman is – control; is under
- Dependent of others
- Fear – suffering, of
- Frightened easily
- Rage, fury
- Restlessness – move; aversion to
- Superstitious

Physicals
- **Head**
  - Pain – blindness, followed by violent headache
- **Throat**
  - Pain – raw; as if
- **Rectum**
  - Diarrhea – alternating with – constipation
  - Flatus – night
- **Skin**
  - Eruptions – Eczema / Urticaria
  - Itching – eruptions – without

- **Back**
  - Cracking – lumbar region – lying on back agg.
- **Generals**
  - Constriction / Tightness
  - Flatus; passing – amel.
  - Food and drinks
    § Fish – agg.
    § Milk – agg.
  - Pain – rheumatic – chill; during

Clinical Clarke[22]
Back – pains in / Bone – pains in / Coryza / Diaphragm – pain in / Dyspepsia / Eyes – affections of / Flatulence / Granular – throat / Headache / **Liver** – pain in / Oedema / Paralysis – nervous / **Pruritus** / Sleep – disorders of / **Spleen** – pain – in / Throat – granular / Throat – sore / Wrist – pain in / **Causation** – milk – effects of

Extracts from the experiments of Dr. A.M. Cushing[34]
§ Remembering that *our most valuable remedies in diphtheria are animal poisons*, and knowing the general fear of being poisoned by eating lobster, I decided to test the poison on myself. I obtained a live lobster and took from the sack just back of the mouth nearly a teaspoonful of a thick, reddish, offensive liquid, the digesting fluid. . . .

- ∮ **Sudden itching** of body and limbs at night, got out of bed and lit the gas to see if there were bugs. . . .
- ∮ Legs lame and painful. Burning pain in legs and feet so I could not go to sleep (mostly below the knees). Feet so hot I had to put them out of bed. As the feet get cool the pain extends up the thighs. . . .
- ∮ Frequent attacks of sudden itching on various parts, worse on limbs. Feet burn . . . Several times a severe sharp pain at the superior spinous process of ilium, left side.[34]

Natural behaviour
Vulnerable whilst shedding the outgrown armour that comes to be too restricting and tight.

Limulus cyclops (Horseshoe crab)

Phylum: Arthropoda.
Class: Merostomata.
Order: Xiphosura.
Family: Limulidae.

Despite their name, horseshoe crabs are more closely related to spiders, ticks, and scorpions than to crabs. They feed on molluscs, annelids, other benthic invertebrates, and bits of fish. Lacking jaws, they grind up food with bristles on their legs and a gizzard containing sand and gravel. Horseshoe crabs are often referred to as living fossils, as they have changed little in the last 445 million years. Forms almost identical to this species were present during the Triassic period 230 million years ago, and similar species were present in the Devonian period, 400 million years ago. Horseshoe crabs are valuable as a species to the medical research community, and in medical testing. The clotting reaction of the animal's blood is used in the commonly employed Limulus amebocyte lysate (LAL) test to detect bacterial endotoxins in pharmaceuticals and to test for several bacterial diseases.

Provings by: **C. Hering, USA (1848); A. Lippe, USA (1848).**

Clinical Clarke[22]
Apoplexy / Cholera / Constipation / Diarrhoea / **Fevers** / Haemorrhoids / **Sea-bathing**, effects of / **Skin** – affections of

Pathogenetic Ward[23]
Acid intestines / **Acne** face / Aorta waves / Beating aorta / Brown spots / Chest full / Cholera expression / Diaphragm impediment / Dislocated hip-joint / Evacuation delayed / Face fever / Facial lines / Gangrene stomach / **Intestines** burning / **Metallic** medicine / Nerves full / Pains indescribable / **Prickling** perspiration / **Suffocative** sternum / Teeth sweet / Warts hands

Mind

- Desires – nothing; desires
- Memory – weakness of memory – names
- **Perseverance** – duties, in performing irksome (*the species is unchanged for millenia*)

Characteristic physicals

- **Ear**
  - Noises in – bubbling
- **Abdomen**
  - Burning heat
  - Flatulency – **Distention, fullness, heaviness, meteorism, tympanites**
  - Flatulency – Flatulence – incarcerated in flexures
  - Inflammation – **Gastroenteritis**
  - Pain – Ileocecal region – cramping
- **Rectum**
  - Cholera
- **Male**
  - Ejaculation – failing during coition
- **Extremities**
  - Eruptions – Hands – herpes
  - Hips – Pain – in right hip
- Numbness – Feet – Sole of
- **Back**
  - Pain – Bending – backward – agg.
- **Skin**
  - Discolouration – red
  - Eruptions – **urticaria**
  - **Formication**
  - Heat – fever; without
  - **Herpes** – of – face / hands
  - Itching – violent
- **Generals**
  - Bathing – sea; bathing in the – agg.
  - Fullness; feeling of – painful – right side of body
  - **Pain – spots; in – burning**
  - Neuralgia – location – Crural anterior

Rubrics based on a repertorisation of a case by Elena Mashalova.[33]

- **Mind**
  - Dancing
  - Escape, attempts to
  - Fear – narrow place, in
  - Fear – suffocation, of
  - Freedom
  - Music – desire for
  - Protected feeling
  - Threatened; feels
  - Dreams – Ocean
- **Generals**
  - **Constriction**
  - **Heaviness**
  - **Numbness**
- *Paralysis* – sensation of
- **Delusions / sensations**
  - *Attacked*; being
  - Crabs, of
  - **Crushed** – she is
  - *Danger*, impression of
  - Drained, sensation of being
  - Fog, invading
  - Influence; one is under a powerful
  - *Intoxicated* – is; he
  - *Invaded*; one's space is being
  - **Safe; she is not**
  - Separated – body – mind are separated; body and
  - **Shell is her protection**
  - Trapped; he is

Natural behaviour

Ability to regrow lost limbs (*cf. Asteria rubens, starfish*). The blood is blue, indicating a high copper content. Hence the remedy has cramps and spasms as prominent features.

Medusa (Jellyfish)

Phylum: Cnidaria.
Class: Scyphozoa.
Order: Semaeostomeae.
Family: Ulmaridae.

Jellyfish and sea jellies are the informal common names given to the medusa-phase of certain gelatinous members of the phylum Cnidaria. Jellyfish are mainly free-swimming marine animals with umbrella-shaped bells and trailing tentacles, although a few are not mobile, being anchored to the seabed by stalks. The bell can pulsate to provide propulsion and highly efficient locomotion. The tentacles are armed with stinging cells and may be used to capture prey and defend against predators. Jellyfish have a complex life cycle; the medusa is normally the sexual phase, the planula larva can disperse widely and is followed by a sedentary polyp phase.

Proving by: **Angelika Gutge-Wickert, Germany (1997).**

Mind

- Ailments from – love; disappointed
- Answering – aversion to answer
- Aversion – children, to
- *Censorious*
- Change – aversion to
- Company – aversion to – desire for solitude
- Conscientious about trifles
- Dancing – amel.
- Delusions
  - *Beautiful – she is beautiful and wants to be*
  - *Hindered; he is*
  - *Work – hard; is working*

- Eating – after – amel.
- *Envy – qualities of others, at*
- Fear – sharks; of (and jellyfish)
- *Hatred – persons – enjoying life, who are*
- Inactivity
- *Independent*
- *Indifference*
- Music – desire for – soft music
- Offended, easily
- Reproaching others
- *Sensitive – beautiful, nice things; to*
- Sleeplessness agg.
- Taciturn

cf. Ars., Urt.

Physicals

- **Vertigo**
  - Motion – head; of – agg.
- **Head**
  - Pain
    - § Beer / Wine – agg.
    - § Pressing pain
- **Eye**
  - Closing the eyes – desire to
  - Lachrymation
  - Pain – Burning
  - Swelling – Lids – edematous
- **Ear**
  - Eruptions – red – swollen; and
  - *Swelling – edematous*
- **Nose**
  - Inflammation
  - Swelling – edematous
- **Face**
  - Eruptions – *vesicles*
  - Swelling – edematous (lips)
- **Mouth**
  - Speech – difficult
- **Bladder**
  - Retention of urine
  - Complaints of urinary organs

- Complaints of genitalia
- **Chest**
  - Eruptions – *vesicles*
  - *Milk – absent / increased*
- **Skin**
  - Eruptions
    - § *Burning / Desquamating / Urticaria – fish agg. / Urticaria – shellfish / Vesicular*
  - *Formication*
  - Heat – Fever; without
  - Numbness
  - *Prickling*
- **Generals**
  - Glands; complaints of the
  - Pain – burning / stitching
  - Seaside; at the – amel.
  - Sleep – after sleep – amel.
  - **Food and drinks**
    - § Fish – agg. / aversion / desire
    - § Milk agg. / desire
    - § Salt – desire
    - § *Shellfish – agg. / desire*

Murex purpurea (Purple dye murex)

Phylum: Mollusca.
Class: Gastropoda.
Superfamily: Muricoidea.
Family: Muricidae.

Purple dye murex is a species of medium-sized predatory sea snail – an edible marine gastropod. Gastropods are one of the most diverse groups of animals in form, habit and habitat. They are by far the largest group of molluscs. Members of the family Muricidae are predators that may use either a secretion to bore holes into shells or the physical force of their proboscis to pry into shelled prey. Many genera use part of their shell to wedge open a clam for feeding. This species produces a secretion which is milky and without colour when fresh but which turns into a powerful and lasting dye when exposed to the air. This species was used by the ancients to produce Tyrian purple fabric dye.

Provings by: **Petroz, France (1840); Hering, USA (1852).**

Mind

- Affectionate – women
- Amorous
- **Anguish – menses – during –** beginning of menses; at the – amel.
- Anguish – pain; from – Hypogastrium
- Delusions
  - Head; floating
  - Melancholy
- Dreams – shooting; himself in head
- Held – amel. being held
- Jealousy
- Lascivious – touch; women become lascivious at every
- **Love – perversity; sexual**
- **Nymphomania**
  - Menopause; at
  - Menses – suppressed, after
  - Metrorrhagia, during
- Restlessness, nervousness; women, in
- Sadness – company – aversion to company, desire for solitude
- Sadness – leukorrhea amel.
- *Sensitive*
- *Shameless*
- Thoughts – disease, of
- *Vivacious* – women
- Weeping – desire to weep – all the time

Female genitalia

- **Cancer** – Uterus
- Conscious – Uterus, of
- Crossing limbs – amel.
- Displacement – Uterus
- Enlarged – Uterus
- Excoriation
- Heaviness – Uterus
- Inflammation – Uterus – chronic
- Itching – leukorrhea; from – menopause; during
- Pregnancy – during; complaints
- Prolapsus – Uterus
- **Sexual desire** – Increased – contact of parts, by least / Menopause; during / Violent
- Ulcers – Uterus – Cervix
- Vaginismus – sensitiveness of vagina; from

Leukorrhea
Acrid, excoriating / Greenish / Yellow – greenish yellow / Menses – after – agg. / Pregnancy agg.; During / Thin / Yellow
Menopause – Pain – menses – *as if menses would appear*

Menses
Before – agg. – Uterus / Clotted / Copious / **Frequent**; too / Irregular / **Protracted** – ten days – ten to twelve days / Scanty / **Metrorrhagia** / Coagulated / Menopause – during

Pain

- **Bearing down**
- **Ovaries** – extending to – Diagonally upward / Ovaries – extending to – upward
- **Uterus** – cutting pain / sore / stitching pain / extending to – upward
- **Uterus and region** – bearing down / pressing on vulva amel. / standing – agg. / Supports abdomen with hands
- **Vagina** – touch – agg.
- **Vulva** – sore

Pathogenetic Ward[23]

Instrument uterus / Sinking epigastrium / Snake ribs / Sore pelvis / Spot pressed / Uterus cutting

Clinical Ward[23]

Burning loins / Chest bruised / **Constriction uterus** / Contused thighs / Cracked skin / Creeping short ribs / **Cutting uterus** / Dilation labia / **Dryness uterus** / Dysmenorrhoea sore place / Enlargement labia / Epigastrium all – gone / Faintness pelvic pressure / Fright indefinite / Gone stomach / Heaviness labia / **Heaviness vagina** / Loins burning / **Loose bones** / Loose pelvis / Pain diagonal / Pain sub-mammary / Pelvis sore spot / Pregnancy looseness / Pressing menstruation / Prostration epigastrium / Pushed genitals / Snake ribs / Sore abdomen / Sore loins / Sore uterus / **Soreness cervix** / Sticking abdomen / Uterus sore / Weight hypogastrium / Weight labia / **Wounded uterus**

Oleum jecoris (Cod liver oil)

Phylum: Chordata.
Class: Actinopterygii.
Order: Gadiformes.
Family: Gadidae.

Cod liver oil is a dietary supplement derived from liver of cod fish. As with most fish oils, it contains omega-3 fatty acids and vitamins A and D. Historically, it was given to children because vitamin D had been shown to prevent rickets, a consequence of vitamin D deficiency. Scandinavian Vikings produced cod liver oil by laying birch tree branches over a kettle of water, and fresh livers were laid over the branches. The water was brought to a boil and as the steam rose, the oil from the liver dripped into the water and was skimmed off.

Proving by: **Neidhard, USA (1872).**

- **Delusions**
  - Identity – errors of personal identity
  - *Insane* – he is insane
  - Mind – out of his mind; he would go

- **Fear**
  - Attacked; fear of being
  - Dark; of
  - Insanity
  - Sudden

Mind
- Affectionate, friendly
- Anxiety – hypochondriacal
- Confidence – want of self-confidence – **support**; desires
- Consolation – amel.
- Mildness
- Quarrelling – aversion to
- Reproaching oneself
- Restlessness – night
- Sensitive – quarrels; to
- Sympathy from others – desire for
- Weak character
- Will – weakness of

Characteristic physicals
- **Cough**
  - Air agg.; draft of
  - Dry
    - § Night – lying – agg.
    - § Sleep – disturbing
  - Laughing agg.
  - Lying – night
  - Paroxysmal – morning
  - Sleep
    - § Disturbing
- Preventing

- **Respiration**
  - Arrested – pain; during
  - Difficult – palpitations; during
  - Painful
- **Head**
  - Pain – Forehead – cough – during – agg. – bursting pain
- **Chest**
  - Palpitation of heart – cough agg.; during
- **Sleep**
  - Sleeplessness
  - Cough, from – lying down, on

Clinical Ward[23]
Aching supra-orbital / **Bursting coughing** / Chill continually / Cold taking / Dead arm / Fluttering sacrum / Hand sacrum / Mind gone / Numbness arm / Periosteum eyebrow / Sacrum support / Split head / Support sacroiliac / Watch occiput

Clinical Clarke[22]
Abscess – cold abscess / Addison's disease / Alopecia / Amenorrhoea / Anaemia / Bone – affections of / Bright's disease / Cold abscess / Dwarfism / **Emaciation** / **Fistula** / **Goitre** / **Hair – abnormal growth of (Hirsutism)** / Heart – palpitation

/ Joints – fistulae and abscess around / Joints – stiffness of / Liver – diseases of / Lumbago / Ophthalmia – scrofulous / Phthisis / Pneumonia / Ringworm / Sacralgia / Scrofulous – ophthalmia / Sleeplessness / Spinal – irritation / Vision – affections of

Temperaments Clarke[22]
Defective nutrition / Face – red / Face – red – in hectic fever / **Milk – children who – cannot take**

Boericke[31]
- Internally, a nutrient and a hepatic and pancreatic remedy. (Burnett.)
- Emaciation, lassitude, scrofulous diseases, rheumatic affections.
- **Atrophy of infants**; emaciation with hot hands and head; restless and feverish at night.
- **Pains in liver region.**
- Tuberculosis in the beginning.

Hering[8]
- Nervous affections, neuralgia, sciatica, lumbago, in emaciated, pale, anaemic persons, with deficiency of animal heat.
- Scrofulosis: diseases of joints; in pale, thin cachectic subjects.
- Rachitis; malacosteon, affecting female pelvis; caries and strumous osteitis.

Oncorhynchus tshawytscha (Pacific salmon)

Phylum: Chordata.
Class: Actinopterygii.
Order: Salmoniformes.
Family: Salmonidae.

The Chinook salmon is the largest species in the Pacific salmon genus Oncorhynchus. They are migratory fish spending one to eight years in the ocean before returning to their home rivers to spawn. They undergo radical morphological changes as they prepare for the spawning event ahead, losing the silvery blue they had as ocean fish – their colour darkens, sometimes with a change in hue. Salmon are sexually dimorphic – the males develop canine-like teeth and a pronounced curve or hook. Studies have shown that larger and more dominant male salmon have a reproductive advantage as female Chinook are often more aggressive toward smaller males. They need adequate spawning habitat – clean, cool, oxygenated, sediment-free fresh water is essential for egg development.

Proving by: **Jeremy Sherr, UK and Israel (2001).**[6]

Fundamental delusions

- Alone, being – world; alone in the
- Beaten; he is being
- Drugged; as if
- Hollow – body is hollow; whole
- Queen; she is a
- Time – timeless and in the present

SRP Rubrics

- Grief – sterility; from
- Speed [= amphetamines] – desire for
- Children – desire to have more children
- Femininity – increased sensation of
- Love – love-sick
- Dreams – nursing newborns

Essence

Arduous Journey, Cycles, Must give birth which = death. Must return home to spawn and get past apex predators to fresh water where they cannot survive. Gives everything for their baby. Travel from the vast open oceans to the source of the river.

Remedy made from Semen, Eggs and Blood

From expensive, luxurious delicacy to over-farmed, ubiquity.

"Salmon sustain the lives of many animals on their **journey**: insects, fish, birds, whales, bears and humans, each waiting their turn on salmon's circular route. And, like nature's clock, salmon **return**, again, and again, and again. Born in the **pureness** of mountain streams, they **feed**, they **nourish**, they **struggle**, they **breed**, and they **die**. Salmon truly resemble the **cycle of life**. . . . I saw salmon jumping the 'ladder' built into the Seattle dam. Exhausted, yet **determined** to push on, they tried, then tried again, until, with incredible **strength** and power of **will**, they cleared the **obstacle** and continued upriver."[6]

Therapeutic indications

Infertility / Endometriosis / Ovarian cysts / Fibroids / Goitre / Slow, exhausting labour

Source words:

Fishy, 'wet fish', slippery, slimy, oyster, mermaid, Neptune, crab, whale, shark, dolphin, shrimp, squid.

Modalities

- **Head**
  - Pain – cold – applications – amel.
  - Pain – mental exertion – agg.
  - Pain – pressure – hard – amel.
- Stomach – Nausea – sleep – after – agg.
- Female – Pain – Uterus – bending double – amel.

- **Extremities**
  - Pain – motion – beginning of – agg.
  - Pain – motion – continued motion – amel.
- Perspiration – Profuse – menses – during – agg.

- **Generals**
  - Ascending – agg.
  - Fasting – agg.
  - Warm – bathing – amel. – hot bath

Provers speaking as one[6]

§ **Sudden, deep belief and conviction that I would find my soul mate or life partner.** . . . Dreams of my soul mate. *Deep, yearning, empty feeling. I feel hollow inside.* Such a deep hunger, but not for food – for something greater, for the other half of myself. . . . **The cycle would continue and separation would follow.** . . . **Deep longing to be pregnant and have children;** I dream about them all the time. How can I last this long without a baby? . . .

§ **Desire to be free and wild.** *I want to die, but the knowledge that I will must return to this world made me feel helpless and trapped.* . . . Feelings of **strength, power** and **speed.** Feel slightly out of control, nervy, like a highly strung race-horse or an athlete about to take off from the starting blocks. As I was walking, *I had a compelling urge to* **walk in a circle.** . . .

§ Extremely **disoriented** when driving in the fog. Got lost and went round roundabouts several times, often picking the wrong way and doubling back on myself. Walked in a circle and ended up in the same place I started from. **I have lost my sense of direction totally.** . . . The bottom of my soul is like all time and all life times, like there is no time and it is just the journey of the soul. It feels like a circle is near to completion. . . .

§ Dream: **"Make baby."** An alien spoke in its language, happy, laughing, easy and comfortable with them both. . . . I felt **wise** and **knowledgeable.** . . .

§ Dream: Many peasant people *dressed in rags*. They all look white. They are carrying sacks of white powder and they are covered in it. They are **crowded together, milling around and going nowhere.** Someone told me that they had come from another place *in search of a better life*.

Pecten jacobaeus (Scallop)

Phylum: Mollusca.
Class: Bivalvia.
Order: Ostreoida.
Family: Pectinidae.

Scallops are one of very few groups of bivalves to be primarily 'free-living'; many species are capable of rapidly swimming short distances and even of migrating some distance across the ocean floor. A small minority live cemented to rocky substrates as adults, while others are more simply attached by means of a filament they secrete called a byssal thread. The majority live recumbent on sandy substrates, and when they sense the presence of a predator such as a starfish, they are able to escape by swimming swiftly but erratically through the water using a form of jet propulsion created by clapping their shells together. They have a well-developed nervous system, and unlike most other bivalves they have numerous simple eyes situated around the edge of their mantles.

No proving: **Clinical observations by Thomas Franklin Smith, USA (1879).**

CASE 7.1 Change in life purpose

Patient: **Female, age 40**

Prescription: **Pecten jacobaeus 200c**

∫ Pulled into a completely new cycle; an intense integration period.
∫ Looking for **support** as I move into new spaces.
∫ Want to run, avoid and **hide** (from difficulties).
∫ Smoking weed, taking mushrooms – **numbing** out.
∫ Feel a call to **open** into and integrate. Want to sit and reflect but reality is about money.
∫ *The flow of life pulls you in different directions.*
∫ Body is catching up, feeling fatigued but internally like everything is going at higher revs.
∫ My default position is to look for **protection**.
∫ Getting rid of the 'people-pleasing' me.
∫ New phase, thinking about **children vs. independence**. Biological clock is ticking.
∫ *Overarching all of it is a **desire to go deeper within myself through intimacy and connection**.*
∫ Desire to love and give birth – the next stage as a human.
∫ But it is not **clear**, it feels **muddy**.
∫ Feel as though there is an inner chaos **bubbling**, but *underneath that is wisdom.*
∫ When singing, my role is as a *channel for the collective.*
∫ **Disconnected** *vs.* **Safe, holding, connection, oneness, trust.**
∫ **Transcending** *feels too scary. So, comes back to **survival**, doing, **fear-based** actions.*
∫ *Sometimes have access to pure **bliss** and joy. Capable of channelling, but it feels massive, so it is scary. **Out of my depth**, not ready for it. **Need anchoring**.*
∫ Want to let go, into my voice and into intimacy and allow that to lead me.
∫ To drop into mystery is way too frightening and unpredictable.
∫ It is like ***grasping, clinging***, becoming ***ungrounded, swirled around***, not *churning, it is just chaos.*
∫ **Can't find my anchoring.**

∫ In reality, it is all **blurry**. I am not *connected* to the moment . . . *checking out . . . (escapism)*.

∫ Chaos means not knowing which action to take (*Irresolution*).

∫ *Want to be OK with being in the void, or* **pulled in a current**. *It is actually exciting and free getting* **pulled in that flow**, *feels spontaneous and* **fresh**.

∫ There is *resistance* to singing, to using my voice (*Earth element*). An inability to get clarity of speech. Resistance is like fear of making a sound, *shyness, tentative,* **closed**. . . .

∫ All coming from the neck, not from anywhere else. **It is like an entity** in its own right (*Animal*).

∫ When I get into a trance that helps the sounds out. It is like I've **shut something down and can't open it**. Just want to find the key for now, this is what I am missing.

∫ Disconnected is like *blackness, can't see it; it is out of view.*

∫ Trance is like sounding without thinking or worrying. *I just am the voice, not the body.* I can feel the *emotion coming through in* **waves** *of feeling.* Like connecting with my ancestors.

∫ When I use my voice and can be a channel, it feels like an **untethering**, pulling out of the shadow.

∫ *It is not ropes, more like horse's tails.* I am **tied to things but there's movement, push and pull** . . . Slowly losing grip.

∫ An anchor is like **holding myself in a place of safety, tethering to something that is serving you**.

∫ But I am *holding myself back*, not being seen or felt. It is like a wall; *guarded and* **protective**. But I want to **surface** emotionally. I am not fully revealed; so am not fully connecting with others. It should feel like a dance, just being in the moment. Like a **merging** with others.

∫ I have an over-active self-doubt muscle! Easily activated into feeling emotional. My little-girl gets tantrummy. *Feel unworthy of being loved, needed or wanted.* Of being too much. . . .

∫ Never want anyone to see me again, **crawl into a hole and never come out**.

∫ *Feel like I want to* **contract**.

∫ Part of me loves the chaos; *like being thrown around in the river.*

Symptoms

∫ Grief / Ailments from disappointed love (repeated) / Weeping suddenly (causeless) / Bumping into things, breaking things, losing things; can't find purse / Disconnected feeling / Company, desire for; community, needs / Panic / Anxiety / Tightness in chest / Emotions, too strong.

The patient was prescribed Pecten jacobaeus based on the characteristic language she used to describe her state. The patient does not spontaneously offer symptoms as such, so following the advice contained in the *Organon,*

I prefer to allow the patient as much freedom to explore their state in their own natural manner.

Animal language
∫ **It is like an entity** in its own right. Transcending *feels too scary. So, comes back to **survival**, doing, **fear**-based actions / the next stage as a human.*

Sea animal language
∫ *Disconnected vs.* **Safe, holding, connection, oneness, trust** / Clear / Muddy / Deeper / Bubbling / Out of my depth / Need anchoring / Ungrounded / Swirled around / Blurry / pulled in a current / Pulled in that flow / Merging / Surface / Transcending

Mollusc language
∫ Crawl into a hole and never come out / Contract / Guarded / Protective / Holding myself in a place of safety / Tethering to something that is serving you / Shut something down and can't open it / closed / Can't find my anchoring / Grasping, clinging / Need anchoring / Out of my depth / **Desire to go deeper within myself through intimacy and connection**

Scallop
∫ **Tied to things but there's <u>movement, push and pull</u>** – *It is not ropes, more like horse's tails /*
∫ Part of me loves the chaos; like being thrown around in the river / Want to be OK with being in the void, or pulled in a current. It is actually **exciting and free getting pulled in that flow**, feels spontaneous and fresh / Ungrounded, swirled around.

Analysis
The scallop can swim "erratically through the water using a form of jet propulsion created by repeatedly clapping their shells together"; so it has much greater freedom than other bivalves that cling obstinately to their rock for support; remaining forever in their comfort zone of protection. The scallop can also tether itself by threads – "A small minority of scallop species live cemented to rocky substrates as adults, while others are more simply *attached by means of a filament they secrete called a byssal thread*".[38]

The patient's situation is that she is struggling with making a transition from being very free and independent into living with a new romantic partner. There is a history of repeated break-ups when the relationships get too difficult. She works as a bodywork healer and combines this with singing to facilitate other's journeys towards a life more connected to the source of 'pure bliss and joy'.

As there are precious few rubrics for the remedy Pecten jacobaeus, use of the repertory would have been difficult in this case.

The only recorded symptoms of Pecten jacobaeus pertain to a cure of humid asthma by Drs Swan and Smith, as mentioned in Clarke's dictionary.[22] There has not been a proving.

Sepia officinalis (Cuttlefish)

Phylum: Mollusca.
Class: Cephalopoda.
Order: Sepiida.
Family: Sepiidae.

Cuttlefish, like other Cephalopods, have sophisticated eyes. Although they cannot see colour, they can perceive the polarisation of light, which enhances their perception of contrast. They have two spots of concentrated sensor cells on their retinas (known as foveae), one to look more forward, and one to look more backward. They have ink stores that are used for chemical deterrence, phago-mimicry, sensory distraction, and evasion when attacked. When faced with a predator, Sepia and other Cephalopods sometimes change and show 4 or 5 body patterns within a few seconds, presumably to confuse or startle the predator. By changing its appearance from moment to moment, potential predators are confronted by quite different looking forms over a short time span. Attempts to threaten or intimidate opponents include creating an illusion of largeness by flattening the body, paling of the skin and creating the impression of possessing multiple eyes and dilated pupils. The blood of a cuttlefish is an unusual shade of green-blue, because it uses the copper-containing protein haemocyanin to carry oxygen instead of the red, iron-containing protein haemoglobin found in vertebrates' blood. Studies are said to indicate cuttlefish to be among the most intelligent invertebrates. They also have one of the largest brain-to-body size ratios of all invertebrates.

Provings by: **Hahnemann, Germany (date unknown); Robinson, UK (1867); Berridge, UK (1871–74); Owens, Wesselhoeft and Allen, USA (1875).**

Cephalopod

Cuttlefish have their feet are around their mouth and their calcareous structure has been internalised, so the creature has **sacrificed protection of home (outer shell) for freedom of movement, opting instead to be a master of disguise and supreme escape artist**. Interestingly, smaller males who 'cross-dress' in order to sneak past the violent intent of the bigger dominant males are more successful in their liaisons with the female cuttlefish, showing the evolutionary imperative of **skilful daring and clever use of camouflage** for this species. Compared to the majority of Molluscs, Sepia no longer survive by clinging to rock – they can be independent and move freely, using jet propulsion and ink clouds to escape from and disorientate predators.

Keynotes
- Disgust of odours (cooked food, husband's odour) agg. during pregnancy
- Domestic duty – overwhelmed and exhausted by the monotony of
- Fear of poverty – leading to industriousness and cares about trifles *vs.* desire for freedom
- Bearing down sensations, sagging, dragging (ptosis)
- Mocking, sarcastic
- Intuitive (especially to weakness of others *cf. Lachesis*)
- Androgyny (combination of masculine and feminine characteristics into an ambiguous form)
- Love for dancing and music
- Senses acute
- agg. after coition ++
- Aversion + Indifference in general(!) – to company, to loved ones, to being touched, to coition
- Joyless
- Introversion *vs.* Exhibitionism (dazzling colour displays)
- Consolation agg.
- Screams unless she has something to hold onto (Uterus – sensation as if clutched)
- Emptiness of stomach when thinking of food (Major remedy in morning sickness)
- Vomiting (bile) during pregnancy
- Thirstless
- Sensations as of a ball, fullness, lump, as if faeces remained *vs.* emptiness & internal organs being forced out
- Prolapse
- Cracked skin, ringworm, blotches, vitiligo
- Circulation – flushes of heat
- Hormonal changes (contraceptive pill, menses, menopause)
- Easy fainting

Sepia polarities from the repertory
- Aversion / brooding / envy / hatred / introspection / misanthropy / sarcastic / repulsive / pessimistic
  vs.
- Affectionate / amorous / benevolent / carefree / curious / dancing / frivolous / laughing / mirthful / positive / vivacious
- Abrupt / ambitious / attacking / harsh / intolerant / passionate / violent / cramping / tension
  vs.
- Abused / dominated / clinging / cowardly / neglected / timid / yielding / flabby / sluggish / puffy

- Affectionate / impressionable / intuitive / maternal / secretive / sentimental / sympathetic / weeping
  vs.
- Avaricious / careful / dutiful / objective / obstinate / responsible / serious

Fundamental delusions
- **Starve; she will / family will**
- **She is being sick and will therefore not work**
  - Express the exhausted burnt-out state of sepia who wants to be left alone. The only way to get out of her responsibilities is to become sick.
- **Alone, being – graveyard; alone in a**
  - What is the feeling behind this delusion? Other rubrics describe a great amelioration from solitude, so perhaps the graveyard is sought after in order to avoid company which requires more effort than the dragged-down Sepia can muster.
  - A graveyard is a place of mourning for lost loved-ones, which is interesting as Sepia can end up feeling indifferent to loved ones, as if they have become lost, if the Sepia state has progressed to the stage of extreme lethargy and apathy.
  - She feels as though she is in a graveyard amongst the tombstones of her family, who have become lost to her, through this extreme bearing-down of duty that her fragile energy levels cannot tolerate.
- **Run – backward; he were chased and had to run**
  - Escape and evasion are the key to Cephalopod survival. Using jet propulsion, they do actually escape backwards! In symbolic terms, moving backwards in the context of being chased, could be felt as a handicap – it is certainly more difficult than running forwards to escape. Although at least running backwards you have your attacker in full sight. In general though, this delusion is an important symbol for those whose tendency is to flee from difficult life circumstances.
- **Strain herself; she could easily**
  - Laxity is a key feature in Sepia – hypermobility – feeling like the abdominal organs are heavy and bearing down, as if they would fall out. The cuttlefish has internalised their calcareous structure so the exterior is incredibly soft and vulnerable. DD Calc.
- **Standing – must stand up – sitting; when**
  - Cannot rest – has to work and keep herself moving. That is the experience of Cephalopods in the ocean. They are constantly under threat and have to be clever and resourceful to survive. There can be no rest – that is an important delusion of Sepia and leads to the worn-out states we see clinically.

Dreams
Astray, going / Body – **deformed** / Business – day, of the / **Carousing** / Continuation – dreams, of – waking, after / **Endless** / Exhausting / Face – **disfigured** / **Falling – height, from a** / Falling – water, into / Ghosts – **fighting with ghosts** / **Lawsuits** / **Lost**; being – forest; in a / Mice / **Pursued, being – run backwards,**

must / Rape – threats of **rape** / **Rats** / Rousing the patient / Running / **Snakes** / Threats / **Vermin** / Vexatious / Visionary

Fears

- **Alone; of being**
- Approaching; of – others; of
- Cancer; of
- Crowd; in a
- **Death, of – soon; that one will die**
- Driving him from place to place
- Fever – during fever
- Friends; of his – meeting his friends; of
- Going out; of
- High places; of
- Humiliated; of being
- Injury – being injured; of – sewing; when
- Job, to lose his lucrative
- Joints are weak, that
- Killing, of – child; her
- **Narrow place, in – vaults, churches and cellars; fear of**
- **Old; of getting**
- **People; of – being alone; yet fear of**
- **Pregnant**; of getting
- Rats
- **Separation**; of – husband; from
- **Sex; of opposite**
- Snakes; of
- **Social position; about his**
- Spiders; of
- <u>**Starving; of**</u>
- Stool – involuntary stool; of
- Thunderstorm; of
- Touched; of being
- Tremulous

Injuring himself – fear to be left alone, lest he should injure himself

Sensations & functions

- **Scream – unless he held on to something, he would**
  - Reveals the intensity of the Sepia state at its worst. e.g. Intense uterine cramps
  - Sensation – as if everything is falling out (ptosis). Function is to hold on tight.
    - § Abdomen
      - *Beaten – together, intestines would be*
      - *Contents, intestinal, would issue through genital organs*
      - *Full – and contents of abdomen would fall out over pubes, bladder were*
      - *Torn – out, intestines were*
      - *Turn inside out, bowels would*
    - § Rectum, anus and stool
      - *Fall – involuntary stool would*
      - *Weight – like a ball in anus*
    - § Female sexual organs
      - *Clutched then suddenly released, uterus were*
      - *Contents of pelvis would pass through genitals*
      - *Crossed to prevent protrusion from vagina, limbs must be*
      - *Force itself out of vagina, something heavy would*
    - § Neck and back – break – in back, something were going to

Camouflage

- Hiding from predators. Covered by spots and freckles which change according to environment in order to camouflage them.
- Dark cloud of ink, over-pigmentation, chloasma, melanin over / under-production.
- The remedy is made from the ink which is used as a **decoy** to **escape** from predators.
- Sepia has internalised its calcareous structure which provides **free mobility** and eyes.
- No skeleton to give them resistance – hence **laxity** is a feature.
- 'Pathological state of relaxation' For example, ligaments more lax in women, hence predominantly female remedy.
- **Soft, vulnerable**, can be eaten by many predators.
- Mollusc-like features – *drawn back to safety of family and partner.*
- They must be **smart and cunning to survive**, using their ink as an **evasive** measure.
- **Solution is to escape quickly, unseen:**
- When attacked, shoots backwards at great speed using water propulsion, emptying ink sac, leaving **dark cloud.**
- Vigorous motion (especially exercise) ameliorates as this stimulates the circulation and tissues.
- **Only one mating season then they all die. Offspring are orphans.**
- In the patient – motherhood is perceived as a threat to independence and they end up feeling coerced into doing things "opposed to their intentions." Kent[18]
- **Retiring and masking** – because vulnerable.
- Can become introverted – socially unresponsive, withdraws from social contact because it is such a great effort to come out of the stupor.
- "In her run-down condition she feels stupid, dull, forgetful; and when over-wrought she feels she must hold tightly to something to keep from screaming." Coulter[15]
- She does not lack love but "simply has no physical or emotional energy left for love. . . . Love does not go forth into affection." Kent[18]

Reproduction

Females are very picky about with whom they mate and which sperm they use to fertilise the eggs. Smaller males who 'cross-dress' in order to sneak past the violent intent of the bigger dominant males are more successful in their liaisons with the female cuttlefish. This characteristic links to the symptom of being averse to the opposite sex.

Exhibitionism

- They use a dazzling visual display of shifting colours to stun and capture their own prey.
- They have strong emotions (like Nat-m.) but when over-exerted or suffering from excesses (particularly sexual) they develop indifference and guardedness, desiring solitude to recover their depleted energy reserves (*cf.* Nux-v.).

Sea Animals 463

This situation in a human context has become most commonplace; mothers opt for continuing their careers alongside family responsibilities. Calc-carb would be gathering everyone around her in the home and embracing the mother role wholeheartedly. **Sepia is torn between the impulse to act independently and the instinct to be the dutiful mother**, which as the repertory tells us, is (at least partially) opposed to her intentions. In nature, the **cuttlefish has only one mating season, leaving her young to be orphans**, and dying soon after. No wonder the remedy is considered sterling in cases where there is aversion to loved ones, family and husband.

Compare with Calcarea, where the inherent fragility of the Mollusc's survival, dependent on clinging to a rock surface its whole life equates to stasis and immovability and improper assimilation. Sepia has a great deal of weakness, irritability and "complete intellectual and emotional indifference and indolence" Gutman[19]

Evasive, Escaping

To be a successful Sepia, they must be quick-witted, decisive, clever, evasive, dazzling, always on their guard – **the sea is a dangerous world of sudden, unexpected attack!** These actions ultimately require a great deal of resources to maintain and eventually lead to the sepia picture in pathology – that of being **dragged down, sagging, nagging and indifferent** to everything around them. They are worn out by the rigours of life's demands – or more specifically, the demands they place on themselves in order to be successful out there in the world, whilst simultaneously fulfilling their duties as a parent.

Hidden, Unseen

Their survival depends on escaping, hiding, being extremely well camouflaged, being picky, rejecting the advances of males. They need to remain unseen and there are many rubrics about desiring solitude and being ameliorated by it. There is something innately evasive about people who respond to sepia in potency. They don't like narrating their symptoms, or even taking medicine – they just want to be left alone to deal with their grief in the only way they know how – to find peace in solitude, away from the nagging demands of their dependents.

They have a fear of being dominated; in nature they reject the dominant males and choose the sneaky, cross-dressing males – the ones who go unseen most successfully, who excel at deception. This is what will aid them in survival in a dangerous world where they **feel vulnerable and at risk of being forced to do things they do not want to.**

Delusion that she is alone in a graveyard

What is the feeling behind this delusion? Other rubrics describe a great amelioration from solitude, so perhaps the graveyard is sought after in order to avoid company which requires more effort than the dragged-down Sepia can muster. A graveyard is a place of mourning for lost loved-ones, which is interesting as Sepia can end up feeling indifferent to loved ones, as if they have become lost, if the Sepia state has progressed to the stage of extreme lethargy and apathy. She feels as though she is in a graveyard amongst the tombstones of her family, who have become lost to her, through this extreme bearing-down of duty that her fragile energy levels cannot tolerate.

Characteristic symptoms
- **Ptosis** in abdominal organs, sensation of drooping and prolapse.
- Characteristic sensation of a ball or lump in the internal organs – ptosis of wall muscles.
- Dullness, of being dragged down, bearing down of sexual organs.
- Forced to act against her own will, down-trodden, brow-beaten.
- Drawn back to partner who dominates her, and family who demand from her (*cf.* Molluscs).
- Desires brisk movement, exercise and amel. by occupation.
- Seeks solitude and craves independence (Cephalopod).
- Melanin increased in endocrine disturbance during pregnancy and menopause and in Addison's disease (function of adrenal cortex impaired).
- Hypo-adrenia is very similar in early phases to Sepia.
- Apathy, dejection, sadness, weeping, apprehension, dizzy spells, fainting attacks, muscles atrophy, eyelids droop, speech retarded, severe backache, headaches, insomnia, constipation, sexual desire lost, aversion to fatty food.
- *Nausea from smell of cooked food – SRP.*
- **Circulation** = congestion, heaviness of legs. Metabolism slowed, stagnation and putrefaction.
- **Ink** is melanine (most widespread pigment of the body).
- Contains: 12% sulphur, hence circulation, venous stasis, liver and skin symptoms – (Psoric miasm – the water version of sulphur). *Nash – nearer to Sulphur than any other remedy.*
- Senses acute – *cf.* Nux vomica.
- Boenninghausen – very excitable when in company. Angry, sensitive, irritable.
- Crave sour flavour.
- Obstinate constipation and haemorrhoids.

Irresponsive
- Shut off in own world – does not care at all what happens.
- Company, aversion to, avoids the sight of people, and lies with closed eyes.
- Company, aversion to, desires solitude to lie with closed eyes.
- Company, aversion to, menses, during.
- Delusions, that she is alone in a graveyard.
- Desire to be alone, but also a fear of being left alone.
- Sense of self – loss of identity – Sea remedies.
- Negative atmosphere, depression, misery.
- Suppressive, hides his emotions, suspicious nature, driven by hidden urges.
- *Can appear like Phos before life bears down on her.*

CASE 7.2 Insomnia

Patient: Female, age 38

Prescription: Sepia 200c

∫ **Our dad was more like our mum** – he would look after us and take us to school.

∫ We spent more time with him. **My mum was not maternal. In a way we lost our mum.** I was quite resentful. **I took on the mum role** – I became a mum. Bit of **resentment** for that. She was away with her boyfriend doing evening courses. That's where our problem lies; she's got the child role and **I've got the mum role in our relationship** (*cf. Milks*), which does not work. . . .

∫ No matter what country, I never feel settled – I think that is my **fleeing** mode; to run away from problems. I always glamorise where I could be; generally I am quite a **dreamy** type, I can often see myself somewhere different. Moving a lot in childhood – never had a place where i thought – i am going to stay here.

∫ Maybe I just don't deal with **pressure?** This isn't where I wanna be (Laughing);

∫ obviously fleeing. Work is so hard I am **drained.** Cos my **daughter is so clingy** she is just on me the whole time so I can't do anything.

∫ *Tell me about about the effect that pressure has on you –*

∫ I just try and **flee.** Used to try and drink a lot of alcohol – that's just running away. Maybe I am quite good at running away.

∫ Pressure gets to me at work – I always want to do my best – **don't want to let anyone down.**

∫ Feel **pressured** – and agonise all day – how do I say no. That makes me anxious, which affects my sleep cos I am anxious about having said no (to an extra shift).

∫ That's the feeling that I can't . . . I can't keep up with the pressure, even if I do my best it is not good enough.

What's the experience of being under pressure – what happens generally when there is pressure?

∫ Someone would **explode** . . . **Feel crushed, heavy.**

∫ I am in no way **confrontational** (spontaneous denial of the animal kingdom), but my mum has just been here – we've been getting on fine. But she does not clean up or anything. I am doing her washing. In my mind, I am **bubbling up** thinking I am going to say something to her. Then I think, no I won't because we'll have an argument, and then I won't be able to sleep. So it is all inside me getting angrier and angrier.

∫ **I never confront anyone.**

How would you summarise your mum?

∫ She has just got multiple personalities – a really breakable side, a depressed side, and an unreasonable horrible side . . . she struggles and is up and down. If you cross her, **you expect her to start a real revenge against you (animal)**. I am exactly the opposite. I was always the responsible one. And I just looked after the babies all day from a really young age.

Note how the animal characteristics have been projected onto somebody else.

	sep.	sil.	lach.	sulph.	phos.	hep.	nat-m.	aur.
	1	2	3	4	5	6	7	8
	14	14	13	13	13	13	13	13
	35	26	32	32	29	28	24	22
1. MENTAL QUALITIES - Money (238) 1	4	2	2	4	2	4	2	4
2. MENTAL QUALITIES - Snakes (204) 1	3	2	4	2		2	2	1
3. MIND - ANXIETY (692) 1	2	2	2	3	3	2	2	3
4. MIND - CONFUSION OF MIND (578) 1	3	3	3	2	2	1	3	2
5. MIND - MEMORY - weakness of memory (406) 1	3	2	3	2	3	3	2	2
6. HEAD - DANDRUFF (81) 1	2	1	2	3	3	1	3	1
7. FACE - ERUPTIONS - acne - rosacea (71) 1	2	2	3	2	1	1		1
8. BACK - PAIN - Lumbar region (465) 1	3	2	2	3	3	2	2	1
9. SLEEP - SLEEPLESSNESS (702) 1	3	3	3	3	3	3	2	2
10. SKIN - ERUPTIONS - boils (167) 1	2	2	3	3	2	3	2	1
11. GENERALS - EATING - after - amel. (127) 1	3	1	1	1	3	2	1	
12. GENERALS - EATING - while - amel. (142) 1	2	1	3	1	1	2	1	1
13. GENERALS - FOOD AND DRINKS - sweets - desire (286) 1	2	1	1	3	2	2	1	1
14. MIND - YIELDING DISPOSITION (73) 1	1	2			1		1	2

Figure 7.2 Repertorisation

Spongia tosta (Roasted sea sponge)

Phylum: Porifera.
Class: Demospongiae.
Order: Dictyoceratida.
Family: Spongillidae.

Spongia officinalis is a commercially used sea sponge. Individuals grow in large lobes with small openings and are formed by a mesh of primary and secondary fibres. It is light grey to black in colour and is found throughout the Mediterranean Sea up to 100 meters deep on rocky or sandy surfaces. They can reproduce both asexually, through budding or fragmentation, or sexually. Individuals can be dioecious or sequential hermaphrodites. The free-swimming larvae are lecithotrophic and grow slowly after attaching to a benthic surface.

Proving by: **Peter Friedrich, Germany (2000).**

Mind

- **Brooding** – condition, over one's
- Confusion of mind – surroundings, of
- **Courageous** – alternating with – **fear**
- Cruelty – seeing or hearing cruelty; cannot bear
- **Death** – dying, sensation as if
- **Despair** – life, of
- Resignation – *senselessness; feeling of*
- Sadness – dwelling constantly on her condition
- Sadness – impotence, with
- Sensitive – cruelties, when hearing of
- Suicidal disposition – perspiration, during
- Weary of life – fear of death, but
- Wretched

Delusions

- Closing eyes; on
- Clothes – uncomfortable
- *Deceived; being*
- Fail; everything will
- Faint; he would
- Identity – errors of personal identity
- *Insane – he is insane*
- *Meaningless; everything is*
- Motion – up and down; delusion of a motion
- **Murdering**; he is – has to murder someone; he

Fear

- Coughing; of – whooping cough; during
- **Death, of – fatal end of disease; of**
- **Death, of – suffocation; from**
- Heart – disease of the heart – organic disease; of
- Suffocation, of – heart disease, in

Bold type Respiratory symptoms

- **Larynx and trachea**
  - Constriction – Larynx – sleep – during
  - Croup – night – midnight – before
  - Dryness – Larynx – perspiration; during
- **Pain**
  - Cough agg.; during – burning
  - Larynx – singing agg.
  - Larynx – swallowing – agg. – sore
  - Larynx – touch agg. – sore
  - Trachea – cough – with – burning
- Sensitive – Larynx – touch; to
- Spasms – Larynx – Thyroid gland; from enlargement of the
- Turning head agg.
- Voice – crowing
- **Respiration**
  - Asthmatic
  - Bending – head – backward – amel.
  - Cold; after taking a
  - Difficult
  - Menses – during – agg.
  - Sleep – after – agg.
  - Talking – after
  - Impeded, obstructed – constriction – Larynx; of
  - Rough – crowing / sawing
  - Touch – throat agg.; touching
  - Turning – head – agg.
- **Cough**
  - Drinking – amel.
  - Dry
  - Drinking – amel.
  - Eating – amel.
  - Excitement
  - Rasping

Chest

- **Oppression**
  - Lying – head low; with the – agg.
  - Heart – lying – head low; with the – agg.
- Orgasm of blood – exertion, least
- **Pain**
  - Cough – during – agg. – dry cough
  - Cough – during – agg. – dry cough – burning
  - Heart – lying – agg.
  - Heart – lying – head low; with the – agg.
- **Palpitation of heart**
  - Night – midnight – after – 1–2 h
  - Night – midnight – wakes up
  - Menses – before – agg.
- **Phthisis** pulmonalis – progressive
- Weakness – exertion agg.; after

Therapeutics Lilienthal[32]

"Laryngo- and tracheo-bronchitis. Croupy, dry, sibilant cough, continuing day and night, in long-lasting, distressing paroxysms, laboured, crowing, wheezing inspirations, sometimes accompanied by râles. On every slight exposure the cough returns violently, with pressing dyspnoea, sibilant rhonchi, and violent, convulsive cough. Dry bronchitis, with terrible, hard, dry, racking cough; much dyspnoea and slight expectoration, agg. in hot room, amel. by eating ever so little; stuffed, obstructed sensation, difficult inspiration, agg. by lying down, amel. by leaning forward and by eating and drinking."

"Contracting pain in heart; heat, suffocation, faintness and anxious sweat; pressure across chest, as from a heavy weight, especially at aortic arch (aneurisma aortae); sudden awaking after midnight, with suffocation, great alarm and anxiety; agg. with the head lying low, at every attempt to lie down."

Stoichactis kenti / Stychodactyla gigantea (Giant sea anemone)

Phylum: Cnidaria.
Class: Anthozoa.
Order: Actiniaria.
Family: Stichodactylidae.

Stichodactyla gigantea, commonly known as the giant carpet anemone, is a species of sea anemone that lives in the Indo-Pacific area. The tentacles and their stinging cells do not react to random brushes with rocks, sand, and other non-fleshy items in their surroundings, and they don't react to contact with certain clownfishes either. Basically the anemones don't recognise these things as 'food'. A clownfish can swim right into an anemone without being grabbed and stung to death. Clownfish and sea anemones have a symbiotic, mutualistic relationship, each providing a number of benefits to the other. The sea anemone protects the clownfish from predators, as well as providing food through the scraps left from the anemone's meals and occasional dead anemone tentacles. In return, the clownfish defends the anemone from its predators, and parasites. The anemone also picks up nutrients from the clownfish's excrement, and functions as a safe nest site.

Extracts from the proving of Sea Anenome by: **M. Burch:**[7]

There is a close relationship to Sepia, with the hormonal problems, low libido, menses affected, skin rashes, tiredness, and antagonism with partner . . . there is a strong affinity with cold symptoms, accidents, and skin rashes. Themes of **dirt, exploitation, prostitution and feeling handicapped.**

Delusions
- *Angels*, seeing
- *Curtain – heavy curtain hangs between her and others*
- Disabled, she is
- Dissolving, she is
- Forsaken; is – care for her; no one would
- Heart – open; is
- Insulted, he is
- *Protection, defence; has no*
- Small – body is smaller

Mind
- Ailments from – abused; after being
- Alone; being – desire to be alone
- Amativeness – want of amativeness – women; in
- Ambition – increased – competitive
- Amorous
- Awareness heightened – body; of – centred in body; feels
- Confidence – want of self-confidence – support; desires – family and friends; from
- Confusion of mind – identity, as to his – boundaries; and personal
- Content – himself, with – harmony with oneself; in
- Dogmatic
- Dwells – happy moments; dwells on past
- Energised feeling
- Fear
  - Age; of one's own
  - Attacked; fear of being
- Introspection
- Love – romantic love; desire for
- Obstinate – resists wishes of others
- Truth – sensitive to people's truthfulness
- Violent

Dreams
Abused sexually; being / Accidents / Adoption / Airplanes – **crash** of an airplane / Amorous / Animals – killing / Arguments / Beach / Blood / Buildings – neglected / Car / Cats – kitten / **Children**; about – **adopting** them – **rescuing**; of – **responsibility** for / **Choked**; being / Churches / Coition / Competition / Country – native country / Criticised; being / Danger / Dead; of the – relatives / Death / **Dirty** – buildings – place / Dolphins / **Drowning** / **Electrocution** / **Encircled tightly, being** / Excelling – mental work; in / **Explosion** – bombs; of / Falling / Family,

own / Father / Fighting; one is / Fish / Flowers / Food / Funerals / High places / Homeless – being homeless / House / Hunger / Hurry / **Imprisonment** / Infection; of an / Injuries / Insane – being insane – man; a / Insects / Insults / Jewelry / **Kidnappers** / Killing / **Kings – royalty** / Knives / Landscape – beautiful / Magic – black magic, **voodoo** / Mammae / Mistakes; of making / Mistakes; of making – remember names; can't / Mortification / Mother / Murdered / Music / **Mythical creatures** / Nakedness / Needles / Nostalgic / **Plundering** / Police / Poverty / Prostitutes / Relatives / Reprimanded – teacher; by / Rescuing; he is / Robbers / **Sea** / **Sexual** / **Shameful** / Singing / Snakes / **Speeding** / Spinning / **Stabbed**, being / Stealing / Strangers – entering house; stranger / Teeth – breaking off – falling out / Trees – cut; being / Walking – country; through open / War / Water – swimming in / Waves – huge wave approaching / Wedding / Wolves

Physicals

- **Head**
  - Heaviness – dull
  - Pain
    - § *Cutting pain – knife; as with a*
    - § *Nail*; as from a
  - Tired feeling
- **Vision**
  - *Blurred – outlines of objects not sharp*
  - Wavering
- **Nose**
  - Sinuses; complaints of – Frontal sinuses
- **Face**
  - Eruptions – herpes – Lips – About
  - Expression – soft
- **Throat**
  - Mucus – thick
  - Obstruction
  - Pain – Lymphatic glands – sore
- **Chest**
- Eruptions – Mammae – itching

- **Female genitalia/sex**
  - Leukorrhea
    - § Brown – menses – after – agg.
    - § Greenish
  - Menses
    - § Milky
    - § *Ropy, tenacious, stringy*
- **Skin**
  - *Eruptions*
  - *Eczema – bathing in the sea – agg.*
  - Itching – waking; on
  - *Rash – stinging, biting*
  - Red – spotted
- **Generals**
  - *Bathing – sea; bathing in the – agg.*
  - Clothes – tight; too
  - *Inflammation – Sinuses; of*
  - Mucous secretions – ropy, tenacious
  - Seaside; at the – agg.
  - Trembling – Internally – weakness; with

Provers speaking as one

ʃ Suddenly I realise I am a mature older person. I feel like this fat, middle aged, complaining, bitching woman. . . . I am sexually frustrated and feel my boyfriend is not interested in the relationship; totally melancholic, love sick like a teenager. I get this strong sensation on the navel, as if my **umbilical cord** was there. . . .

ʃ I am doing much more things alone, **not so needy or clinging**. . . . I had a very strong resentment of actually having to care for people. **I felt powerless.** . . .

§ There is an invisible curtain between other people and me. . . . *Detachment, it is no problem if I die.* . . .

§ I'm immediately hyper, the world is wonderful. **I feel peaceful**, the pace is right, everything goes fine. My life is extremely **harmonious** these days and has no tension even where there are **conflicts**. . . .

§ I feel **self-pity**, depressed, no self-confidence, **handicapped**. I'm so **small**. I'm **trapped** in my little world. . . . I'm fed up with myself, this depressive cap on me, this **limited** world and experience. It is like a big **stormy dark sea** going nowhere, being nowhere, just gloomy. I don't laugh. I want to be big strong attractive, not this **pile of shit of suffering** and no fun. . . .

§ I am being inside in my own world, my own self, **shutting off from the rest of the world. I avoid hurt and touch, being in my own self, dark self, depressive state, not doing anything just lying around.** . . .

§ I **retreat, interiorise**, inner focus. I forget about meeting my secret love, no use. . . . I had sudden desire to **rest, retreat**, and feel sleepy. The desire is to be in the dark and just close the eyes. The pain of the bones in the maxillas became more intense, heavy, sore, and then **invaded the whole shell**, then draws up as if somebody is pulling your whole head up . . . with something heavy and dark like a **heavy dark shadow or cloud**. It is concentrated and focused on the top of the head chakra and leaves through there like an upward chimney. It leaves this shadow and then all feels much lighter![7]

Common sensations of Cnidarian remedies ₑᵥₐₙₛ[21]

- Burning, stinging. Pins and needles, electric currents, tingling, throbbing, pulsing.
- Feels like jelly, weakness, collapse of structure, numbness, empty.
- Itching, crawling.
- Dislocation, dismemberment, disorientation, disabled.
- Beaten.
- Swelling, enlargement, elongation.
- Squeezed, pinched, compressed, constriction, pulled, drawn backwards, pressed downwards.
- These can naturally include real pains and also delusions as to the nature of the body.

CASE 7.3 Spaced out, directionless

Patient: Male, age 48

Prescription: Stoichactis kenti 1M

∫ The effect that confrontation has on me (*animal*); firstly **turns me to jelly**. (*Cnidarian*)

∫ Then I am left in the completely **spaced out, can't think**-familiar sensation. . . .

∫ There was **lots of confrontation at home** when I was a kid. (*animal*)
∫ Dad would come home pissed and late – dreading that time of day.
∫ Now I am so **sensitive to conflict** amongst people.

Talk some more about the effect that confrontation has on you –
∫ Like a **stunning feeling** in the back of the neck and head; it is almost **concussive**.
∫ The acute event that lead to **general spaciness – is like concussion**.
∫ The confrontation thing – the anticipation of there being confrontation is just stunning – it really unsettles me, and I get the sensation of fear in Hara (stomach area).
∫ It is a fight – fear of fight. (*animal*)

What is it to be stunned?
∫ **Rendered inactive, electricity and being electrocuted, shocked.**
∫ **Being inactive – that's a lot of my problem – is inactivity.**
∫ Not knowing . . . underactive.
∫ Underlying sense of there being an incoming event that will render everything pointless. For example, going home when I was 6 – knowing dad turns up pissed and there being more arguments. **That dis-settling in the home gave me no personal base to step on solid grounding to be able to have sense of self and direction.** (*not enough earth and abandonment as a child*)

What is the opposite state to all this?
∫ Stability – with everything I've got in my actual surroundings; home, money, tools. Being able to function with the reality of that. Feeling secure. (*Earth polarity*)
∫ Simplest sense of wellbeing. I guess **I am almost under a constant threat** (*animal*) of it not being right or there being no point.
∫ **No solidity in my sense of self** – in all the music that I play, I don't know any songs – I don't have any melodies. That does not mean that much to me cos I am so unbalanced musically. I don't have any memory to be able to . . . Or have never tried.
∫ I'm not singing any particular song – thats what I am doing in my life. (*directionless*)
∫ I don't own any songs, can't remember – cos of **spaciness**.
∫ The spacey feeling is like a spanner in my works of being able to learn and remember.
∫ Confrontation – Shock! Fright. **Being stunned.**
∫ Opposite – my mind had gone into stunned mode.
∫ Blank sheet, just . . . I've used an ice analogy before – like traction of the mind.
∫ Like being on ice – no grip.
∫ Like flicking the computer off.

∫ Anaesthesia for the mind rather than body.
∫ Nothingness, a void.
∫ There's a definite tension to it, of being very ill-at-ease in it.
∫ **It is not a safe place to be. . . .**
∫ *Can you describe a safe place?*
∫ Having one's wits about oneself. . . . Being prepared for whatever might happen.
∫ Anticipatory re: something likely to happen.

Synthesis of the case:

Stunned, inactive, concussed, like jelly. Under constant threat; Avoids confrontation, wants grounding, security, solidity.

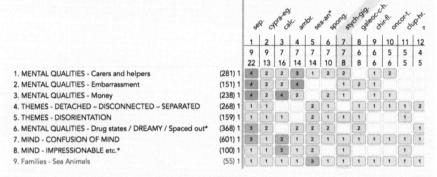

Figure 7.3 *Repertorisation (filtered to Sea Animals)*

Characteristic symptoms and dreams in the case
(from a reverse repertorisation)

- Accident-prone
- Ailments from – abused; after being
- Awareness heightened
- Confidence – want of self-confidence – support; desires
- **Confusion of mind**
  - Drugs; as if under
  - Identity, as to his – Boundaries; and personal
- **Delusions**
  - Forsaken; is – care for her; no one would
  - Injury – about to receive injury; Is
  - Insulted, he is
  - Protection, defense; has no
- Driving – desire for driving – fast
- Dwells – childhood, on his
- **Fear**
  - Accidents, of
  - Attacked; fear of being
  - Fight, wants to
- Indifference – opinion of others; to
- Laziness
- Love – romantic love; desire for
- Mistakes; making – speaking, in – spelling, in
- Observer – being an

- Orientation; sense of – decreased
- Pities herself
- Quarrelsome
- **Sensitive**
  - External impressions, to all
  - Pain, to
  - Rudeness, to
  - Sentimental
- Thoughts – father; of her
- Violent

Dreams
  - Abused; being
  - Animals – killing
  - Electrocution
  - Strangers – entering house; stranger

Urolophus halleri (Round Stingray)

Phylum: Chordata.
Class: Chondrichthyes.
Order: Myliobatiformes.
Family: Urotrygonidae.

Round stingrays strongly segregate by age and sex, with the females staying in water deeper than 14m and males and juveniles in shallower habitat. The juveniles feed on polychaete worms and small benthic crabs until they are 14cm across. As they mature, their diet shifts towards bivalve molluscs. They are daytime foragers that are most active in the warm temperatures of summer and fall. Using their pectoral disc and mouths, they dig large pits to uncover buried prey which plays an ecologically important role, as they also uncover prey for smaller fish. Female round stingrays emit a localised positive electric field from near the spiracles behind each eye, which serves to attract males. The males will bite at the area, with successful contact necessary for copulation.

Proving by: **Todd Rowe, USA (1998).**[12]

Delusions
- Appreciated; she is not
- *Betrayed*; that she is
- Detached; is
- Division between himself and others
- Floating – air, in
- Fragmented; she is
- *Lost*; She is
- Persecuted – he is persecuted
- *Personality – disintegrating, is*
- Shabby
- Superhuman; is – control; is under superhuman
- Talking – part of body is talking to another part; one
- *Transparent* – he is
- Unreal – everything seems unreal

Mind

- Anxiety; sudden, paroxysmal
- Censorious, critical
- Clairvoyance
- Confusion of mind – dream, as if in a
- Day-dreaming
- Detached
- Estranged – family; from his
- Fear; animals, of
- Fear; snakes, of
- Grounded – not grounded
- Humiliated; feeling
- Injustice; cannot support
- Suspicious
- Thoughts; persistent – violent
- Withdrawal from reality

Dreams

Amorous / Animals / Boyfriend – old boyfriend / Dancing / Floating / Friends; old / Ghosts, spectres; pursued by / Journeys / Men / Murder / Obstacles, of / People – seen for years; people not / **Pursued, of being** / Reunions, of / Torture, of / Water / Wedding

Physicals

- **Vertigo**
  - Turning; when – head; or moving the
- **Face**
  - Eruptions – *herpes* – Lips – About
- **Throat**
  - Anxiety and apprehension in throat
  - Lump; sensation of a – swallowing – agg.
  - Pain
    - § Cold – drinks – agg.
    - § *Warm – drinks – amel.*
  - Swelling – sensation of
- **Female**
  - *Uterus and region – night – bed agg.; in – bearing down*
- **Chest**
  - *Pain – Mammae – stitching pain – milk would appear; as if*
- **Back**
  - Pain
    - § Lying – amel.
    - § Menses – before – agg.
    - § Extending to – Hip
- **Extremities**
  - Itching – Forearms
  - Restlessness – Feet – night
- **Sleep**
  - Sleeplessness – cares; from
  - Waking – night – midnight – after – 3 h
- **Generals**
  - Bubbling
  - Faintness – tendency to

Proving Themes

Suspiciousness / **Betrayal** / Injustice / Humiliation / Disconnected / **Disintegration** / Alone / **Confusion between dream and reality** / Psychic abilities / Floating / Flying / Explosive violence / Shabby

Proving report[12]

- "**Betrayal** of relationships . . . suspiciousness, feeling of **injustice** and even [unfeeling] **violence** . . . **two men tried to rape me** and I killed them with a broom – there was no feeling . . . **Nurturing and Connection** . . . Dream: she was in a classroom with a bear and the teacher and other students were animals

– the teacher was at first **nurturing** but then became **impatient** and angry. . . . The theme of betrayal also arises around theft. This was best illustrated by one prover who had something stolen and said **stealing makes your heart dirty**. . . . The sexuality in this remedy was focused around **illicit sex and homosexuality**. There was also **confusion about sexuality**. In addition, there was a strong theme of rape."

- "Provers saw **sexuality as torture** in several dreams. The female stingray is often **abused** with many scars by the male stingray. The reverse side of this came out in one male prover who saw **women as very powerful** and in control of everything . . . the **female** stingray **separates** from the males for most of the year and lives a **solitary** existence. She returns to mate briefly on an annual basis. The reunions for stingrays are only for sexual purposes. The weddings [had] a quality of **shabbiness**. One prover had a dream where her daughter was **sexually tortured** on her wedding night."

- "The theme of **disconnection** was strong. This is similar to Sepia, although the **disintegration** goes beyond this recalling Baptisia. This also took on the form of confusion. In one prover, the **confusion was so strong**, that she tried to end the proving early because her **dreams felt too real**. . . . Provers noted that they **felt pregnant during the proving but without any emotion** about it . . . birthing babies in their dreams and the wish to **cocoon in a safe warm place**. There was also a wish to care for other's babies."

- **Curative responses**: "It may be useful in fibromyalgia coupled with fatigue. One prover had a substantial improvement in her fibromyalgia. This continued at the six month follow up. Another prover had chronic nightmares with spirits being after her and being lost in her house which resolved with the proving. At a six month follow up this symptom remained cured."

Summary

*Stingray can be compared to Sepia, and other ocean remedies. The **disconnection**, **rape themes and psychic abilities** all recall Sepia. Many of the physical and general rubrics also contain the remedy Sepia. Menopausal symptoms.*[12]

Venus mercenaria (Hard clam)

Phylum: Mollusca.
Class: Bivalvia.
Order: Veneroida.
Family: Veneridae.

The clam is a sedentary filter-feeding creature with a heavy and protective shell. They strain out the edible microscopic organisms and other nourishing particles contained in water. When undisturbed, they lie partly buried in the sand or mud with the ligament up and the shells slightly apart. Their mantle has scattered sensory cells which probably respond to touch and light. When a clam is irritated, the foot and mantle edges are withdrawn, and the 2 valves close very tightly – or 'clam-up'.

Proving by: **Raeside, UK (1960–61).**

Essence
Similar to Calc Carb. Mollusc themes: soft hearted inside / harder exterior, threat outside / protection of home, shutting out horrible things. Ailments from having to move house. Buries her head in the sand. Burdet[25]

Psychological Aspects – Julian[26]
- Lack of co-ordination of thoughts (*cf.* ambr.)
- Sensation of **boredom** with fear of crying for no reason.
- Feels **cut off** from the world, travelling on a bus bores him.
- Drunk feeling in the morning.

Source words
SHELL: protection, 'I stay inside', 'my house is important to me', 'in my shell', 'soft and vulnerable inside', 'hard exterior', spiral, 'I close up', 'half and half' (= bivalve), 'I build a wall', 'I withdraw', 'I hide', 'I close a door on it', 'I go into a cave', Intrusion by drilling, breaking, intruding, crushed, smashed. Burdet[25]

Modalities
- **Head**
  - Pain – Forehead – mental exertion agg.
  - Pain – Forehead – sleep – going to sleep; on – agg. – pulsating pain
- **Stomach**
  - Nausea – eating – after – agg.
  - Constriction – eating – amel.
- Abdomen – Pain – menses – during – agg.
- Extremities – Pain – Ankles – motion – amel.
- **Generals**
  - Pain – pressure – agg.
  - Food and drinks – cold drink, cold water – desire – evening – amel.
  - Motion – amel.

REPERTORY ADDITIONS FOR SEA ANIMALS
(to existing rubrics in Synthesis[17]):

- **MIND**
  - ABANDONED
  - ABSENTMINDED – dreamy
  - AILMENTS FROM
    § abused; after being
    § anger – suppressed
    § death of loved ones
    § domination
    § grief
    § love; disappointed
    § responsibility
    § sexual excesses
  - ANGER – easily
  - ART – ability for

- ○ AWARENESS HEIGHTENED
- ○ BLISSFUL FEELING
- ○ BROODING
- ○ BUOYANCY
- ○ CLAIRVOYANCE
- ○ CONFUSION OF MIND
  - § identity, as to his
  - § identity, as to his – boundaries; and personal
  - § identity, as to his – sexual identity
- ○ CONNECTION; SENSE OF
- ○ CONSOLATION – agg.
- ○ CONTENT
- ○ CURIOUS
- ○ DANCING
- ○ DELUSIONS
  - § alone, being
  - § dissolving, she is
  - § division between himself and others
  - § floating
  - § floating – air, in
  - § flying
  - § light = low weight – is light; he
  - § lost; she is
  - § mind – out of his mind; he would go
  - § pressed down by a great force
  - § protection, defense; has no
  - § safe; she is not
  - § separated – world; from the – he is separated
  - § time – exaggeration of time
  - § trapped; he is
  - § unreal – everything seems unreal
  - § victim; she is a
  - § vivid
  - § weight – no weight; has
  - § weight – pressing down from above
- • DEPENDENT OF OTHERS
- • DEPERSONALISATION
- • DESTRUCTIVENESS
- • DETACHED

- • DISCONNECTED FEELING
- • DISGUST
- • DREAM; AS IF IN A
- • DULLNESS
- • DWELLS
  - ○ past disagreeable occurrences, on
  - ○ recalls – disagreeable memories
- • ELATED
- • ESCAPE, ATTEMPTS TO
  - ○ run away, to
- • ESTRANGED
  - ○ friends and relatives
- • EUPHORIA
- • EXHILARATION
- • FEAR
  - ○ alone, of being
  - ○ disease, of impending
  - ○ happen, something will – family; to his
  - ○ insanity
  - ○ misfortune, of
  - ○ narrow place, in
  - ○ pain – of the pain
  - ○ poverty, of
- • FEARLESS
- • FLOATING SENSATION
- • FORSAKEN FEELING
  - ○ isolation; sensation of
- • FREEDOM
- • GRIEF
- • GROUNDED – not grounded
- • HATRED – persons – offended him; hatred of persons who
- • HELPLESSNESS; FEELING OF
- • HIDING – himself
- • HOME – desires to go
- • HORRIBLE THINGS, SAD STORIES AFFECT HER PROFOUNDLY
- • HUMILITY
- • IDEALISTIC
- • IDEAS – deficiency of
- • IMPRESSIONABLE
- • INDEPENDENT
- • lack of independence
- • INDIFFERENCE
  - ○ duties; to

- ○ family, to his
- ○ loved ones, to
- INSECURITY; MENTAL
- INTROSPECTION
- INTUITIVE
- LASCIVIOUS
- LOATHING – life
- LOVE – exalted love – humanity; for
- MEDITATING
- MENSES – before
- MERGING OF SELF WITH ONE'S ENVIRONMENT
- MILDNESS
- MIRTH
- MOOD – repulsive
- MOTHER COMPLEX
- MUSIC
  - ○ agg.
  - ○ amel.
- MYSTICISM
- NAIVE
- NYMPHOMANIA
- OBSTINATE
- ORIENTATION; SENSE OF – decreased
- PATIENCE
- PERSEVERANCE
- PESSIMIST
- PLEASURE
- POSTPONING EVERYTHING TO NEXT DAY
- PRESSURE; EXTERNAL
- PROTECTED FEELING
- REMORSE
- RESPONSIBILITY – taking responsibility too seriously
- SADNESS
  - ○ alone – when
  - ○ menopause, during
  - ○ menses – before
  - ○ menses – during
- SECRETIVE
- SELFLESSNESS
- SENSES – confused
- SENSITIVE – music, to

- SENSUAL
- SIGHING
- SPIRITUALITY
- STARTING – dreams, in – from a dream
- STRANGER – presence of strangers – agg.
- SWIMMING – desires
- SYMPATHETIC
- SYMPATHY FROM OTHERS – desire for
- THINKING – aversion to
- THINKING – logical thinking – inability for
- THOUGHTS – sexual
- TIMIDITY – bashful
- TRANQUILLITY
- UNIFICATION – sensation of unification
- UNSYMPATHETIC
- VIOLENCE
- VIOLENT
- VIVACIOUS
- WATER – loves
- WEEPING
  - ○ amel.
  - ○ easily
  - ○ menses – during
- WILL – weakness of
- WITHDRAWAL FROM REALITY
- YIELDING DISPOSITION
- **VERTIGO**
  - ○ FLOATING, AS IF
  - ○ NAUSEA – with
- **HEAD**
  - ○ CONGESTION – Brain
  - ○ EMPTY, HOLLOW SENSATION
  - ○ WAVING SENSATION
- **VISION**
  - ○ BLURRED
  - ○ FOGGY
- **EAR** – STOPPED SENSATION
- **EXTERNAL THROAT** – GOITRE
- **MALE GENITALIA/SEX**
  - ○ ERUPTIONS – Penis
  - ○ ITCHING – Penis

- PERSPIRATION
- POLLUTIONS
- **FEMALE GENITALIA/SEX**
  - ABORTION
  - LEUKORRHEA
  - MENOPAUSE
  - MENSES
    - § absent
    - § clotted
    - § copious
    - § intermittent
    - § irregular
    - § painful
    - § suppressed menses
  - METRORRHAGIA – menses – between
  - OVARIES; COMPLAINTS OF
  - PAIN
    - § Ovaries
    - § Uterus
    - § Vagina
  - SEXUAL DESIRE
    - § diminished
    - § violent
  - STERILITY
  - TUMORS – Ovaries – cysts
- **CHEST**
  - INDURATION – Mammae
  - MAMMAE; COMPLAINTS OF
  - PAIN
    - § Mammae
    - § menses – before – agg.
    - § sore
  - SWELLING – Mammae
- **BACK**
  - HEAVINESS, WEIGHT
  - PAIN
    - § Coccyx
    - § Sacral region
- **DREAMS**
  - FAMILY, OWN
  - FISH

- FLYING
- FRIENDS
- HOUSE
- JOURNEYS
- MOTHER
- MURDER
- SEA
- VIOLENCE
- VISIONARY
- **SKIN**
  - DRY
  - ERUPTIONS
    - § herpetic
    - § psoriasis
    - § rash
    - § urticaria
    - § vesicular
  - HEAT – fever; without
  - ITCHING – burning
- **GENERALS**
  - APOPLEXY
  - BUBBLING
  - FLABBY FEELING
  - FLOWING
  - FOOD AND DRINKS – salt – desire
  - FULLNESS; FEELING OF – Internally
  - HEAT – flushes of
  - INDURATIONS – Glands
  - LASSITUDE – morning
  - LIE DOWN – desire to
  - MOTION – desire for
  - MUCOUS SECRETIONS – watery
  - PAIN – compressed; as if forcefully
  - PRESSURE – agg.
  - ROOM – full – people agg.; of
  - SHOCK – electric-like
  - SLUGGISHNESS OF THE BODY
  - SWELLING – sensation of
  - ULCERS – Glands
  - VIBRATION, FLUTTERING, ETC.

References – Sea animals

1 Morgan J. *The Proving of Pearl taken from the common Mussel*. Tunbridge Wells, 1997. (Accessed in RadarOpus.)

2 Grimes M. *A Homeopathic Proving of Galeocerdo cuvier hepar – Tiger shark liver*. Seattle WA: Alethea Book Co; 2000.

3 Norland M, Fraser P. *The Homeopathic Proving of the Atlantic Herring*. Stroud, 2008. Available online at: *https://www.homeopathyschool.com/the-school/provings/herring/* (Accessed 23rd April 2020.)

4 Schadde A. *Listening to Stone, Wood and Shell – Cypraea eglantina*. Munich: Homoeopathic Medical Publishers; 2004.

5 Sonz S. *Hippocampus kuda, A Proving of Sea Horse*. New York NY. Available online at: *https://nyhomeopathy.com/provings/hippocampus-kuda* (Accessed 23rd April 2020.)

6 Sherr J. *The Homeopathic Proving of Oncorhynchus tshawytscha – Pacific chinook salmon*. 1996. Malvern: Dynamis Books; 2013. Available online at: *https://homeopathyforhealthinafrica.org/product/oncorhynchus-tshawytscha* (Accessed 23rd April 2020.)

7 Burch M. *Stoichactis kenti – Sea Anemone Proving*. Cambridge MA: Inner Health Inc; 2006.

8 Hering C. *Guiding Symptoms of our Materia Medica*. Philadelphia PA. (Originally published 1879.) (Accessed in RadarOpus.)

9 Hughes R, Drake J.P. *Cyclopedia of Drug Pathogenesy Vol. 1–4*. New Delhi: B. Jain Publishers; 2013. (Originally published 1886–91.) (Accessed in RadarOpus.)

10 Buck H. *The Outlines of Materia Medica*. (Accessed in RadarOpus.)

11 Mangialavori M. *Koiné seminar* Vol. 1. *Remaining in a safe environment: the sea remedies*. Bologna: Matrix; 2004.

12 Rowe T. *Urolophus Halleri a proving of Round Stingray*. Phoenix AZ: AMCH Publishing; 1998.

13 Herrick N. *Animal Mind Human Voices – Lac delphinum*. (Unabridged edn). Grass Valley CA: Hahnemann Clinic Publishing; Unabridged edition; 1998.

14 Gray A. *A Homoeopathic Proving of Chironex Fleckeri – Box Jellyfish*. Sydney, 2001. (Accessed in RadarOpus.)

15 Coulter C. *Portraits of Homeopathic Medicines* Vol. 1. London: Quality Medical Publishing; 1997.

16 Sherr J, Neu R. *Q Repertory of Medical Qualities*. Hompath; 2014. Available online at: *https://hompath.com/Qrep-Jeremy-Sherr* (Accessed 23rd April 2020.)

17 Schroyens F. *Synthesis 9.1* (Treasure edn). Ghent: Homeopathic Book Publishers; 2009 (plus author's own additions).

18 Kent JT. *Lectures on Homeopathic Materia Medica* (4th edn). Philadelphia PA. (Originally published in 1916.) (Accessed in RadarOpus.)

19 Gutman W. *Homoeopathy – The fundamentals of its philosophy the essence of its remedies*. New York NY: The Homoeopathic Medical Publishers; 1978.

20 Ortega P.S. *Notes on the Miasms*. Mexico City, 1946. Available online at: *https://pdfcoffee.com/ortegapdf.com-pdf-free.html* (Accessed 23rd April 2020.) (Also accessed in RadarOpus.)

21 Evans J. *Evolution of the senses: Cnidarian remedies*. London: 2013. Available online at: *http://www.interhomeopathy.org/evolution-of-the-senses-cnidarian-remedies* (Accessed 23rd April 2020).

22 Clarke JH. *Dictionary of Practical Materia Medica* (Vols 1–3). Mumbai: B Jain; 2005. (Work originally published in 1900.) (Accessed in RadarOpus.)

23 Ward J. *Unabridged Dictionary of the Sensations "as If"*. Noida Uttar Pradesh: B Jain Publishers; 1995.

24 Phatak SR. *Materia Medica of Homeopathic Medicines*. Maharashtra, 1997. (Accessed in RadarOpus.)

25 Burdet C. *I bury my head in the sand: a case of Venus mercenaria*. Bristol: 2013. Available online at: *http://www.interhomeopathy.org/i-bury-my-head-in-the-sand-a-case-of-venus-mercenaria* (Accessed 23rd April 2020.)

26 Julian O.A. *Materia Medica of New Homeopathic Remedies*. Beaconsfield: Beaconsfield Publishers Ltd; 1984.

27 Lucas J. *Proving of the Erythrinus fish*. Saddleworth, 2007. (Accessed in RadarOpus.)

28 Grimmer A, Currim A.N. *The collected works of Arthur Hill Grimmer M.D.* Connecticut: Hahnemann International Institute for Homeopathic Documentation; 1996.

29 Adam A. *Sea remedies: a vast little-explored treasure source of healing potential*. Bristol; 2013. Available online at: *http://www.interhomeopathy.org/sea-remedies-a-vast-little-explored-treasure-source-of-healing-potential* (Accessed 23rd April 2020.)

30 Vervarcke A. *Rare remedies for difficult cases*. Ghent, 2016. (Accessed in RadarOpus.)

31 Boericke W. *Pocket Manual of Homeopathy and Repertory*. Mumbai: B Jain Publishers; 1980. (Originally published in 1901.) (Accessed in RadarOpus.)

32 Lilienthal S. *Homeopathic Therapeutics* (2nd edn). Warsaw: Palala Press/ABE; 2015. (Originally published in 1879.) (Accessed in RadarOpus.)

33 Mashalova E. *A Leap into the Sea: The Experience of the Source of Limulus Cyclops*; 2016. Available online at: *https://Hpathy.com/clinical-cases/a-leap-into-the-sea-the-experience-of-the-source-of-limulus-cyclops* (Accessed 23rd April 2020.)

34 Cushing A.M. *Medical Advance – 1888, Vol XX, Vol XXI – No. 5*. (Accessed in RadarOpus.)

35 Yakir M. *Wondrous Order – Systematic Table of Homeopathic Plant Remedies*. Israel: Narayana Verlag; 2017.

36 Gibson D. *Studies of Homeopathic Remedies*. Beaconsfield: Beaconsfield Publishers; 1987.

37 Tyler M. *Pointers to the Common Remedies*. Mumbai: B Jain Publishers; 2003. (Accessed in RadarOpus.)

38 Vermeulen F. *Source and Substance*. California, 2019. (Accessed in RadarOpus.)

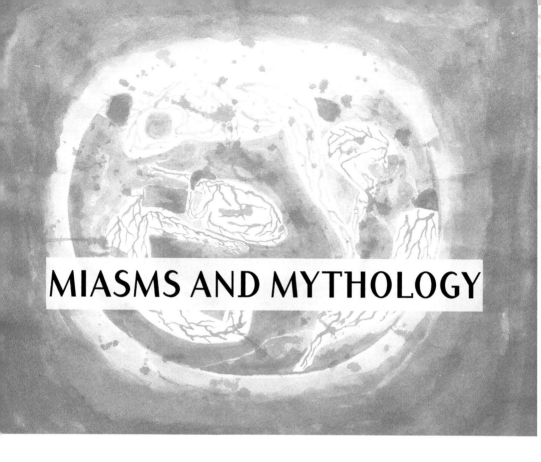

MIASMS AND MYTHOLOGY

These miasmatic modes are based on Rajan Sankaran's teaching. They are, at their most basic level, archetypal energy patterns ranging from very rapid, intense and generalised symptoms to slow, insidious and pathological (acute to syphilitic).

ACUTE TO SYCOTIC

Acute Miasm

The Acute miasm corresponds to the fight or flight response, and is the body's instinctive choice for defending itself because it is highly effective at ensuring survival so long as the vitality of the person can withstand and tolerate the intensity of the inflammatory process. Somebody who responds to life according to this miasm is apt to fly into panic, fear and anxiety over seemingly innocuous events, to which they may respond by fleeing or becoming aggressive. It has a very primal energy pattern, typified by the remedies of the Solanaceae – bell. and stram. and also lyssin. In the latter, the rubric – anger followed by quick repentance – is a very good example of the kind of reaction an acute miasm manufactures. First, there is the exciting cause which brings about panic – even predicting the time of death in the case of Aconite – then there could be a reaction of trying to escape or facing and fighting off the danger. When the threat has passed, the person can quickly return to their normal, more balanced manner, unless the miasm has become so strong over the person's vital force that they get stuck in this heightened adrenal state all the time. This could happen because the person is oversensitive to both external and internal impressions, or that they are locked into a situation which repeatedly 'pokes' them on their area of susceptibility.

In the acute remedies, it can be easy to confuse them with the syphilitic end of the spectrum as they can appear to have similar themes of violence, fear, death and annihilation. The difference is that the syphilitic miasm is much heavier, and the signs more pathological – leading to actual tissue degeneration and necrosis. In the acute miasm, a person will bounce from one extreme to the other – from light to dark, hot to cold, and the states although highly polarised, are more fleeting rather than of a chronic duration. One can see this as being reminiscent of Hermes – a winged messenger and the Greek god who can move between realms, a god of boundaries who can descend to the Underworld, where he takes mortals to their death, carrying messages from Olympus to Earth. He can enter what appears the syphilitic realm of Hades – death, decay and destruction – but he always returns unscathed. This is similar to the nature of Acute episodes, which appear life-threatening, intense and with sudden violence, but as long as the vital force has enough potency, will usually result in survival. Acute remedies therefore seem to oscillate between the heavenly realm of Fire and the Dark forces of elemental Air.

Typhoid Miasm

The Typhoid energy pattern lies between the rapid pace and shallow depth of the Acute miasm and the constant low-grade struggle of the Psoric miasm. When the body is healthy and following its instinctive vital process, the Acute miasm is the best way to deal with a stressor; it combats the problem quickly and without sacrificing a particular organ to the inimical agent. It acts swiftly, flying into battle like the god of War; Ares, or the Zodiac sign Aries. But, it expends a lot of energy and if somebody is overexposed to situations that touch their sensitivity, their vital power will diminish. Then they will move into another miasmatic expression that represents a partial retreat from the front-line, sacrificing the first line of defence and erecting a protective barrier to ensure survival of the most important parts of the kingdom.

Also known as the subacute miasm. Remedies in this miasm were originally used for typhoid fever – that is high, unremitting fever often associated with prostration from violent diarrheas or other infections. The infections are slightly less rapid in their onset (like all our descriptions of Bryonia) than the remedies in the acute miasm. . . . The patient feels himself to be in an urgent, life-threatening situation requiring his full capacity to survive. The patient is willing to use any means to return to a secure position: Violence, scheming, flight, lying, etc. . . . The feeling is, "If I can just get through this crisis, I have it made and I can rest." He seeks rest and a secure position.[6]

I find Nux Vomica is a very useful remedy with which to characterise the Typhoid rhythm. Nux works very efficiently to achieve their goals; they are driven and ambitious, using stimulants to keep themselves going. Eventually all this effort (the Psoric component of struggle can be seen here) leads to anger, irascibility and brain fag from having too many irons in the fire – not being able to switch off from thoughts about their tasks. They become hurried, quick to anger and have the delusion that someone is in their bed and there isn't enough room for them in it. They want to reach a position of comfort, as does Bryonia who also prattles about work, but their place of repose has been stolen. When the sub-acute pattern relapses, there is a sense of crisis that has to be dealt with right now, it will require a lot of effort.

Sankaran[2] mentions crisis as being very much of the Typhoid essence One of my patients who was prescribed Nux vomica said,

> *Need to keep pushing – project manager – keep managing myself. Right, did that – whats the next thing? Quite fast and busy, hectic – It is a lot of pressure – so I'm spinning loads of plates – and I'm consumed by it. I'm one of those people who appears calm and capable – so i get asked to do more – feeling overwhelmed with life – i'm not managing it all. Generally i feel a bit racy inside, there has been a niggling feel – that feeling like – after a roller coaster ride – its not really severe – its exciting, scary, thrilling, fearful, not sure what to expect – like the thrill of being out of control; that jump in your stomach – going really really fast.*

The Greek god Ares is a good counterpart for the Typhoid miasm. He is very eager to fly into battle, full of blood lust and violent rage – he is the god of War. His nature is simple, and he is driven by the more primitive urges of sex and violence. He was caught in the sexual act with Aphrodite, ensnared by a golden net forged by Hephaestus, and ridiculed for his rather unsubtle approach – warmongering and debauchery being his two well-known attributes. This is very similar to the Choleric Pole on the Mappa Mundi.

Psoric Miasm

The Psoric miasm, Hahnemann's gift to the Homeopathic community, lays the foundation for all the other miasms. In this way, it can be seen as the bedrock of human suffering, so it can be useful to look at mythology here as well. Prometheus is an interesting figure with which to relate to the Psoric miasm. He was a Titan god, whose love for humankind led to mischief that would bring down the wrath of Zeus; he stole fire from Olympus and gave it to the human race. In his rage, Zeus offered mankind the gift of Pandora's box, out of which came all the sufferings and toils of mankind, and at the bottom of which lay hope. This ties in rather nicely with the hopeful struggle of Psora. Prometheus himself was banished and chained to a rock where an eagle would come and peck out his liver by day, and by night he would regenerate owing to his divine immortality. The theme we can take from this story is that there is always struggle and toil for those with a Psoric miasm, but there always remains the possibility of hope lying at the bottom of Pandora's box. Mankind and Prometheus are both punished, but they will both still survive.

The miasm expresses itself in the form of hypofunction, or lack and in this way it has an opposite quality to sycosis. The ability to properly assimilate becomes impaired, leading to a lack of nutrition and delayed development, as in the case of Calcarea and Lycopodium. Psorinum represents the heart of this miasm and has a strong delusion of poverty, a feeling that everything will fail – he feels so poor that even his body parts don't belong to him! There is of course great itchiness, and crawling sensations with weakness, debility and a sense of being unwashed or polluted. Sankaran[3] describes Psora as an

> . . . intense struggle with a problem from the environment. This problem is nonspecific in the case of Psorinum; it can be a religious problem, a problem about money, a problem about love. . . . It has an undifferentiated character.

It is the situation of a simple peasant, who toils the land ceaselessly for scant financial reward, and yet he is that 'salt of the earth' type who has few concerns about wealth and status (as would the sycotic person). Psora is like the first line of defence after the power to throw an acute has diminished. There is a resignation to the fact they must now struggle on with limited capacity, but it has not got so bad for them to lose hope of overcoming the problem by maintaining their efforts. They can still see the hope offered at the bottom of all the hardships inflicted by Pandora's box.

With Psora comes the illusion of separateness; Kent equated it with original sin. As the manifestations of the disease itself are on the boundary of the self, the skin and mucuous membranes, the formation of the ego and the illusion of being separate are contained within the myth of Psora. According to Plato, human beings were once complete, spherical individuals, containing both the male and female anatomy – they wheeled around happily until Zeus became angered and split them asunder. This illusion of being separate leads to the desire to form bonds with others in order to feel complete again. It is the absolute bedrock of the human condition and feeds the delusion of the egoic mind. In this way, Psora can be seen as having something in common with the mineral kingdom; lacking completeness by oneself so needing to form a bond to compensate for that weakness. I think this correspondence demonstrates that both Psora and Minerals are the building blocks of more complex natural structures. I can see a relationship between Psora and the Earth aspect of the Mappa Mundi, where there is a drying up or solidifying process – wanting to find a place within the structure. Ailments manifested in the Earth realm are less serious than the Fire / Air polarity.

Sycotic Miasm

The Sycotic miasm impels the individual to keep up appearances, maintain the facade or veneer of their image. They don't like others to see the shameful aspect of themselves which is being kept under wraps, like the Conifer that grows so abundantly on the exterior that the interior is starved of light and goes into a state of decay. This brings the other theme to light; that of over-growth and excess, which can be seen in the extremes of behaviour in Medorrhinum; from Piety to Partying! Zeus (Jupiter) was the patriarchal God who ruled Olympus, whose reign was benevolent, and who was a symbol of masculine strength. He was an extremely unfaithful partner to Hera, and who had many sexual conquests with both mortal and divine women, giving rise to the birth of a plethora of different sons inhabiting the earthly and godly realms. There are some overlapping themes here with Sycosis, which is connected with the fig-wart growths of gonorrhoea, the disease you get from an unprotected sexual encounter. Jupiter is also a massive planet which ties in with the Sycotic trait of growth, excess, overdoing it.

This tendency to overgrowth can also be seen in physical attributes, such as excessive hair, full lips and big facial features, with the tendency also being to put on weight. Sankaran[2] adds the idea of accepting the situation as it is, because they know they cannot struggle against it anymore. In psora there would still be a struggle, but with sycosis there is a hiding away of the inner weakness (guilt, shame or ugliness). As long as they can cover it up, the coping mechanism is more or less working. They do this by compensating. For example, there is a fixed feeling inside of being fragile and sensitive to external influences – they cover this up with bravado and confidence (medorrhinum). In Thuja, they imagine that nobody can love them if they knew the ugly person they feel themselves to be – they compensate by maintaining a very fixed image of themselves as being very honest, caring and kind. This becomes brittle and fragile the longer it goes on for, and there is a feeling of being split – antagonism with oneself.

Sycosis seems to have a broad spread across the Mappa Mundi where one can see aspects of the Phlegmatic temperament in the fixed idea of weakness in himself that makes him of a yielding disposition; opposing the Choleric aspect of masculine strength and bravado to cover up his inner weakness.

Malarial Miasm

Lies between the Acute and Sycotic.

Like the Typhoid miasm, there is a periodicity to the Malarial miasm as it oscillates between the fixed phase (of sycotic origin) and the acute flare up, which feels tormenting, as if the person is persecuted and harassed as by a mosquito. Sankaran[2] says it goes between excitement and acceptance, and these can be seen as the more positive expressions of the acute and sycotic. Migraine headaches fall into this category, with periods of acceptance, covering up the weakness or fragility through habits and routines, making sure they don't eat or drink things that might trigger the migraine. If they overdo it (sycotic) or eat the wrong food, or have a stressful day at work, these trigger off the acute side of the miasm to vent off some of this build up of tension. In this period of flare up, the person is utterly overcome, they often must lie motionless in a dark room to avoid aggravating the intense disturbance of the migraine. The situation Sankaran[2] gives for this miasm is like the employee of an irate boss – you're stuck and dependant (sycotic) on the job, but also feel persecuted, harassed and undermined by them.

Nat-m has this experience in the realm of Row 3; issues of the relationship. Natrum has a stage 1 expression of feeling as though they absolutely need the other person to make them feel secure and whole (acute), whereas muriaticum has a stage 17 expression of feeling betrayed, let down and used by their partner. They react to this by withdrawing, brooding, hiding the turbulence of their emotions, and seeking a tumultuous ocean, or a wild love affair with which to excite / rouse themselves again (sycotic). However, the drama inside will eventually seek an outlet that could be somatised (for example, migraine) in order to vent the pent-up emotions inside. The myth of Aphrodite's forced marriage to the lame smithy god Hephaestus has some resonance with this miasm. As a dependent upon Zeus, she was forced into this dull marriage (fixed, acceptance); but she had many passionate liaisons (excitement) with Ares to make up for this boredom.

Ringworm Miasm

The Ringworm miasm is characterised by an unequal struggle, whereby despite all your efforts to overcome the problem, eventually you realise it is bigger than you and you resign yourself to succumbing to its greater power. Sankaran[3] goes on to say "I have understood the main feeling of this nosode to be that the task at hand is just beyond where the person can be sure of success. The main action of the prover or the patient is therefore trying to do something, trying to accomplish a task. He starts with a kind of lack of confidence, becomes hopeful, tries to accomplish the task and struggles at it. At some point however he decides that it is not going to work. . . . So he gives it up, and accepts that he has to live with it . . . the pathology and symptoms all come and go in **phases**. There is often a history of fungal infection. . . . The symptoms never really become acute or destructive, and the person feels that he will must live with the problem, although it would be better to try and get rid of it. He struggles periodically but when he fails, he just accepts it."

The ringworm miasm is evident in almost everybody, it is ubiquitous where there is a tussle between striving toward one's goals and giving up in the face of hardships that feel too strong to surmount. We're all able to identify with this pattern, and it seems to be very fitting for the generation dubbed 'the millenials'; a group now in their 30's who are often still living with their parents, unable to earn enough money to get onto the property ladder and establish themselves fully in the adult world. They were born into an era of growth and possibilities, were told they should all go to University to get a good education and be guaranteed a good career, but the economic crash (a force much bigger than any individual) has put paid to these expectations, bringing things to a standstill. Within this pattern, one can see the initial period of hope and struggle and effort to get good enough grades to enter University. The struggle continues during this period as one tries to establish themselves in the wider world, proving their acumen and diligence to their course of study. After university, there is often a period where the individual returns home whilst they search for work, and there may be periods of striving to get job interviews – competing with many others – before accepting defeat and resigning themselves to a job that does not really test their capacities or bring satisfaction. The resignation comes after the initial period of hopeful striving has run its course; when the limited resources of energy have been used up.

The Ringworm experience is of a striving towards a goal that is almost within reach but not quite. You never quite make it before your capacity runs out (Dreams – unsuccessful efforts). There is an obstacle in the way which is bigger than you, so unlike the Typhoid type – who has the strength to make a really big effort to overcome the problem, the Ringworm type has to accept his limitations and periodically give up on his goals. It is impossible to sustain the effort. Here we see that the vital force is diminished further than in the Typhoid or Malarial miasms, both of which have an acute element, representing the highest level of health; it is the body's front-line defence against attack and does not sacrifice any parts of the organism to the disease. Instead, the energy of this miasm lies between Psora and Sycosis – alternating between struggle and resignation, between hope and a fixed feeling of weakness that one has to cover up and hide.

There is a correlation between this miasm and the waxing and waning phases of the moon – each month you have the hopeful beginning of the journey towards the completion of full moon, and then you have the period of introspection and looking back when one recuperates and attends to the need for nurture of the lunar self. During the waxing phase, the person feels more hopeful as they move towards completing their task, this correlates with the taking up of new projects, having the energy to get things going, being motivated, sowing the seeds. This phase is associated with the goddess Artemis. She is a youthful goddess of the hunt, who has a bow and arrow – a weapon that enables you to meet your target from a great distance. This is like seeing your goal, and then having the energy and purpose to get straight to it, as would an arrow fly through the air to pierce its target.

After this follows the period of the waning moon, when all the efforts need to subside to allow for rest and recuperation and looking longingly to the past that was so full of promise. The goddess of witchcraft – Hecate – is associated with this phase of the moon. She was Persephone's escort to and from the underworld as marking the shifting of the seasons. When a person's vital energy cannot make a sustained effort (shifting like the seasons) and is perceived as holding them back, they can become indifferent to their environment – resigned to their failings and give up what they once began so hopefully. This correlates with the pace, depth and intensity of the ringworm miasm. It is an everyday kind of miasm – it frustrates the sufferer but does not lead to such isolation and despair as the heavier miasms, because it is not life threatening.

This role of Artemis also seems to fit in with the Lac-humanum picture very neatly, given the very direct link to the source of the bond between mother and child following birth. Problems at this early stage of connecting with one's mother may indicate the remedy so long as it fits the totality of the case. With the connections to the Moon it seems appropriate that the Mappa Mundi placement for this miasm should be in the realm of Water, with its tides controlled by lunar phases. It is also opposite the fixed and durable quality of Earth (relating to Psora) followed by exhaustion and giving up (Sycosis) – there is no sustained effort within the changeability of elemental Water.

There is a typical family environment where one can paint a Ringworm miasm situation. There's the Dulcamara mother, who is domineering and obsessive over little details especially with her Calc-silicata son's progress at school, whose grades keep getting worse. A lot is expected of him and yet his achievements probably don't amount to all that much. He goes on living with his parents well into his 30's. It is like the situation of the "millennial" I already mentioned; they're unable to get on the property ladder due to limited success in their careers and the discrepancy between wages and house prices. It is more like snakes and ladders (Sankaran[2]). Calc-sulph is listed under fear of snakes!

A lot may be expected of these young people, as they were born in the go-getting atmosphere of the 1980's. Within Calc-sil, there is the desire to achieve success according to his family's principles, maintaining the image and reputation of his good family (Sil.) combined with the hesitancy of Calcarea in the workplace – feeling unsure of oneself and staying passive, inert and observing others before feeling sure enough to give it a go oneself. The father in this scenario could be Kali-Sulph – a combination of the upright dogmatism of the Kali sense of duty to the family, combined with the scorned and rejected Sulphur, who needs to make a lot of effort to keep up appearances and compensate for his bruised ego.

Another situation of this miasm is like the one Sankaran[4] describes of joining weight watchers – trying so hard for a period of time to change your diet and lose some weight with exercise, before eventually relapsing and bingeing on a load of cakes and chocolate. Sankaran[2] also places several Sulphuricum salts into this miasm – Calc, Kali and Mag-s are all equated with Ringworm. He mentions appearance, ego and effort to prove oneself as being key themes of suphur –

The Magnesium sulphuricum woman has the feeling that in order to get the support that she needs, she has to make a big effort, do many things, appear proper, etc. She feels the need for appreciation by those on whom she depends for love, care and nourishment.

Burnett[9] mentions Sulphur and Tellurium as well as Sepia (alongside Bacilinum) in the efficacious treatment of Ringworm (the fungal infection itself). The ink from which Sepia is made contains a lot of Sulphur, whilst Tellurium is in the same column as Sulphur in the periodic table, corresponding to stage 16. Keywords of this stage according to Sankaran[2] are –

- No capacity,
- No energy,
- Incapable,
- Not possible to work,
- Indifference,
- Neglectful,
- Forgetful.

These really resonate with the waning phase of the ringworm miasm, when all efforts have been exhausted, and the fear of not being able to achieve the goal becomes overpowering, forcing the sufferer to give up hope. This lasts until the next phase begins and their confidence returns – the exuberance of the Sycotic miasm, or Jupiterian influence can re-ignite the ambitions.

Recap

Up to this point, the miasmatic range has gone from the sudden, intense panic and violence of the Acute, through the hopeful struggle of Psora to the resigned acceptance of a fixed limitation belonging to the Sycotic miasm. In between have been stops to the Typhoid, Malarial and Ringworm miasms which are all compounds of these 3. I can see a correlation between the personal planets in Astrology and these 6 miasms – namely:

- **Mercury** – Acute – winged messenger, moves between the underworld, earth and heavens.
- **Mars** – Typhoid – flies into battle without thinking of consequences. Rash, bold, impatient.
- **Sun** – Psora – Apollo remained eternally youthful Sun god. Prometheus stole fire and opened Pandora's box, containing hope but creating struggle and toil.
- **Moon** – Ringworm – phlegmatic, waxing and waning, connecting to feminine image: Lac-h.
- **Venus** – Malarial – the excitement of love affairs with Mars but stuck in boring marriage with lame Hephaestus.
- **Jupiter** – Sycotic – Zeus – promiscuity, power and cruelty alternating with benevolence.

The heavier, more isolated and increasingly desperate and disturbing states belonging to Cancer, Leprosy, Tuberculosis, Aids and Syphilis have more of a correlation with the outer "transpersonal" or generational planets. Respectively, these pertain to the Underworld, the previous Titan dynasty and the turbulent ocean in Greek mythology:

- **Saturn** – Cancer – Kronos – hard taskmaster, demands structure and imposes limitations.
- **Uranus** – Tubercular – Creative, revolutionary, erratic, sudden changes, idealism.
- **Neptune** – Aids/ Leprosy – Dissolving of form, self-sacrifice, no boundaries, addiction
- **Pluto** – Syphilitic – Destruction of form, Underworld, transformation, death, criminal, genius

CANCER TO SYPHILIS

Cancer Miasm

The cancer miasm can be seen as being a tri-miasmatic state, combining elements of Psora, Sycosis and Syphilis. There is the Psoric element of struggle that has been amplified to such a level that the individual feels as though they must make a superhuman effort to overcome the task. They set themselves a goal that is so far out of reach it is almost impossible to get to without a near impeccable performance, they are striving for nothing less than perfection, and so they are pushed to great lengths, and take on a lot of responsibility from a young age. We can see how this could come about in a home environment that demands a certain standard of behaviour, where the spontaneity of the child is suppressed in favour of manners and achievement. The tumour itself is a result of a pro-liferation of cells (Sycotic excess) that continue to grow, replicating themselves, ignoring the code of healthy cells so they end up destroying existing structures (Syphilitic destruction of form). This polarity between conformity and rebellion can also be seen in the cancer miasm; if somebody is heavily suppressed for a long period of time, either they will want to break free from this restrictive structure, or their body will develop pathology that expresses this breaking free from the structure such as when a tumour metastasises.

The Myth of Kronos, who castrates and emasculates his own father, before becoming ruler of the Titans, fits with the archetypal pattern of the cancer miasm. He is the youngest of Gaia's (Earth) children. Ouranus, his father, is deeply dissatisfied with much of their offspring and thrusts them back into the womb of Gaia. Here we can see the oppression of the paternal figure, and the ensuing rebellion where Kronos (the youngest) takes up the (superhuman) challenge of overcoming his father and taking his place. He goes on to a long reign over the Titans, maintaining authority by eating his own children so they cannot overpower him the way he did to his own father. Thus, the cycle is repeated, and the theme of suppression is continued until Zeus eventually over-throws his father. The more you exert a suppressive force, the more anger will be built up against the oppressor, leading to rebellion and warfare. This is the battlefield of cancer – waging war on your own body to defeat the revolution-ary cells of the tumour.

Saturn in the astrological chart is where one has set goals to achieve; they are usually out of reach, requiring ambition to reach them and leading to frustra-tion when one comes across an obstacle that seems to limit your capacity. This is where your resources are tested, and your achievements measured against the rest of society – have your efforts come up to the desired standard, what will others think of your standing in the world? Saturn is a hard taskmaster, there is often a lot of self-criticism with a strong Saturnian mark – like the father who does not offer praise, only criticism. This can propel the individual into working harder, perfecting their routine until they can perform the superhuman task. Classical music and Ballet are both good examples of the demands of the cancer miasm – perfection in performance, extreme dedication to form, needing ambition and steely nerves to take centre stage and see off competition from your peers, having to learn and perfect your craft from a young age that means the innocence of childhood is often sacrificed.

Tubercular Miasm

The Tubercular miasm can be seen as a type of Pseudo-Psora, where the struggle is so intense, hectic and destructive, that the person feels oppressed and needs to break away as soon as possible. It is even more revolutionary than the cancer miasm, which has a slower kind of pace to it. Perhaps because there is more involvement from the syphilitic aspect and none of the fixed nature of Sycosis present in the energy? In the tubercular energy pattern, the desperation and desire for rapid change is so great, so keenly felt, that the individual will feel claustrophobic when anything stays the same for too long, they'll create chaos in their lives just to break away from the restraints of habit, routine and structure. They want to go through life in the fast lane – the disease was called consumption because of this rapid nature of consuming the patient. Many musicians who burn up their creativity so quickly that they end up dying in their 30's were probably in this miasmatic group – Mozart, Hendrix, Cobain.

One can think of the Bacillus that ends up trapped in the tubercles of the lung; the body's white blood cells cannot get there, so fibroblasts are sent to entomb the unwitting bacteria in scar tissue, which calcifies and forms bone so that escape is rendered impossible. This is also remarkably similar to the experience of the insect in Drosera, where they're caught in the worst scenario – any struggle only worsens their situation, hastening their eventual demise. There is also the theme of lost homeland – the situation of having to flee from your own beloved country because of oppression – retaining a nostalgia for the past whilst also needing to chase after new experiences, and visit far flung corners of the globe. The person who stays on a perpetual gap year, travelling – doing a season here and a season there, seeking adventure and constant movement, never staying still for long enough to get settled / bored of routines.

Uranus is the planetary aspect that shares these themes – its sphere of influence on a person's life is associated with drastic, unpredictable and erratic change. Change that cannot be predicted, totally reorganising the person's world around them so it is almost unrecognisable. Some people thrive off these changes, and channel the Uraniun energy from which it stems. Mozart was an Aquarian and therefore ruled by Uranus – he was a child prodigy, incredibly precocious, traversing the whole of Europe as a performer by the age of 8. He had to work incredibly hard (Psoric struggle) to earn any money because his ideas were so ahead of their time, and he put many people off through his wild personality and taste for scatological humour. He had 4 planets in Aquarius and moon square to Uranus so this tubercular energy was very strong indeed in his case; one could almost say he was a very pure archetypal expression of it, and he was thought to probably have died from the disease, when it was first coming to prominence in Europe.

Tuberculinum Nucleus

- Trapped, suffocated, only way out is by intense, hectic activity
- Innocence, romanticism for the past. Desire to embrace the new but always comparing it back to the idyllic homeland (Neptune)
- Affinity to insects (Drosera)
- Fear of immediate death
- Great restlessness and fervent activity required in order to survive
- Sense of being caged or entombed (as by the fibroblast around the bacillus)
- Lungs are suffocated – space taken up by fibrosis
- Desire for open air
- Exploring the new – innovative, creative, explorer, adventurer, unsettled, constant change, never satisfied, unfulfilled longing
- Precocious restless child

Leprosy Miasm

Leprosy Miasm – shunned, the great unwashed; cast out by society. He is estranged and cannot be redeemed, so must accept his lot as an outsider and beg for the kind acts of others to ease his suffering. Like the tubercular miasm, there is too a feeling of great oppression within the leprosy miasm, but his reaction is to retreat away from society, becoming an outcast. There is more resignation to the inevitable sense of being cast out for one's sins, feeling dirty and hunted down like a criminal. The leprosy miasm evokes a despair of recovery nearly as profound as that of the syphilitic state. The violence seems to be more directed inwardly at the self – shutting himself away, tearing and biting at himself.

The feeling of being unfortunate has some parallels with the Malarial state, where he also feels unfortunate, persecuted or tormented by his oppressor. The difference being that this has a periodicity in Malaria, with periods of leniency from the tormentor. In Leprosy, this is a constant feeling, with little hope of survival or even changing the situation for the better.

Sankaran[3] writes:

> The main feeling in the leprosy miasm is similar to the tubercular miasm, only much worse. The feeling is that even with intense, rapid, hectic activity to come out of this destructive process, there is very little hope. In terms of pathology . . . there is the tuberculoid type which, though progressive, has a better prognosis than others – there is hope. At the other end, there is the lepromatous leprosy which is rapidly progressive and destructive, resembling syphilis. There is a feeling of tremendous oppression.

In the disease itself, the body isolates a single part and sacrifices it for the good of the whole organism – the affected limb decays and eventually withers away entirely. So there are the dual themes of isolating, and decaying. This miasm creates an energy pattern that is devastating to healthy conditions, giving rise to feelings of utter self-condemnation and loathing, feeling as though everyone were utterly revolted by the mere sight of them, disgusted at their very presence (Del – friends – lost the affection of, he has). There is a kind of paranoia that everyone else feels that he is putrid, that if they come too close, they will also become infected. Here it has a strong affinity with the Aids miasm.

Perhaps the astrological symbol most closely associated with leprosy is Chiron – the immortal son of Kronos who was rejected by his mother upon discovering he was a centaur – he was outcast as a child and was always on the periphery of the other Centaurs who were far more bawdy and violent than he. He was also mistakenly wounded by a poisoned arrow from Heracles that left him with a wound that would never heal (although he couldn't die owing to his immortality). Eventually, to seek an end to the suffering inflicted by this wound, he offered to sacrifice his immortality to exchange places with Prometheus who had been tied to a rock in Tartarus all this time since trying to deceive Zeus. Like leprosy, there is no chance of survival, so the only option left is to accept the situation and sacrifice yourself to the inevitable.

The positive aspect of this type of self-sacrifice, and contained in the myth of Chiron, is the wisdom of detachment; becoming free of the tension of opposites within the egoic world view. When there is nothing left to lose, your position on the periphery can take the form of the wise elder, sage or shaman who offers advice, guidance and healing to others. Chiron saves Prometheus from his suffering, and is known as the 'wounded healer'. The Mappa Mundi position most fitting for this myth / miasm is the Melancholic aspect, which has the dynamic of closing in, shrivelling, drying up and contracting.

Aids Miasm

Aids – boundaries have broken down completely – the ego is dissolved. Free flow from without to within, there are no defences anymore. This leaves the person open to invasion and attack, but also to love and connection. Free love and homosexuality. Also the theme of barriers – latex and condom as a protection against HIV. Sexual torture and domination – in the case of Falcon. Very severe, so as to give the individual the feeling that they belong totally outside the group – they just do not belong with normal beings who haven't experience such hardships as them. The world they live in has been harsh and cruel, so they see themselves as being on the outside, outcast and dirty. In a similar way to the Leprosy miasm, these individuals are tainted by their disease label – they have been given a death sentence – it is inevitable, only a matter of time, and they carry such a stigma that they are alienated from the rest of society.

The idea of taboo practices is contained within the miasm as well – someone who practices anal sex, or who injects intravenously is much more likely to contract the disease. There is also a conspiracy theory that Aids came about because of testing in Africa through vaccination that led to the Simian version of the disease transforming across from one species to another. This is a new age where boundaries even between species do not exist; there is, as Peter Fraser has outlined, a correspondence with the technological age – where all information and communication is in digital form and can be sent without wires to anywhere in the globe.

National frontiers no longer have any bearing on travel – people move freely between border controls. Immigration is huge. Threats can get into the country incognito, in the form of rogue terrorist agents who can bypass the normal defences (body's immune system in Aids) and blow up a bomb next to the country's headquarters. Thus there is a feeling of being defenceless from attack, shunned from society, but also having your own group (the gay community) where there is a free-flowing love and mutual appreciation for each other. Neptune is the Astrological symbol for this miasm, being the dissolver of forms. There is an idealism, with themes of self-sacrifice, seeking oblivion through addiction and an overwhelming tide of oceanic-feeling contained within the image of this planet. It connects with the collective unconscious, where one escapes from the rational mind back into the oneness of spiritual practice, as Aids dissolves all the boundaries setup by the healthy immune system to maintain the physical container of the ego. But it is easy to get lost in the great ocean, and losing oneself is a key theme for Neptunian individuals – they can get very lost and alienated from society, seeking solace in alcohol, drugs or day dreams.

Syphilitic Miasm

Lastly, the Syphilitic miasm – the final nail in the coffin. There is no last chance now – basically the feeling is that they're doomed, and if they're going down then it isn't going to be without a considerable amount of fighting back. This can equate to psychotic states, where there is an unfeeling kind of maliciousness to the person, who can be cool and calculated in their revenge. It is unlike the hot temper of Mars and more like the cool, subterranean wrath of Pluto or Scorpio. Hades, lord of the Underworld, with whom there can be no bargaining, when your time has come, he is going to take you to your death.

Astrologically, Pluto presides over the deepest periods of transformation in your life – where everything seems to be taken away, where events are so strong that you must submit to fate and let go of control. There is an element of chaos, destruction and obliteration inherent in this miasm, but there is also the polarity to this – which is that once everything material has been stripped away, you're left with an opportunity to be reborn without all the trappings and attachments of having an ego. The form is destroyed, so you can now allow the un-manifested, the no-thing to be part of your life. There is such a strong power to Pluto and the Syphilitic miasm – it can be equated with a laser-like vision, a narrowing, and refining down to the essence of the matter (as Jeremy Sherr points out).

There may be chaos surrounding the person, but in their chosen area of expertise they can have a quality close to genius, a kind of attention to detail that cannot be disturbed. This is like the effect of Syphilis on the tissues of the body – slowly eating into the bony structures, chiselling and refining rather than the growing outward action of sycosis. It is looking inward, and specialising in the oneness rather than the many, like the way that Mercury amalgamates with other metals by eating its way into them.

References

1 Norland M, Johnson G, Snowdon J, Mundy D, Sherr J. *Lectures notes*. Stroud: School of Homeopathy; 2012–2016.

2 Sankaran R. *Sankaran's Schema* (2nd edn). Mumbai: Homoeopathic Medical Publishers; 2007.

3 Sankaran R. *The Soul of Remedies*. Mumbai: Homoeopathic Medical Publishers; 1997.

4 Sankaran R. *The Substance of Homeopathy* – Naja tripudians. Mumbai: Homoeopathic Medical Publishers; 2005.

5 Fraser P. *The Aids Miasm – Contemporary Disease and the New Remedies*. Bristol: Winter Press; 2002.

6 Morrison R, Herrick N. *Miasms of the new millennium*. Grass Valley CA: Hahnemann Clinic Publishing; 2014.

7 Jung C G. *Memories, Dreams and Reflections*. Basel: Fontana Press; 1995.

8 Meineck P. *Classical Mythology: The Greeks (The Modern Scholar)*. Pince Frederick MD: Recorded Books/RB Media, 2004.

9 Burnett JC. *Ringworm: Its Constitutional Nature and Cure*. London: Forgotten Books; 2018. (Originally published in 1882.) (Accessed in RadarOpus.)

INDEX

Index

Index